"This book usefully approaches ecological/embodied cognition as a project rooted in several philosophical traditions and is a fresh and significant proposal in the area of the ontology of cognition."

Lorenzo Magnani, *University of Pavia, Italy*

The Ontology of Ecological Cognition

This book provides the first explicit examination of the underlying ontology of the ecological/embodied cognition philosophical project. More specifically, it examines the locative concepts used by defenders of representationalism and the more environmentally oriented, ecological/embodied views on cognition.

The book's main argument is that ecological/embodied cognition is embedded in various philosophical traditions. It establishes that there is a lack of clarity in how we conceptualize locative relations in contexts having to do with cognition. The book tackles questions of what it means that internal representations are internal, that the external world is external, that the extended mind is extended, how we should understand the claim that cognition and consciousness are in the head, or, alternatively, in the environment. Additionally, it addresses what it means that cognition enacts an environment, which is likely the most controversial claim made in some branches of embodied cognition. The goal of the book is to capture the essential traits of cognition thought of as an ecological phenomenon – as a factor determining a specific locus – and thereby elicit how cognition takes part in the creation of the world as we know it.

The Ontology of Ecological Cognition will appeal to scholars and graduate students working in philosophy of mind, cognitive science and metaphysics.

Konrad Werner is Professor of Philosophy at the University of Warsaw, Poland. He is the author of *The Embodied Philosopher: Living in Pursuit of Boundary Questions* (2022) and numerous papers published in journals such as *Synthese*, *Topoi*, *Erkenntnis*, *Journal of Consciousness* Studies, *Constructivist Foundations*, among others.

Routledge Studies in Contemporary Philosophy

Philosophy Across Borders
Perspectives from Contemporary Theory
Edited by Emma Ingala and Gavin Rae

Phenomenologies of the Digital Age
The Virtual, the Fictional, the Magical
Edited by Marco Cavallaro and Nicolas de Warren

Naturalism and Its Challenges
Edited by Gary N. Kemp, Ali Hossein Khani, Hossein Sheykh Rezaee, and Hassan Amiriara

Scripts and Social Cognition
How we Interact with Others
Gen Eickers

The Philosophy of Environmental Emotions
Grief, Hope, and Beyond
Edited by Ondřej Beran, Laura Candiotto, Niklas Forsberg, Antony Fredriksson, and David Rozen

Rethinking Self-Control
Matthew C. Haug

The Rise of Polarization
Affects, Politics, and Philosophy
Manuel Almagro

The Ontology of Ecological Cognition
Konrad Werner

For more information about this series, please visit: www.routledge.com/Routledge-Studies-in-Contemporary-Philosophy/book-series/SE0720

The Ontology of Ecological Cognition

Konrad Werner

Routledge
Taylor & Francis Group
NEW YORK AND LONDON

First published 2025
by Routledge
605 Third Avenue, New York, NY 10158

and by Routledge
4 Park Square, Milton Park, Abingdon, Oxon, OX14 4RN

Routledge is an imprint of the Taylor & Francis Group, an informa business

ISBN: 978-1-032-94642-9 (hbk)
ISBN: 978-1-032-94641-2 (pbk)
ISBN: 978-1-003-58099-7 (ebk)

DOI: 10.4324/9781003580997

Typeset in Sabon
by SPi Technologies India Pvt Ltd (Straive)

To Jerzy Perzanowski (1943 – 2009). In grateful memory

Contents

Preface

The call for a new ontology of cognition has been coming from many directions for quite some time. To cite a spectacular example, Niels Bohr explicitly wrote that while in the classical conception of the world the distinction between *subject* and *object*, and thus the conception of observation (including scientific observation, which was Bohr's primary concern), had been fixed as referring to two clearly delineated domains, in light of the findings of quantum physics the line should be redrawn. For the latter makes it really problematic "how objectivity may be retained during the growth of experience beyond the events of daily life" (Bohr 1963; quoted after Honner 1982: 12).

On the other hand, in theoretical biology, Humberto Maturana famously proclaimed that "everything said is said by an observer" (Maturana & Varela 1980: 8). This might seem to suggest that, unlike Bohr, he took the notion of observation for granted, but nothing could be further from the truth. The observer who makes distinctions in the biological realm, e.g., between a living creature and its environment, is *itself* a living creature, and therefore the *subject/object* distinction cannot be taken for granted and instead turns out to be *a product* of the ever-changing process of living.

Maturana's approach is further developed by Francisco Varela, Evan Thompson and Eleanor Rosch in their seminal book "The Embodied Mind" (1991). Much of the book draws on this inspiration – the cognizing subject (system) and its environment are structurally bound together in a process of co-determination, so that it's impossible to refer to a cognitive system without considering its environment, and it's equally impossible to refer to an environment without specifying whose environment it is.

Today's *Zeitgeist*, manifested in developments such as enactive theory, embodied cognition, or the extended mind hypothesis, among others, clearly points to the idea that cognition, in its many forms and at every stage of development, from sensorimotor coordination to scientific observation and measurement, is not just a matter of recording what's *out there*; instead, it is constituted (made *what it is*) by a particular kind of engagement with the world. In this sense, it's *ecological*. The task of a new ontology of cognition, then, is to provide the most general characterization of this ecological engagement. It aims to articulate what all these listed terms actually stand for. In what sense is the cognitive system bound to an environment? What is this environment? How does the cognitive bond with *an environment* differ in its most fundamental way from other bonds with the world?

This book is primarily driven by the aforementioned developments in theoretical biology and enactive theory, leaving parallel work that would delve into the field of philosophy of physics to others better prepared for that job. The book thus provides at least partial and tentative answers to the aforementioned questions of cognitive systems, environments and their relationship, and calls for further work in what I propose to call *the ontological foundations of ecological cognition.*

But first, what is *ontology* as such – this is something we need to introduce briefly here before diving into the actual investigation.

*

My understanding of ontology is based in particular on the seminal work of Roman Ingarden (1964), followed by Jerzy Perzanowski (1990). They in turn draw on early conceptual/logical analyses by Edmund Husserl (1901), Stanisław Leśniewski (1916), and others. For comparison, see, for example, Smith and Mulligan (1983), Burkhardt and Smith (1991), Poli (1996), Smith (2003), Hofweber (2005), Rescher (2008), Fine (1996), Arp et al. (2015).

Thus, I take ontology to be the central philosophical discipline whose goal is to analyze the most abstract *categories* that organize the world as we know it (an endeavor that goes back to Aristotle; see, e.g., Chisholm 1996; Jansen 2007). It therefore does not employ any *specific* conceptual framework (as understood by Ajdukiewicz 1934 then followed by Carnap 1950 and others) from the sciences or everyday discourse (for which Carnap 1950 famously criticized philosophy), but rather, metaphorically speaking, reveals (or at least aims to reveal) the *architecture* of the entire conceptual edifice that we construct, both in scientific knowledge and in everyday thought. It's like an attempt to draw attention to *the scaffolding* on which all specific conceptual frameworks hang; thus, to a factor that makes these specific frameworks possible. As such, it also uses concepts, for how else could it proceed, but these concepts are quite specific (they are *boundary concepts*, as I argued in Werner 2022b).

General ontology deals with categories such as OBJECT, PROCESS, EVENT, PART and WHOLE. The references of these categories are further POTENTIAL or ACTUAL, PRIMARY or SECONDARY. Moreover, going back to Aristotle, we can try to distinguish between MATTER and FORM in each case. Some objects, processes, etc., are PARTICULAR, while others are UNIVERSAL; some are MATERIAL, while others may be INTENTIONAL or IDEAL.

Applied ontologies deal with specific phenomena, e.g. the ontology of the social domain deals with GROUPS or INSTITUTIONS, and the ontology of the biological domain seeks to define categories such as ORGANISM or SPECIES.

At the center of this book is the ontology of cognition, which deals with concepts such as COGNITIVE SYSTEM (or MIND), COGNITIVE RELATION or COGNITIVE PROCESS, and of course the aforementioned SUBJECT–OBJECT bond. And this is the focus of this book. Embodied cognition and enactive theory, in my opinion, have the potential to bring a new (but not without antecedents in the history of philosophy, as we shall see) ontology of cognition. That is, the most abstract, and thus most fundamental, *architecture of all our conceptualizations of cognition*. Unveiling at least part of it will be my goal.

From a variety of ontological vocabularies and approaches, I take the one that seems most appropriate for the task, given the talk of environments and the dependence of cognition on its placement in a particular milieu – that is, the ontology of location, broadly construed (including elements of the ontology of boundaries; see Smith 1996), or *locative ontology*, as Perzanowski (1993) has called it.

*

This book summarizes several years of my work, and therefore owes much to a large group of people, institutions and circumstances. The beginning of the process and its completion stand out as the most important. As for the former, my interest in locative ontology, which is part of a larger formal-ontological tradition, began with my brief but consequential collaboration with Jerzy Perzanowski, who supervised me during my first year of doctoral studies and, as one of the greatest ontologists of our time and a bigger-than-life personality, largely shaped my approach to philosophy. His untimely death, however, set me on another path, which would not have been possible without the helping hand of Perzanowski's closest friend and student, Janusz Sytnik-Czetwertyński. Then, as part of the Department of Cognitive Science at the Jagiellonian University in Kraków, under the careful supervision of Józef Bremer, I began to work in the field of philosophy of perception, philosophy of mind, and on this path I came across the works of Francisco Varela. The latter, along with Perzanowski's formal ontology, would be the second major source of insight. This book is largely a combination of the two.

As for the conclusion of the process, major parts of the book were written during my nearly year-long visit to the University of Pittsburgh, sponsored by the Polish National Agency for Academic Exchange (PPN/BEK/2019/1/00325), where I spent a wonderful and productive time, thanks in large part to the extraordinary hospitality of Colin Allen to whom I extend my sincere thanks. I also thank Edouard Machery – attending his seminar on the concept of representation helped me a lot.

In between, I was able to develop some of the ideas in the book during a year-long visit to Columbia University, thanks to my conversations with Achille Varzi, whose works have been instrumental in my work.

I would also like to thank Katarzyna Paprzycka-Hausman, the entire team at my Department of Epistemology, Faculty of Philosophy, University of Warsaw; Sebastjan Vörös from the University of Ljubljana, and Ludger Jansen, to whom I owe my most recent research stay at PTH Brixen, Italy, where these words are being written.

I am grateful to the Routledge editors for their support and, above all, for their openness to this philosophical project.

Last but not least, my sincere gratefulness to my loved ones, family and friends for their invaluable support.

*

This book is the final product of the research project carried out at the University of Warsaw (2019–2022) and supported by the National Science Centre (Narodowe Centrum Nauki), Poland, grant no. 2019/33/B/HS1/01764).

*

The book includes and develops selected fragments from the following papers of mine:

- Enactment and construction of the cognitive niche: toward an ontology of the mind-world connection. *Synthese* 197, 2020: 1313–1341 https://doi.org/10.1007/s11229-018-1756-1
- Structural coupling and the puzzle of surfaces: ontology of boundaries from the minimally cognitive perspective, *Adaptive Behavior* 29 (6), 2020: 601 – 615 https://doi.org/10.1177/1059712320937475

1 Minds and Places

The Need for a Locative Ontology of Cognition

1.1 Out of our heads, but where to?

"Keep *in* mind that …" is a phrase that our parents, friends or collaborators use when they want something to sink *in*, to be remembered, and thus stored inside some cognitive depot. But does it actually make sense to say that something is "*in* mind," "*inside* the mind" or, more generally, that minds can be conceived of as *bounded loci*, where specific sorts of entities can be stored, kept, located, etc.? This is one of the questions this book shall attempt to address.

Over the last century, and in particular in the last 30 years, many thinkers have rejected this manner of conceptualizing the mind. Alva Noë, for example, invites us to consider what he believes to be an entirely different scenario:

> Stop and notice that you can believe in consciousness […] without believing that there is a place, or a moment in time, when and where consciousness happens or comes to be inside of us.
>
> (Noë 2009: 3)

> Consciousness is not something that happens inside us. It is something we do or make (…) Consciousness is more like dancing than it is like digestion
>
> (Noë 2009: xii)

Leaving aside the fact that Noë speaks of *consciousness*, which is not necessarily equivalent to *mind*, he suggests that a more fundamental change is required in how we conceptualize our cognitive functioning at the most general level. This means that in order to better understand the nature of cognition, we need a change in ontology – a new ontology dealing with places, regions, environments; boundaries, and relations such as *being-in* or being *contained*, being *internal* or *external*, etc.

DOI: 10.4324/9781003580997-1

While semantic externalism famously came up with the slogan "meanings just ain't in the head" (Putnam 1975), there is a discernible trend within contemporary philosophy of seeking a more sweeping externalism, so that in the end no cognitive entities, processes or functions can be regarded as being solely "in the head." This would not only indicate that cognitive functions are not where they were thought to be for centuries, but, following Noë's suggestion, that the concept of location is not at all applicable to the domains of cognition, perception, thinking, or consciousness. Simply put, mind *is not* a place.

On the other hand, the concept of location cannot be dismissed altogether, since the above-mentioned externalists sought to demonstrate that while mind itself is not a place, it must nevertheless be *placed* somewhere – in the world, or in some environment. There is an abundant current of philosophical ideas functioning under various umbrella terms, all of which advocate for a more ecological, thus environment-oriented, approach to cognition, consciousness and perception. A provisional list, in no specific order at this stage, would include: the ecological theory of perception proposed by Gibson (1979), Noë's (2004) sensorimotor theory of perception (frequently referred to as sensorimotor enactivism); multiple theories of direct perception which deny that there is such a thing as representational content stored in our minds (frequently referred to as relationism), defended by a variety of scholars such as Martin (2010) or Brewer (2007); the enaction theory (frequently referred to as autopoietic enactivism) of Varela, Thompson and Rosch (1991) followed by Thompson (2007) or, in a different spirit, by Di Paolo (2005). The enaction theory is linked to Noë's proposal, but deriving more from two other intellectual currents, each of which has its own separate place on this list (see e.g. De Jesus 2015 for more details): Merleau-Ponty's (1962/2005) naturalist phenomenology of perception, and the biological approach to cognition (e.g. various studies on the evolution of cognition and minimal markers of cognition; see e.g. Godfrey-Smith 2016; or earlier von Uexküll 1926; Maturana & Varela 1980). Finally, we also have the extended mind hypothesis of Clark and Chalmers (1998) which also brought some biologically informed views to the table, such as niche theory (e.g. Lewontin 1983; Laland & Sterelny 2006) and the "scaffolded mind" hypothesis put forward by Sterelny (2012).

As we can see even from this introductory list of references, this is an immensely broad tent, and it would be quite impossible to present all of these views here in a way that would do justice to the conceptual detail of each. It may be well to start by establishing what these allegedly novel externalist concepts of mind and cognition oppose, as well as what their alternatives entail. To set up a provisional discussion framework for this chapter, and thus to a degree for the whole book, I shall use a distinction which bears a certain affinity to Shaun Gallagher's (2017) differentiation between "cognition-in-the-head" and "cognition-in-the-world." I propose to draw a more general distinction between mind-*as*-a-place and mind-*in*-a-place. According to the former, the mind (or the cognitive system more broadly) is *a locus*, thus it makes sense to say that something is *in* it, while the latter proposes that the mind is itself necessarily *a located* phenomenon, thus it must be *in* something.

My initial diagnosis is, therefore, that we are witnessing a major transition from the more traditional mind-*as*-a-place paradigm to a newer mind-*in*-a-place paradigm. Understanding what this transition entails is an issue of paramount philosophical importance.

1.2 The missing conceptual link

According to George Lakoff (1987) and Mark Johnson (1987), we used to treat our bodies as containers, since "perhaps the most basic things we do are ingest and excrete, take air into our lungs and breathe it out" (Lakoff 1987: 271), and also as entities contained within something else. Hence, the idea of containment "defines the most basic distinction between IN and OUT" (Lakoff 1987).

Generally speaking, containers are determined by two factors. First, by the fact that they are entities whose function, with respect to other entities, is to provide the latter with an *address*. For example, my table is in the room, the room is in the building, and the building, where I am writing this, is in Pittsburgh. The relevant literature in linguistics (see sections 1.4 and 1.5) teaches us that amid the variety of locative relations expressed by prepositions such as "in," "on," "over," "under", our intuitive notion of containment is initially articulated through "in." Therefore, a container is above all a type of entity that other entities can be *in*.

On the other hand, certain uses of "in" may not pertain to location. When I say that a room is *in the building*, it may also mean that the room is *part* of the building, and parthood is an entirely different relation. We shall have to unpack this (see Chapter 6).

Finally, while there is a locational aspect to both "in the room" and "in Pittsburgh," there are also some differences between the two. While the first can be understood as a physical location, location within a portion of physical space (in the common sense of the term), this is by no means clear with reference to the latter. If Pittsburgh were moved by some powerful gods, say to Florida, with me still in it, I would remain *in* Pittsburgh, yet I would be in a different physical location, a different climate zone, etc. Therefore, perhaps we should also posit something like location within an institution (the City of Pittsburgh in this case; see). All that being said, being-in and containment turn out to be quite intricate relations.

The second factor is that containers have boundaries. It makes sense to distinguish a container's *interior* from its *exterior*. If I am in the room, I am not in the kitchen; if I am in Pennsylvania, I am not in Ohio. Hence, it seems that the boundary of a container works to separate two domains or areas. But is this always the case? Chapter 6 shall bring some answers.

Following Lakoff and Johnson's observation, as we look around us, plenty of entities fit the container schema – not only our bodies or the bodies of other animals, but also numerous things, both natural and man-made, such as caves, burrows, cabinets and mugs. Unsurprisingly therefore, we are naturally inclined, according to Johnson (1987) as well as Lakoff (1987) to model our minds in a similar manner, as *containers* of some sort.

Ubiquitous as it is, the container schema, but also other more general notions of location and boundary, have attracted the interest of philosophers and logicians. Along with formal theories of parthood, initiated by Leśniewski (1916/1992) and Leonard and Goodman (1940), based in part on the work of Husserl (1901/2000), a more disciplined scrutiny of boundaries was first proposed by Whitehead (1929) and Clarke (1985). Additionally, abstract theories of location emerged in linguistics with the work of Herskovits (1986), Vandeloise (1991), and in philosophy thanks to Perzanowski (1993) and Casati and Varzi (1999). Together, these various currents form the body of a logico-philosophical discipline dubbed *mereotopology* by Smith (1996). Here, following Perzanowski (1993), I would prefer to speak of various *locative ontologies*. This is because location is a key factor in this particular investigation – *parthood* and *boundary* can be studied in their own right, but the job assigned here to these concepts is to facilitate a proper theoretical grasp of what Lakoff and Johnson regard as the "container schema."

This book is predicated on the belief that a more scrupulous examination of locative-ontological terminology, in particular of the concept of containment as well as related notions, would be beneficial to philosophical investigations of the nature of mind and of cognition. In other words, it is my contention that identifying the locative ontologies underpinning various conceptualizations of cognition would lead to a better understanding of the conceptualizations in question, and in particular, of the shift we are now observing from mind-*as*-a-place to mind-*in*-a-place. Clearly, this shift has been articulated in explicitly locative terms; however, the terms themselves remain to be clearly defined.

The goal of this book, however, is not merely to provide such conceptual clarification. It is much more constructive than that. The book concludes with a positive proposal as to what a new locative ontology of the mind and cognition might look like, doing justice to the core tenets of both the mind-*as*-a-place and the mind-*in*-a-place paradigms.

In this introductory chapter, I would like to substantiate the claims I have just made. In other words, to demonstrate why a more elaborate ontological investigation is necessary if we are to properly understand and harness the full potential of this current paradigm shift.

1.3 Ryle, Popper and Putnam: Analytical critics of the mind-as-a-place paradigm

In 20th-century philosophy, it was Gilbert Ryle (1949) who first explicitly noted that since people observe things, processes and events in their physical surroundings, they are inclined to believe that what happens in their minds consists of entities which, although clearly unlike these material things, still belong to the category of *objects*, *processes*, *events*, etc. Thus, there must also exist mental objects, mental processes, etc. which are different in kind, *qua mental*, from physical objects and physical processes, but not that different *qua objects* or *qua processes*. According to this argumentation, mental processes also need a locus, since all objects and processes do. Based on encounters with familiar things, it may seem perfectly reasonable to some people that since our bodies are containers, our minds must also be containers, just filled with other kinds of entities. The container schema provides the most fundamental "architecture" of our conceptualizations of mind and of the mind-world relation. Needless to say, Ryle unambiguously described this way of conceptualizing the mind as a categorial mistake.

The Rylean reading of the mind-*as*-a-place paradigm proposes that this view is not a deliberate, even if only provisional, *solution to a problem*, but rather the spontaneous, mostly tacit product of a mental habit. Ryle argues that when scrutinized, the latter exhibits serious logical flaws, and should therefore be abandoned. Although Lakoff and Johnson do not attempt that much to correct this habitual way of conceptualizing the mind, Ryle is on the same page as them by maintaining the "mental habit" interpretation.

Karl Popper is also in this camp, abandoning what he termed the *bucket theory of mind*. It says that "our mind is a bucket which is empty, or more or less so, and into this bucket material enters through our senses" (Popper 1972: 61). Yet there is one subtle difference. Popper did not refer to mental habits (or not only to them), but seemed to contend that the bucket theory, as a specific philosophical conception of knowledge (emerged as part of empiricism), was the wrong *solution*, or at least a flawed answer to an otherwise serious problem. So, unlike Ryle as well as Lakoff and Johnson, Popper upheld what I would roughly call a "solution approach" rather than the "mental habit approach" to the mind-*as*-a-place view.

This difference is momentous because one cannot search for the rationale underpinning a mental habit, whether arguing in favor of it or against, or even seeking a compromise position – these rational investigations are quite implausible when dealing with a habit. They may be legitimate pursuits with regard to a deliberate position, thesis or concept. I believe that Popper was fundamentally right to address the bucket theory as *an answer to a problem*, not an automatic extrapolation from the domain of material things to the domain of the mental. Whether that answer was incorrect, as he insisted, or not, is another matter.

But what exactly does the bucket theory state and who formulated it first? Its fundamental tenet, according to Popper, is that the mind passively receives data from the world, like a bucket being filled with liquid. In sharp contrast to what the bucket theory says, gaining new empirical knowledge is, Popper argues, anything but putting new pieces of data into a container. Instead, as he famously said (consciously or not restating the view held by Plato; see 1.6), the mind works like a searchlight, guiding active observation. The minded subject is not a passive recipient of data, but an active seeker of information.

Yet it is still not entirely clear what motives lie behind the bucket theory and, more broadly, the mind-*as*-a-place paradigm. Seeking answers, we shall likely encounter the analysis proposed by Hilary Putnam, who in this respect follows William James and Edmund Husserl. We learn from him, in my understanding, that the real deep-seated rationale for targeting the mind as a locus had to do with a certain fixation on the idea of a *boundary* delineating the mind from its exterior, i.e.,

> the famous picture, the dualistic picture of the physical world and its primary qualities, on the one hand, and the mind and its sense-data, on the other, that philosophers have been wrangling over since the time of Galileo.
>
> (Putnam, 1987: 6–7)

If Putnam is right, the keystone of the mind-*as*-a-place paradigm, which has prevailed over the last couple of centuries, is the "invention of the external world," which we owe to Galileo (see Husserl 1970), and therefore also the relevant "invention" of the *internal* world of impressions or sense-data. These "inventions" were then continued and philosophically examined by Descartes and the British empiricists.

But what is so inventive about the *internal–external* division, which seems to be an intuitive given, and not some philosophical fiat? This is a very subtle moment. It is indeed quite intuitive to draw a line between *me* and what is *not me* or *not part of me*. Yet this intuition does not make it clear what this line is, how it works, or what it potentially delineates. Thus, each further precision in this regard is no longer a mere commonsense intuition, but a theoretical *decision*.

Putnam explains that this decision had to do with the "epistemic ideal of achieving a view from an 'Archimedean point' – a point from which we can survey observers as if they were not ourselves, survey them as if we were, so to speak, outside our own skins" (Putnam, 1990, p. 17). Reaching the "Archimedean point" would mean occupying the ideally objective position – external to all subjective influences and limitations. So, the *internal–external* division is really about how we understand knowledge in the most proper sense of the term.

This Galilean ideal of objectivity, his understanding of knowledge and thus his "invention of the external world" was given an explicit metaphysical basis by Descartes. The otherwise intuitive inner-outer line began to be thought of as an absolute demarcation between two essentially different realities: the external realm of mechanical entities and the internal domain of thought.

Of course, this idea had been anticipated by many traditions, most notably Platonic and neo-Platonic, but it was Descartes who gave it a clear conceptual framework based on a scientifically informed internal–external dichotomy. How so? First of all, we need to consider his studies in optics, which adopted the atomistic paradigm of his time and largely contributed to the future corpuscular theory of light. He provided a mechanistic account that identified light with a specific kind of motion, and thus, in line with Kepler's earlier studies, a mechanistic account of visual perception (see McDonough 2015). So, given what Descartes knew from his scientific research, the pursuit of thinking must have appeared to be of a very different nature from what he observed on the physical side of human cognitive functioning, so to speak. Moreover, thinking was accessible only to the thinker, i.e., to use Augustine's model, from within the "inner self." Hence, from this point on, the internal–external line was not just an intuitive posit separating two functionally distinct realms within a single reality, but a genuine metaphysical chasm between two kinds of substance.

Arguably, Descartes himself was quite puzzled by this result, which is clear in his *Meditations on First Philosophy* (Descartes 2008); i.e., in the intellectual struggles honestly reported there. And yet he had to accept this outcome, driven as he was by his own analytical method, and also probably by his desire to comply with his own methodological commitment to clarity and distinctness. In short, Descartes' first-person method of analysis saw thinking as a fundamentally non-physical endeavor, one that, even if it was indeed carried out by physical machines (brains and nervous systems – Descartes himself was one of the pioneers of brain research), could be carried out without a physical carrier, "since they can at least be produced separately by God" (Sixth Meditation 78; Descartes 2008: 55). Now, insofar as thinking was a particular cognitive process, it required a vehicle. Again, given the Augustinian model of the inner self, the postulation of some kind of internal locus for the thinking substance may have seemed conceptually inevitable.

But one thing must be made clear. My intention here is not to criticize Descartes for his alleged mistakes, which is quite common in externalist circles today, usually in book introductions and without paying attention to the historical context. I will return to Descartes' legacy in the later sections of this chapter and in Chapter 2, and add some more nuance.

To summarize this in a more general manner: to a large degree, how we *actually understand* the mind-*as*-a-place paradigm is determined by our understanding of the *internal–external* boundary, which supposedly delineates the realm of the mind from the rest of the world. As we shall see further on, this allegedly intuitive line is by no means a trivial philosophical concern. On the contrary, it can be given many different meanings, thereby determining our most abstract locative conceptualizations of cognition (locative ontology of cognition).

1.4 Peculiarities of "in"

The container schema and the locative relations constituting it, such as being-in or being-out, and respectively qualities such as being internal or external, may appear to be rather trivial and unproblematic. Therefore, whether we side with Ryle, Lakoff and Johnson, and Popper, or with Husserl and Putnam when it comes to alleged causes of the prevalence of the container schema in philosophy, the *schema itself* is not an issue. We know what it stands for – one might assume. However, I will now demonstrate that this is not the case.

Given that at least some critics of the mind-*as*-a-place approach appeal to the alleged intuitive sense of being-in, therefore attention should be paid to how we intuitively conceptualize locative relations. The purpose is of this section is to unveil a variety of meanings attributable to the relation of being-in. I believe that only once this variety is unfolded can we start to see being-in, especially as it applies to mind and cognition, as an issue worth tackling.

However, by "intuition" I do not mean my own subjective feelings, but rather what linguists define as the meanings attributable to ordinary uses of locative phrases. The latter include locutions such as "I'm *in* the room," "My laptop is *on* my desk and a book is placed right *near* the laptop," etc. Out of the variety of locative relations expressed in natural language(s), here I shall be exclusively concerned with "in," for reasons already sufficiently made clear.

The linguist Claude Vandeloise points out that it is an essential function of spatial relations as they manifest themselves in ordinary speech "to situate objects that the discourse participants hope to find or contact in some fashion" (Vandeloise 1991: 13). In his view, in step with Lakoff and Johnson, the preposition "in" primarily refers to containment – it "imposes one obvious condition on the object: it must be a potential container" (Vandeloise 1991: 6). However, *being a container* cannot be fully described in geometrical terms only. For example, there may be no structural difference whatsoever between a stone or a pebble and its paper model, insofar as their geometry is concerned, meaning that the geometrical representations of their shapes – edges, angles and curves – are identical. And while it may seem to us that the paper model is empty inside, which renders it a potential container, and the pebble is filled with matter, in fact both are filled: while the pebble is "filled exactly with a pebbly meaning," as the poet Zbigniew Herbert once beautifully put it,[1] the paper model is also filled with physical contents, e.g., air. Thus, the *emptiness* which characterizes containers is not a property that can be defined in physical terms, even if certain kinds of physical substances, gases or liquids, are more likely to be regarded as potential loci, which would pose some difficulty in the case of the "pebbly meaning." So, if the emptiness characteristic of containers cannot be described in either geometrical or physical terms, a different vocabulary is needed.

Now consider the following examples:

- the fly is in the box
- the fly is in the glass
- the moth is in the dark corner of the room
- the pen is in the box
- the pen is in the cup
- the wine is in the glass

First think of the difference between the fly being in the box and the pen being in the box: while a part of the surface of the pen coincides with a part of the surface of the box, there is no such coincidence in the case of the fly. Therefore, if one prefers to define being-in in terms of the coincidence of surfaces, it cannot work as a universal characteristic. More precisely, it is possible to posit that *x is in y* if all the boundaries of *x* coincide with some boundary (boundaries) of *y*, which could be imagined as *x* being wrapped up by *y* like a birthday present. Yet, the *fly in the box* shows that there can be no coincidence at all, while the being-in relationship clearly does occur.

Two further problems arise when we compare the case of the *pen in the box* with that of the *pen in the cup*. First of all, we would likely say that the pen is indeed in the cup, despite only *a part* of the pen actually being in the cup. But imagine that someone puts a much thicker, two meter-long stick into this same cup and the whole structure is propped up against the wall, so as not to collapse – are we also willing to say that the stick is *in* the cup, or perhaps we would prefer to say that just one *end* of the stick is in the cup while the rest is not? If so, then how long must an entity *x* be to justify the claim that *x* is in the cup and what length makes it necessary to say that only a *part* of *x* is in the cup? Naturally, there is no definite answer to this question, but there is a lesson to be drawn from both cases.

Once again, we learn that something else, not just the geometry of a potential container and a potential occupant, determines being-in or not-being-in. According to Vandeloise, as long as the cup modifies the external forces acting on the pen, for example, gravity, keeping the pen on the table, and constrains its freedom of movement by surrounding at least part of it, we can likely speak of containment, thus being-in. Therefore, in the case of the long stick, only part of it is contained, because another part of it is causally constrained by the wall and not the cup.

Whether or not Vandeloise's proposal can be generalized, an initial conclusion is that we may need a more *functional* approach to location in order to account for the variety of being-in relations. Think of the case of the wine in the glass, which also illustrates this point nicely. Once a quantity of wine is in the glass, moving the glass means moving the wine as well. As Sinha and Jensen de Lopez (2002) and Tyler and Evans (2003) remind us, containers do not merely contain "but also constrain the movements of their contents" (Tyler & Evans 2003: 30). Therefore, containers *do* something with their occupants.

Another interesting example is put forward by Annette Herskovits (1986). Imagine a pearl on top of a pile of pearls, which reaches higher than the bowl containing them (Figure 1.1A).

As pointed out by Herskovits, language users usually say that the pearl on top is *in* the bowl, yet geometrically this is not at all true. Try to disregard all the other pearls and focus on the arrangement comprising only the top pearl and the bowl: there is no containment whatsoever, strictly speaking, not even a partial one (Figure 1.1B). This example shows that when it comes to our natural grasp of the meaning of containment, functional and situational aspects sometimes prevail over geometrical ones.

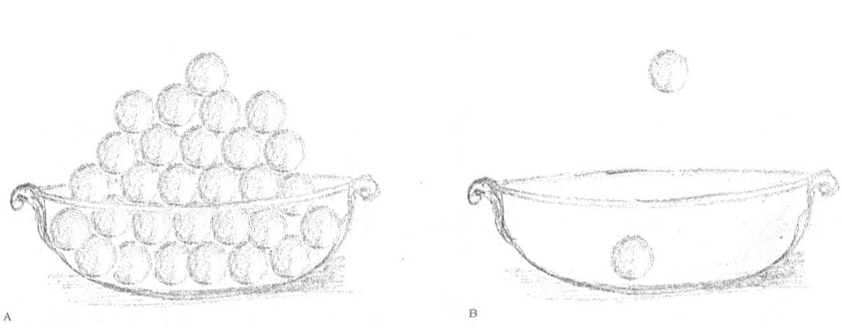

Figure 1.1

Cases such as the latter led Herskovists and others to draw a distinction between the geometrical and functional senses of "in," with the former being defined by context-free factors such as measurable relations between shapes, i.e., angles, curves, lines and the latter defined predominantly by functional, situational and thus context-dependent factors. We shall take this distinction to heart, since speaking of the functional sense of being-in makes room for a more abstract account of the mind-*as*-a-place paradigm.

Going back to the *pen in the cup* case, another thing to notice is that containers may be partially open. The same goes for the cases of the *wine in the glass* and the *fly in the glass*. Therefore, despite the fact that the distinction between open and closed entities is otherwise quite crucial, entities of both kinds can equally well serve as containers.

But consider the context of the *moth in the dark corner*: it seems to be fully defined by functional and situational factors, for the dark area has no clear-cut boundaries. So, if the notion of containment makes any sense here, the container is fully open. One might say that there is no container at all, nonetheless the moth *is* somehow non-incidentally in a specific segment of the world, not just anywhere. However blurred the distinction between the dark area and the illuminated one is, it remains crucial to the moth. As a result, we must say that there is no clear-cut, context-free "geometry" of the lighter versus darker division in the room; however, the moth can sensibly be regarded as non-accidentally located *in* the dark corner and constrained by this placement.

There are further cases like the ones sketched out above, but the examples provided suffice to show that the locative relation of being-in is by no means trivial. Therefore, even if we assume that Lakoff and Johnson or Ryle are right in that we intuitively extrapolate everyday cases such as the ones discussed above to the domain of cognition, it remains undecided which sense of "in" is actually in use here. This is not a philosophical issue in and of itself, but it should, I believe, spark philosophical reflection.

1.5 What it is like to be "in mind": Some intuition pumps to begin with

The variety of meanings attributable to "in" unveiled above renders the mind-*as*-a-place paradigm potentially quite complex. For it turns out that there is no *a priori* need to take being-in as a relationship which encompasses and encloses an entity within clear-cut, geometrical (not to mention physical) boundaries, which goes against what the bucket theory of mind suggests. According to the bucket theory, an entity cannot be partly in the cognitive system, and partly outside it. But why? Perhaps it would sound somewhat outlandish to suppose that an entity could be in a state of partial placement in the mind, but is this impression not due to a tacit *a priori* assumption about the nature of the locative relation in question? Why not try out partial containment, for example?

It is not my intention to solve a philosophical problem by appealing to natural language. However, I do contend that instead of denouncing such imaginative constructs in ordinary speech we should take a radically different approach: elicit and analyze them, as they can move forward (but not replace) the pursuit of philosophizing. For example, if the mind is conceived of as a container, then let us explore the variety of ways in which one thing could be said to contain another. This will make us realize that the "bucket theory" as rendered by Popper is not the only way of conceptualizing how the mind and containment may relate to each other. In this manner we obtain imaginative tools which may be called, following Dennett (2013), "intuition pumps," propelling our theoretical effort toward novel technical posits.

Let us concede that "intuition pumps" are imaginative exercises designed to warm up our conceptual creativity. I put them in the form of questions. So, here are the first two, based on what we have said so far about the meaning of "in":

> First intuition pump: *Is the mind a locus defined functionally or geometrically?*

If we adopt the functional understanding, the bucket theory turns out to be too concerned with an allegedly clear-cut distinction between the interior of the mind and its exterior. For while this dividing line is supposed to be clear and free of any situational factors, it may actually depend on context. As a result, one might argue, the bucket theory mistakenly focuses only on the internal side. Meanwhile, thinkers such as Andy Clark, as we shall see, would advocate for a cognitive system with a more functionally defined interior, to the effect that "human minds and bodies are essentially *open* to episodes of deep and transformative restructuring in which new equipment (both physical and 'mental') can become quite literally incorporated *into* the thinking and acting systems that we identify as our minds and bodies" (Clark 2008: 30–31; my emphases; see also Clark 2003).

However strange it sounds at first glance, Clark invites us to imagine being-in-the-mind as something closer to the *pearl-in-the-bowl* case cited above; thus, the possibility of an entity that is "geometrically" outside the system and remains *in* the system in some other sense. It is "functionally" *in* insofar as it partakes in what that system is doing.

Going further, and harking back to the *pen-in-the-cup* example, we obtain:

> Second intuition pump: *Is the mind an open (wholly or partially)-container like a vessel, or a closed one, like an egg or a cocoon?*

The idea of a closed container was introduced by behaviorism which famously modeled the cognitive system as a black box. One might say that it is the paradigmatic instantiation of the bucket theory. Interestingly, cognitive science built upon the concept of a physical computational system (see Chapters 2 and 3) began as an effort to look inside the box and nail down its *internal* machinery, while keeping the box heuristic itself in operation. In contrast, we shall see that, e.g., James Gibson's (1979) proposal sees the mind as being in a sense *open* to informationally rich environments, but the fact that a container is open is not at odds with the container schema itself. The latter realization shall prove crucial later in this book.

Further intuition pumps are inspired by further work on the linguistics of "in." Andrea Tyler and Vyvyan Evans (2003) propose a general schema for the relation of containment which they refer to as the "proto-scene" for the preposition "in." They point out the functional aspect, saying that containment "has consequences for both the [contained] and the [container]. [2] For instance, the surrounding [container] will often offer physical protection from outside forces and hide [the contained] from outside view [...]. Thus, the spatial configuration is not conceived as neutral, but as meaningful and consequential" (Tyler & Evans 2003: 25).

The proto-scene posited by Tyler and Evans (2003) describes the basic "architecture" of *being-in* – of what I shall call a *bounded locus*. Further on, they devise a list of developments of the proto-scene, that is to say, a sequence of different meanings of "in" derived from this initial schema. Below some of them are invoked; i.e., those that may be found interesting when it comes to the puzzle of how the mind-*as*-a-place view can/should be understood.

The In Situ Sense: This adds a new aspect to the proto-scene, namely containment here is not incidental or momentary. The contained entity remains in the container for some time and for some reason. In other words, "in" exhibits a more deep-seated situation which the contained entity is involved in. This is the sense in which we say, e.g., "He is in prison" or "He is in hospital." There is a significant difference between being *in hospital* and merely being *in the building* that happens to house a hospital or a prison.

Going further, Tyler and Evans propose:

The Disappearance Sense: e.g. "The wine quickly *soaked in*."

This develops the idea that containers obscure access from outside, here by effectively making the contained entity indistinguishable from the container. Therefore, it strengthens the In Situ Sense and can also be tacitly the case when, for example, someone asks, "Do you see the toy?" and the answer is of the form "No, he has just put it *in* the box." Here "in the box" is not merely about location (as if the question were "Where is the toy?") but rather about *accessibility*.

Taking the two senses together, we obtain the notion of an *occluder* which is a combination of the In Situ and the Disappearance senses. As a result, here is the next intuition pump.

Third intuition pump: *is the mind an occluder or not?*

It seems that at least part of the mind-*as*-a-place tradition takes the mind as an occluder of sorts. This, in a sense, is what Husserl and Putnam elicited about the Galilean and Cartesian fixation on the *internal–external* division as well as the subjective–objective chasm. Take one of the classical philosophical conundrums, namely knowledge of other minds (see e.g., Russell 1912), which has come to the fore in more recent years in the form of Chalmers's (1996) thought experiment with zombies. In the end, the puzzle in both cases is whether we can know anything remotely reliable (not to mention certain) from a third-person standpoint about someone else's first-person mental contents which are essentially occluded from view.

But the idea of the mind as an occluder has a flip side, as it were: it is not only the case that the contents poured into the mind are protected from external access, but also that the external world may also, in principle, be occluded from the mind. In other words, if we conceptualize the mind in this way, we end up with the question of modern idealism, namely whether or not there *is* any external world; and if so, whether we can know anything about it. Here we meet some great names, beginning with Descartes, through Berkeley and Hume, up to Russell and Moore.

In contrast, Dan Zahavi, for example, reminds us that according to Husserl, "all types of re-presentation (...) are derived acts that refer to a proper presentation (...) which is the mode of givenness where the object is given directly, originally, and optimally" (Zahavi 2003: 29). Here we are explicitly invited to reconsider the mind as a factor that not only does *not* occlude anything, but, at the other extreme, actualizes a certain presentation, thus working in the opposite way. And in step with the latter intuition, here is another derivative sense of "in" proposed by Tyler and Evans:

> *The Perceptual Accessibility Sense*, e.g. when we say "I have it in view" or "Susan always tries to stay in touch." Here "in" refers to situations *in* which an entity becomes accessible, uncovered, available.

A similar use of "in" is when we say that something is "in the light" and "in the open," meaning that the thing is illuminated and can therefore be seen, or that the thing is not separated from its environment by any barriers.

Thereby we arrive at another pivotal intuition pump:

> Forth intuition pump – *Is being in the mind more like being hidden in the box or more like being in view or being exposed?*

The point made by Husserl, at least in Zahavi's interpretation, is that being-*in*-the-mind, contrary to the entirety of the Cartesian tradition as it is usually understood, can refer to the *exposure* and *presentation* of an entity, not its occlusion. If we reflect on this possibility for a moment, it turns out that this idea is by no means unprecedented in the history of philosophy. Recall these lines from Plato's *Republic* 508 b–e (Book VI) which we shall hark back to later on:

> And the power which the eye possesses is a sort of effluence which is dispensed from the sun?
>
> Exactly.
>
> Then the sun is not sight, but the author of sight who is recognised by sight?
>
> True, he said.
>
> And this is he whom I call the child of the good, whom the good begat in his own likeness, to be in the visible world, in relation to sight and the things of sight, what the good is in the intellectual world in relation to mind and the things of mind.
>
> (…)
>
> And the soul is like the eye: when resting upon that on which truth and being shine, the soul perceives and understands, and is radiant with intelligence; (…)
>
> Now, that which imparts truth to the known and the power of knowing to the knower is what I would have you term the idea of good, and this you will deem to be the cause of science, and of truth in so far as the latter becomes the subject of knowledge (…)
>
> (Plato 2021)

Therefore, if we follow this intuition pump, the mind is fundamentally concerned with *actualizing* certain aspects of the world so that they *can be cognized*. The mind is in the business of *making the world manifest itself* thus and so.

Further on, Tyler and Evans propose:

> *The State Sense*, e.g., "I am in pain" or "We are in a state of war." This refers to being in a certain state, thus to the location in a state of affairs or in a situation.

So "in" does not have to refer to things or objects. It can also refer to entities belonging to different categories, e.g., the arrangement of things, states of affairs, situations or relational networks.

Having the State sense of "in" in mind, we can see that even if Ryle is right when he claims that people spontaneously (and naively) conceptualize the mind by taking the world around them as a template, that template offers more than just one pattern. Therefore we obtain:

> Fifth intuition pump – *If something is said to be in the mind, does it mean location in another object, or in a certain state?* In other words, is *being in the mind* more like *being in the box*, or more like *being in a state of war*, or to use a more pleasant and also quite telling example, like *being in conversation*?

The Cartesian tradition leans toward the former option, arriving at the behaviorist idea of the mind as a black box. In contrast, some of the posits proposed by enactivism, as we shall see, would suggest that the term "mind" may not stand for an *object* at all, but rather for a certain dynamic (re) arrangement of objects, made by embodied agents. This thought proves quite crucial and shall be articulated later on in terms of cognitive niche construction.

Warmed up by the above imaginative exercise, let us go back to philosophy proper.

1.6 Structures of location and the pursuit of intelligibility: Plato's insights

Needless to say, by invoking historical figures such as Galileo and Descartes, critics of the mind-*as*-a-place paradigm attempt to lead us down a treacherous path: that of examining history, but without the proper preparation for such a momentous journey. We should not heed this invitation, in the sense that all the claims made here, all the interpretations provided below, can at best be seen as introductory thoughts. However, it does seem reasonable to highlight just how broad the scope of the problem we are about to tackle is historically. Initial attempts to provide a historical context were already made in the previous sections. Perhaps instead of actually setting off on a historical journey we could make a sort of roadmap and circle a few major points on it. We shall let our fingers do the walking, merely indicating some of the must-see sights along the way.

I shall adopt the "solution approach" to the mind-*as*-a-place paradigm, inspired by Popper. While we already have some idea of what its critics say about its origins, I believe it is useful to do justice to the other side of the argument as well. The question to be provisionally answered here is: what was (and still is) the rationale for the mind-*as*-a-place paradigm as it emerged in philosophical reflection?

To frame the following paragraphs and justify the required effort, let me state that rationale upfront: the reason for the emergence of the mind-*as*-a-place view was not a preoccupation with a specific ontology of the mind. Nor was it a preoccupation with any specific notion of location that the mind should exemplify. Instead, the mind-*as*-a-place view(s) stemmed from a need to account for an apparent fact which manifests itself in our everyday experience. Namely that we humans *are not only agents or doers; we are also thinkers, meditators and understanders*. This does not in principle imply being a walled-off fortress, but it does mean being able to *retreat from* the open, so to speak, to *the safe space of an inner self*, understood in any way one wishes, but in some sense "kept safe" from the goings-on of the world. This does not necessarily mean being a passive recipient of whatever the world delivers via the senses, but it does mean being able to stop and distance oneself from these various interactions and activities in order to *reflect* on them. Finally, it does not necessarily mean being a bucket filled with purely subjective impressions or sense data which can have no existence outside of this bucket, but it does mean being able to process some contents behind the closed doors of our inner, reflective lives.

This is all somewhat vague, but it could hardly be any different at this stage. Let me reiterate: we are discussing a type of first-person phenomenological or reflective observation, made not only by philosophers, although philosophers were at the forefront of the effort to do justice to this observation as part of our most general conceptualization (thus ontology) of the world and of the mind-world connection.

It is not easy to point to the first instance of the mind-*as*-a-place paradigm as such, but perhaps one of its first formulations comes from Plato. That said, his attitude toward it was by no means outright endorsement. Indeed, it may be that he should instead be added to the camp of its critics. This is because Plato clearly rejects the empiricism of his contemporaries, and therefore something akin to the bucket theory of his time. Inspired by Homer, in the *Theaetetus* he depicts the perceiving subject as a wooden horse, hollow inside, merely fed different sensations. Plato uses this metaphor to ridicule the empiricist account of perception. It would be hard to imagine a more biting depiction and explicit rejection of the bucket view. In *Theatetus* 184 d we read:

SOCRATES: Yes, my boy, for no one can suppose that in each of us, as in a sort of Trojan horse, there are perched a number of unconnected senses, which do not all meet in some one nature, the mind, or whatever we please to call it, of which they are the instruments, and with which through them we perceive objects of sense.

And then in 186 a–c:

SOCRATES:	And would you say the same of the noble and base, and of good and evil?
THEAETETUS:	These I conceive to be notions which are essentially relative, and which the soul also perceives by comparing in herself things past and present with the future.
SOCRATES:	And does she not perceive the hardness of that which is hard by the touch, and the softness of that which is soft equally by the touch?
THEAETETUS:	Yes.
SOCRATES:	But their essence and what they are, and their opposition to one another, and the essential nature of this opposition, the soul herself endeavours to decide for us by the review and comparison of them?
THEAETETUS:	Certainly.
SOCRATES:	The simple sensations which reach the soul through the body are given at birth to men and animals by nature, but their reflections on the being and use of them are slowly and hardly gained, if they are ever gained, by education and long experience (Plato 2008)

It would seem, however, that Plato does not oppose the idea of perceptual input, i.e., the in–out distinction suggested by the wooden horse model. Or perhaps this was not an issue that drew his attention at all. What he strongly rejects is the hollowness of the container. Sensations are not enough, he says, since we need a machinery to integrate these scattered inputs – a machinery capable of creating a comprehensive world-view from these atomized givens. Hence, he argued, it is imperative that we introduce a soul or a mind. The backbone of Plato's theory of mind is something like a representational system capable of processing the incoming data. In this context, it is not entirely clear whether Plato would have rejected a container model as such, or just pointed to the necessity of having a cognitive machinery within it.

Leaving this interpretative puzzle aside, it appears that, first of all, the bucket theory might already have existed in antiquity, and second, that the philosophers of that time might have been discussing potential refinements to the bucket model, which might also have created room for a more abstract mind-*as*-a-place model (which we see clearly in the neo-Platonic tradition, see below); finally, that the cited fragment from the *Theaetetus* indicates an early correlation of two ideas: first, that cognition somehow relates to structures of location, in a general manner, thus to places and boundaries, and second, that it involves not only the mere gathering of incoming data, but also – crucially – making sense of these data, thus making sense of the world, i.e., the pursuit of *understanding* (see also Lagerlung 2007).

A complementary picture emerges from Plato's *Republic*, which was already cited above, in which the sun represents the highest idea – the Good – which makes the universe *intelligible*, just as the sun makes the world visible. The highest idea (*Republic* 508 e) "imparts truth to the known and the power of knowing to the knower" (Plato 2021).

The problem of *understanding* and *making sense* of the world, rather than merely collecting stimuli, stands out in Plato's critique of empiricism and his overall reflection on the conditions of *intelligibility*. Note that this metaphorical image also has an intuitive locative interpretation, for it is natural to say that something is *in the light*, and analogously, if the Good is thought of as making the world intelligible, it can also be said that something is *placed in* a specific "light," say in the light of the highest Reason. Reason, therefore, clearly establishes a certain *place* – a "space of reasons," as Wilfrid Sellars (1956) and John McDowell (1994) might say.

1.7 The origins of the inner self: The insights of Augustine and Descartes

All that being said, the locative commitments of Plato, when it comes to the pursuit of understanding, are not entirely clear, and their proper interpretation would require some more effort. Yet there is another ancient thinker whose commitments in this regard are quite clear and whose influence on modern thought seems paramount when it comes to how we conceptualize mind. This is in large part due to his influence on Descartes. I am of course referring to Augustine of Hippo.

Philip Cary opens his brilliant book (2000) with the following statement:

> For the most part, we in the West still take it for granted that we can talk about an inmost self and conceive of it as an inner world, a sort of private realm where we are most at home and most ourselves. Many still find this concept indispensable, as if we human beings would lose sight of some important part of ourselves without it. Yet such talk is hardly universal or necessary for human life. [...] Human beings can describe themselves in emotional, ethical, and religious terms without recourse to the conception of a private inner world. Indeed, before Augustine everyone seems to have found it natural to do so, having no notion that there was an alternative.
>
> (Cary 2000: 9)

One thing especially stands out in this fragment. It enables us to recognize that the idea of an *inner self*, of the mind as a private sphere, thus a special *private locus*, is precisely that – *an idea*, an intellectual construct, and not a brute fact simply manifesting itself, as chairs or tables do. In a sense, it is always refreshing to realize that even something that we take for granted, as a given, has actually been created. As such, the idea can of course be rejected, but not simply as the outcome of a mistaken, reflexive habit. If it is to be rejected, it must be rejected on rational grounds, since there was a rationale for it in the first place, and any alternative proposed must deal with this fact. The Popperian solution approach, therefore, seems to have more historical weight than the Rylean habit approach, for if Cary is right, before Augustine no one had quite targeted cognition in terms of containers.

That being said, the above rationale needs to be spelled out clearly. It turns out that Augustine's reason for developing the notion of an inner self was not merely a desire to wall the self off from the external world. Instead:

> (…) inwardness involves more than a concept of the self; it is concerned with the divine, the eternal, the ultimate. From its inception, inwardness meant seeking a glimpse of the soul's inner relation to its divine origin.
> (Cary 2000: 10)

Therefore, even if the notion of containment (the bucket, as Popper would term it) is one way of interpreting Augustine's thoughts about the inner self, arguably it is neither at the core of his reflection, nor a goal in and of itself. In other words, Augustine does not seem to care whether the self is predicated on containment or another locative relation. Instead, his core concern seems to be that the mind is a "safe space" of self-knowledge, moral knowledge, and most importantly, of divine ideas which ultimately make all knowledge possible.

This reference to God is crucial. Yet from the standpoint of this book, the goal is not some sort of philosophical theology, but the following idea: just as with Plato's highest Good, the reference to divine ideas reflects the fact that as reflective thinkers engaged in the pursuit of intelligibility, we must think of the mind as something capable of making that pursuit *possible*. Insofar as insight requires some degree of receptivity and temporary retreat from worldly engagements, any conceptualization of the mind must involve some sort of safe space or refuge where this peculiar moral and epistemic endeavor can be realized. Whether or not the mind is a container or another kind of locative structure is a secondary issue that Augustine himself does not problematize.

To get a better sense of what is at stake, let us refer to a contemporary thinker who is correctly recognized as one of the founding fathers of the mind-*in*-a-place paradigm: Maurice Merleau-Ponty. He provides us with one of the best articulations of what likely motivated Augustine, and perhaps already Plato. To my knowledge, the literature on embodied cognition has paid no attention to this insight. In the *Introduction* to his *Phenomenology of Perception*, Merleau-Ponty closely examines the concerns of phenomenology and writes:

> Reflection does not withdraw from the world towards the unity of consciousness as the world's basis; it steps back to watch the forms of transcendence fly up like sparks from a fire; it slackens the intentional threads which attach us to the world and thus brings them to our notice.
> (Merleau-Ponty 1962/2005: XV)

The above can be reformulated as the following claim: even as embodied, living creatures we have the capacity to loosen or relax our intentional bonds, as it were, which is a very peculiar cognitive achievement – the fundamental cognitive endeavor that makes us (humans) what we are – creatures capable of reflection, but it is also a capacity that requires that certain conditions first be satisfied. Augustine's inner self is a specific proposal concerning those conditions, and while modern cognitive science paints a different, more scientifically accurate picture of the subject, the question of how to account for the "slackening" Merleau-Ponty refers to remains open. Any decision to abandon the traditional Augustinian mind-*as*-a-place posit still has to provide an alternative.

Now, as the story of the inner self develops and builds upon Augustine, we must reconsider Descartes, who is widely recognized as Augustine's follower, while at the same time working in a completely different environment, in the midst of a scientific revolution that he himself contributed to in large measure. It was Descartes who, as already noted above, was the first to have devised the notion of mind as a specific realm, sharply delineated from the "external world," and thus – according to empiricism, not that much Descartes himself though – best represented as a closed container filled with ideas.

Descartes' use of the locative framework is somewhat reluctant, which is also worth noting. First, if Ryle or Lakoff and Johnson were right in their claim that we imagine the realm of mind simply by extrapolating our imaginative models of ordinary things, it should have occurred naturally to Descartes that the mind is a container – an idea that would additionally be reinforced by his achievements in the field of optics and physiology of perception. Meanwhile, he writes:

> Nature likewise teaches me, through these very feelings of pain, hunger, thirst, and so forth, that I am not present in my body only as a pilot is present in a ship, but that I am very closely conjoined to it and, so to speak, fused with it, so as to form a single entity with it.
> (Sixth Meditation 81; Descartes 2008: 57)

It would seem, therefore, that he is aware that the container schema is somewhat problematic as a descriptive tool designed to grasp the actual dynamics of cognition, and therefore it is doubtful that he was strongly inclined to consider the mind as a container or indeed to approach the mind-body relationship in these terms.

Perhaps the bucket theory arose neither from a mental habit, as Ryle would argue, nor from a strong theoretical conviction, as Popper suggested, but was just a provisional postulate, for lack of a better option. The conceptual framework for cognition was not sufficiently developed at that time to enable thinkers such as Descartes to attempt to advance a more nuanced locative narrative of the mind. A pivotal notion in this more nuanced narrative, I would argue, is that of "environment," which we now possess in our theoretical toolbox, but which Descartes and his empiricist followers clearly lacked.

Regardless, just as Augustine before him, Descartes does not seem overly concerned with what the correct locative "architecture" of the mind actually is. He also puts emphasis on the question of how *knowledge* is possible and searches for an ultimate placement or foundation for it. As obvious as the latter statement is for an epistemologist, it comes as somewhat of a surprise for the philosopher of mind. Answering the question of *what* a mind is, which today exists as a question in its own right, was for Descartes secondary to the issue of how the mind could encapsulate ultimate, irrefutable knowledge. It would seem that for Descartes, as for Augustine, whatever the mind is, it must necessarily be something capable of playing the crucial role of *a receiver of ideas emanating from* God. In fact, for Descartes, the one core idea – that *of* God – anchors the whole construct of knowledge via the notion of divine trustworthiness. And clearly, such knowledge, grounded in God, is his main concern. As such, the mind cannot be a bodily substance, Descartes argues, and therefore it must constitute some *locus* awaiting God's intellectual gift. Yet what *kind* of locus it is was not a question which, in my view, was a major concern for Descartes.[3]

Popper was therefore right, whether deliberately or not, not to attribute the bucket theory to Descartes. Instead, his criticism was aimed at empiricism above all, and thus at the founding fathers of modern philosophy such as Hume and Locke. Indeed, *their* vocabulary suggests that the mind functions as a container for a peculiar sort of entities which have no existence outside of this container. Perhaps then, British empiricism is the proper source of the bucket theory. Whether or not that is true, one thing is clear: given what we know about Plato, Augustine and Descartes, figures who had paramount influence on how we think of the mind, the mind-*as*-a-place paradigm is not essentially about containers. Rather, it is about providing an account of how the intellectual exercise of "slackening our intentional bonds," of pursuing intelligibility, works. Whether this exercise must take place in a container or in a different locus remains an open question.

Empiricists took the containment option at face value, or perhaps we should say that they took the bull by the horns, and delivered a new account of the mind. Finally, there was something that could actually be recognized as an exemplification of the bucket theory of mind, of the model of mind as a container. For example, when John Locke says that "external objects furnish the mind with the ideas of sensible qualities, which are all those different perceptions they produce in us" (Locke, *An Essay Concerning Humane Understanding* 2.1.5; Locke 2004; my emphasis), the concept of *furnishing* clearly appeals to the notion that something is being *put in* something else. So, external entities causally affect our sense organs and this is *the only basis* for more complex knowledge structures:

> In that all our knowledge is founded; and from that it ultimately derives itself. Our observation employed either, about external sensible objects, or about the internal operations of our minds perceived and reflected on by ourselves, is that which supplies our understandings with all the materials of thinking.
>
> (Locke 2004)

However, the problem of understanding remains pivotal, as we shall see in Chapter 2. While for Descartes there is *at least one* input arriving in the mind that is inherently meaningful in and of itself – the idea *of* God coming *from* the mind of God – the only "materials" we can fill the empiricist "blank slate" with are sense impressions, lacking any intrinsic sense or meaning (as later argued by Kant, who used the term "blind" to describe them). Meaning is, therefore, according to empiricism, *imposed on* the data received by the subject, who is capable of using them to construct knowledge. Meanwhile, the belief in *inherent* meaning, attributable *to what comes* to the mind *from* without, was a default position in premodern times and to some extent still for Descartes.

Stephen Toulmin made a remarkably insightful comment on this issue. He wrote that "in the Ancient's view, human beings formed part of a single comprehensive cosmos along with physical and biological Nature." This means that "by their nature, the human reason and the universal logos has a close affinity or analogy" (Toulmin 1981; quoted from Ben-Zeev 1984: 331).

Ergo, the point is that for both ancient and medieval thinkers, everything we live in is a domain governed by some inherently meaningful factor, to put it in the most general terms. Therefore, the inputs coming to us from the world must convey some content on their own, and the proper goal of an individual mind is firstly not necessarily to *represent*, but to *participate* in a larger worldly sense (arguably the notion of representation may still be useful, but some sort of participation must precede it).

It is worth noting that, surprisingly or not, this idea of the inherent meaningfulness of sensory inputs makes a comeback in Gibson's (1979) ecological psychology (grounded in some of Husserl's insights) which puts forward the concept of affordances, stating that perception is the context-dependent acquisition of certain action-related "offers" present within the perceiver's species-specific environment. In a certain sense, the same idea underpins the enactive theory, but this claim requires further elaboration (in due course below).

Coming back to Descartes, the transition from his doctrine to Locke and Hume is quite pivotal due to the fact that on the one hand Descartes was a participant in the scientific revolution of his time, which led him toward a more atomistic and mechanistic (in the sense of Galileo) approach to nature and sensory perception, while at the same time he was still embedded within the pre-modern idea of the mind as being fundamentally a receptacle of divine ideas. This pre-scientific presupposition must have led him to the idea that even if the mechanistic model did apply to the mind in some way, at least at the most fundamental level, the mind had to be something *capable of awaiting divine input*, i.e., inherently meaningful content (particularly the idea of God) – an idea that does not need to be glued together by *our* cognitive mechanisms, but rather needs to be properly *understood*. And waiting for this input was Descartes' *res cogitans*.

Meanwhile, the emerging scientific picture of the world and of perception unequivocally suggested that at the end of the day mind itself was also a mechanism processing physical stimuli, a mechanism among many others within physical reality, with no place for some mysterious participation in a greater "meaning."

I shall stop here, for while it is desirable to have some historical awareness, even if somewhat imperfect, it is also a risky endeavor, as I mentioned earlier. We should also be clear where this introduction should end and a proper in-depth investigation should begin. I feel that we have reached precisely that point. Chapters 2 and 3 will be devoted specifically to unpacking the idea of a computational/representational system, its philosophical roots, and it will take the locative-ontological perspective, thereby setting off into the proper investigation this book is devoted to.

Let me, therefore, wrap up this section before moving on. The very purpose of our little historical tour was, first, to point out that the locative "architecture" we are examining, i.e., the mind-*as*-a-place view, does not have to be referred to as habitual, contrary to what Ryle claimed and what Lakoff and Johnson's analysis of natural language suggested. Rather, insofar as philosophical analyses are concerned, it was an *answer* to *a problem*.

Second, the problem, solved (or not) by the mind-*as*-a-place position, was not something akin to "what is the proper locative account of the mind and of the mind-world relation", but rather something like "how should we account for our cognitive functioning, given the fact that we are capable of understanding that the world we live in makes sense to us." Allow me to recapitulate my main point so far: I argue that the most fundamental motivation for the mind-*as*-a-place paradigm – which is *in no way* equivalent to the bucket theory rendered in terms of containment – was the recognition that we are not only doers and recipients of stimuli, but crucially also thinkers and understanders, creatures capable of "slackening" our intentional bonds with our surroundings, and so of rationally reflecting on our engagement with the world.

Third, contrary to what Popper claimed, the mind-*as*-a-place position was not, or at least *not necessarily*, about containment (in other words "buckets"). The latter notion emerged relatively late.

1.8 Cartesian cognitive science

Some might claim that citing the mind-*as*-a-place paradigm and the bucket theory is a convenient way of rounding up the different views we come across when studying the history of philosophy but that it applies imperfectly to our own time in which the real debate concerns much more fine-grained issues relating to the notions of computation and representation. For example, how given representational content is realized within neural networks or what kind of role representations play within the cognitive system (Ramsey's famous 2007 "job description challenge" which I shall address in Chapter 3), etc. These are the empirical, as well as theoretical, concerns of modern cognitive science, and whether those working on them happen to imagine the representational system in locative terms or even in terms of containment is quite irrelevant, one might argue, to the theories they pursue.

However, the issue is not the imaginative capabilities of any researchers. If the mind-*as*-a-place view was not a product of habitual thinking, contrary to what Ryle (1949) claimed, but a certain conceptual decision made by a number of pivotal researchers, there is no reason to assume that their contemporary counterparts are free from any such commitments. Further on, this commitment may also impact how the already-mentioned scientific or meta-scientific debates are framed. Noë makes this point, for example, claiming that the field is still very much determined by the in–out dichotomy. According to him, the "fundamental assumption of much of the research on the neuroscience of consciousness is that consciousness is itself a neuroscientific phenomenon. It takes place inside us, within the brain" (Noë 2009: 5). People working in neuroscience, according to Noë, "tend to think that consciousness [...] must be something that happens somewhere in the human brain, just as digestion must take place in the stomach" (Noë 2009: 4).

Mark Rowlands is of a similar opinion when he points out that "[t]raditional attempts to study the mind are based on the idea that whatever else is true of mental processes – perceiving, remembering, thinking, reasoning, and so on – they exist in brains (Rowlands 1999: 2).

This approach constitutes what Rowlands refers to as "Cartesian cognitive science." He is aware of the dangers involved in using such a broad term, since various important differences between specific conceptions may thereby be attenuated, yet he insists on this categorization:

> We do not need to worry about the details of this dispute. What unites these differing faces of Cartesian cognitive science is an unquestioned – indeed seemingly banal – assumption: whatever else is true of mental processes, whether they are abstract formal processes or patterns of activity in a neural network (or both) – they are processes that occur inside the head of the thinking organism. Cognitive processes – the category of mental processes with which cognitive science is concerned – occur inside cognizing organisms, and they do so because cognitive processes are, ultimately, brain processes (or more abstract functional roles realized exclusively by brain processes). It is this unquestioned assumption that makes Cartesian cognitive science Cartesian.
>
> (Rowlands 1999: 2–3)

One might ask whether representationalists themselves see this issue in a similar way, for there is a risk that anti-representationalists simply misread their opponents. However, Nicholas Shea seems to be quite clear when he openly claims that the utility of the notion of representation lies in addressing the question of "how do mental states manage to be about things in the external world?" (Shea 2018: 5), and more specifically "how do beliefs and perceptual states manage to be about an object that is right in front of the thinker (the pen on my desk), when the object is out there, and the representations are inside the thinker?" (Shea 2018: 9). The mind-*as*-a-place approach, openly building upon the analogy with organs inside the body, is also clearly evident in the following quote from Fred Dretske:

> We are accustomed to hearing about biological functions for various bodily organs. The heart, the kidneys, and the pituitary gland, we are told, have functions – things they are, in this sense, supposed to do. [...] The same seems true for sensory systems, those organs by means of which highly sensitive and continuous dependencies are maintained between external, public events and internal, neural processes.
>
> (Dretske 1995: 63)

Still, someone could claim that I have merely quoted some of Shea's introductory remarks or a generic statement from Dretske, thus ways in which the issue is framed in more intuitive– in this case locative – terms, while these terms themselves have no *real* bearing on proper representational theory; that they are just figurative rhetorical devices, overused and overinterpreted by anti-representationalists. Therefore, a complaint could be directed at many advocates of the mind-*in*-a-place approach, insofar as they make sweeping generalizations, such as those cited from Noë and Rowlands. It could be argued that such general claims do not necessarily engage with the details. This sort of criticism is formulated by Gładziejewski and Miłkowski, for instance, who note that "[s]ome modern antirepresentationalists employ a sort of trivializing argumentative strategy" (Gładziejewski & Miłkowski 2017: 337).

This complaint may indeed be fair, which is why I will delve into much more detailed, fine-grained issues in Chapters 2 and 3. That said, if we are to be more specific, we must not only restrict our attention to a specific formulation of representationalism, but also introduce some additional constraints.

Theories referring to representations form such a broad tent that it is unclear whether any general reference to "representationalism" could include them all. In fact, not all of them problematize what representations are, as if assuming that the term is perfectly clear and unproblematic in and of itself. For that reason, the mere use of the term "representation" is not sufficient to put someone in the representationist camp, insofar as representationalism can be thought of as a genuine paradigm.

Therefore, as for the announced specification, I shall first take the notion of a *representational system* understood *mechanistically* as my main focus in this book (see Chapter 2). I will, therefore, first be discussing certain systems, i.e. complex objects capable of exercising certain functions; second, systems in which some mechanisms can non-trivially be regarded as performing *the function of representing*, meaning that some internal state/object *x* represents (stands for) an external state/object *y*. Both of these characterizations shall be unpacked in greater detail in Chapters 2 and 3.

The notion of representational system was arguably the conceptual backbone of cognitive science as it emerged starting in the 1950s until the 1970s (see Chapter 2). The question is whether it makes sense to speak of *a locative footprint* of the representational system (mechanism), i.e. whether the representational system *determines a specific bounded portion of space*, a certain *bounded locus*. In this context, let me again cite Rowlands, for he describes an important trend:

> [...] in early cognitive science, the emphasis was very much on the "programs" or cognitive "software"; early cognitive science understood

> itself as engaged in the task of providing abstract formal descriptions of cognitive processes. However, from the mid-1980s on, this emphasis gradually gave way to a renewed emphasis on "hardware" in the form of *connectionist* or *neural network* approaches: approaches to understanding cognition based on neurally realistic models of its underlying architecture. Neural network models base their accounts of cognition on a hardware that is explicitly (if roughly) modeled on the brain.
>
> (Rowlands 1999: 2)

If he is right, at the very beginning of the cognitivist revolution, when a more abstract approach – which came from the foundations of mathematics and culminated in the idea of the Turing machine – was still in the air, one could claim that the representational system did *not* necessarily have any locative footprint, being in fact a certain abstract model. However, once cognitive psychologists took the lead in cognitive science and then passed on the torch to neuroscientists, this abstract system became somewhat more embodied, concretized. Finally, a number of researchers, perhaps most importantly Ruth Millikan (1984), but also Dretske (1981) in a somewhat different manner, began to think of representational systems as biological phenomena, realized by concrete organisms within specific environments – an idea subsequently expanded upon by Peter Godfrey-Smith (1996), Brian Skyrms (2010), Tyler Burge (2010), and others.

It must, therefore, be clear that in this book by *representational system* I shall mean not an abstract computational model, but actual, biologically embedded machinery utilized by concrete animals. This is what I call the *biological constraint* of the philosophical investigations to be rolled out in this book.

Thus, for now the discussion of representationalism shall be framed by two concepts (a third shall be added later on): that of representational systems as clusters of mechanisms, and that of biological constraint, in the sense just given.

Nevertheless, Rowlands's term "Cartesian cognitive science" should be used with caution, and, as I suggested earlier, our reading of Descartes requires some more nuance. On the one hand, Descartes himself, although rightly regarded as one of the founding fathers of the scientific study of light, perception and the brain, would not agree that "cognitive processes are ultimately brain processes" (Rowlands 1999: 2). And his so-called dualism was not the main reason, in my view. The main reason was that although he did not think of cognition as a form of engagement with the environment, because he lacked the concept of the latter (for which, of course, he cannot be blamed, given the historical context; see also Chapter 2), he was nonetheless concerned with a different kind of engagement, namely the kind of engagement that made room for the idea of God.

For although a nexus of brute physical mechanisms, beginning with the mechanics behind the retinal image, served as the causal basis of knowledge, it was, in Descartes' view, this divine idea that ultimately made knowledge possible. This creates a tension in his conception of the subject, since there must be something capable of receiving the idea, leading to what we now call dualism. However, a broader view of Descartes' work makes it rather unlikely that he explicitly aimed to confine cognition to a bucket-like subject. So to talk about the identification of cognitive processes with brain processes as the "unquestioned assumption that makes Cartesian cognitive science Cartesian" (Rowlands 1999: 3) is unwarranted and somewhat misleading.

On the other hand, while modern cognitive science belongs to a certain intellectual tradition, with Descartes as a major player, it is not dogmatically, as Rowlands and Noë seem to suggest, aligned with the bucket theory or the like. We will see this particularly in relation to Allen Newell and Herbert Simon (see Chapter 2). Therefore, as with the reading of Descartes, more nuance is needed in the process of unpacking the locative ontology behind what Rowlands called Cartesian cognitive science, assuming, as I do, that this umbrella term makes some sense. I will try to do this with reference to the concept of representational system.

1.9 The locative footprint of representational systems

Someone might argue that the biological constraint trivializes the question of whether a representational system determines a locus, since animals obviously have a locative footprint. They clearly occupy a certain unique, bounded portion of the world and contain other entities within them – to start with, their own functional building blocks, i.e., their organs. Yet upon closer inspection this turns out to be false. Of course, any organism occupies a specific portion of space and serves as a locus for its own components, sometimes (as in the case of complex individuals like animals) including other organisms, such as symbiotic bacteria. However, this does *not* automatically imply that the animal *as a representational system* constitutes a locus, meaning a locus determined by the animal's pursuit of *representing* its surroundings, rather than by its metabolism or motor functions.

Let me clarify this last point to the extent possible at this early stage of the investigation, for we shall get a better grasp of locative concepts in subsequent chapters and stepwise. Here I provisionally propose that *a locative footprint* specific to a system is understood as a bounded locus determined by certain *specific* criteria as to what gets into the said system and what does not. In Chapter 6, I shall provide a more technical characterization of a bounded locus based on the relevant literature.

Going back to the point about biological constraint, having a locative footprint is clearly part of what constitutes organisms. Furthermore, if we suppose that an organism is composed of various functionally distinct subsystems, which is a theoretical fiction adopted as standard in biology (e.g. we speak of the cardiovascular system, the urinary system, the respiratory system; while they obviously cannot exist independently, it is useful to distinguish them functionally), we can also provisionally assume – for the sake of the argument – that the machinery of representation somehow belongs to such subsystems, most likely as a subpart of a broader cognitive/sensorimotor system.

Now, all the systems constituting a particular organism obviously *operate in space*, for how could it be otherwise if they are all mechanical and physicochemical complexes? Yet, and this is the crucial point, *not* all of them determine *their own* system-specific bounded loci or their own *specific criteria* for deciding whether something is *in* or *out*. It is not necessary for a system *s* partaking in the organism to determine its own *s*-specific locus. Instead, *s* can operate in the loci determined by the living creature's other subsystems or in the locus determined by the organism as a whole. So, *operating in space* is one thing for *s*, but *delineating this space* in the unique *s*-specific manner (providing it with boundaries cutting off specific loci) is a different thing altogether, and while some of the organism's subsystems do the latter, others likely do not. At the end of the day, while being *placed* in a location trivially applies to anything in the realm of macroscopic entities such as living creatures, the pivotal issue is whether or not a given system draws *its own* specific boundaries, thus defining *its own specific locus*. For example, the integumentary system clearly defines a certain bounded locus, in all likelihood the one we think of first when we ask ourselves what makes an animal a located entity. It is also crucial for the living creature's ability to remain in a state of thermodynamic disequilibrium with its surroundings. Therefore, the integumentary system determines a specific place for everything that is enclosed by the physical barriers of the body. According to the *criteria* set by my integumentary system, my liver is clearly in, while the cookie I am holding in my hand is clearly out. However, this is not the entire story if we wish to determine the locus of the organism, e.g., an animal, as a whole, especially when we are dealing with complex organisms that have bodies. Note that it is by no means obvious whether the place occupied by what we refer to as a "dog" is identical to the locus determined by its physical barriers (see Werner 2020a; more in Chapter 6). To use a straightforward example: the cavity from the dog's mouth to its anus is *in principle not enclosed* by the barriers in question (certain muscles of the mouth and anus in some sense close the cavity, but insofar as the dog's basic blueprint is concerned, it is still *a cavity*). However, the location of this cavity should certainly be taken into account when we speak of the locative footprint of the *dog* as a whole (see Casati & Varzi 1994 on cavities and holes as peculiar beings). Now what happens when the dog eats the cookie we just mentioned? It is still outside its physical barriers strictly speaking, yet the processes of digestion, beginning with the secretion of chemicals that catalyze the cookie's decomposition, seem to introduce *different criteria* of what is *in* and what is *out* which are not identical to the criteria employed by the integumentary system. For example, if the liver cannot process a certain toxic substance added to the cookie, it is not allowed to move any further, although the toxin is clearly, and unfortunately, *inside* the organism as defined by its physical barriers. On the other hand, urine is also stored for a while inside the bounded locus defined by the integumentary system, but it is not inside the bounded locus defined by the digestive system any more – it is a waste product. Finally, think of the immune system, which is a crucial case discussed in the literature on what is known as biological individuality (see Pradeu 2012). It is said that the immune system determines *its own* criteria of what is part of the organism and what is not, boiling down to immune tolerance. Ergo, we could also state that the immune system determines what can get *in* and what must stay *out*. It thereby defines a certain *immune system-specific bounded locus*, clearly different from the loci established by the integumentary and digestive systems.

In contrast, consider the endocrine system. While its locative aspect is obvious, it makes use of the locus/loci defined by other systems and does not define *its own* locative footprint. In other words, determining the criteria of being *in* or *out* is not part of what it does. Of course, someone might argue otherwise. Admittedly, some cases are more controversial in this respect. For example, does the cardiovascular system define its own bounded loci? I shall not make a determination on this. The claim regarding the endocrine system was also rather weak and merely illustrative. It is sufficient for my purpose to acknowledge that while determining a certain bounded locus is certainly a function of some subsystems that are parts of bigger systems such as organisms, it may not be a function of others.

This is enough to substantiate the point that by committing to the biological constraint we do not automatically take the representational system as determining a bounded locus/loci, since – crucially – what is being asked here is not whether or not the system in question merely *operates* in specific loci (this is obvious). The question is whether the representational system *determines its own system-specific* bounded locus. In other words, whether the representational system takes for granted the locative *in–out* distinction drawn by other systems composing the biological individual as a whole, or introduces *its own* criteria.

I shall be arguing for "yes," which will then be developed into a specific locative ontology of the cognitive niche. The latter is exactly the kind of locus that cognitive systems (not limited to representational systems) construct, according to the proposal laid out in this book. Meanwhile, it is crucial at this early stage to take note of the fact that answering "no" to the question of whether the representational system has its own locative footprint can actually mean two completely distinct, or even opposite things.

The first "no" has just been hinted at in the above paragraphs, where I introduced what it means for a system to have (or not have) its own system-specific locative footprint. This "no" implies that the locative footprint of the representational system is identical either to the locative footprint of the nervous system, perhaps supplemented with some other systems, or to the locative footprint of the animal as a whole. The principal point is that the bounded locus attributable to the representational system does not extend beyond the limits of the overall locus of the organism, even if the latter is somewhat more loosely defined and elicits debate in the literature. I shall argue against this claim in due course.

The second possible "no" comes, unsurprisingly, from the proponents of the mind-*in*-a-place model. They would not only reject the very idea of a representational system as such, but more specifically – what is crucial at this point – they (or some of them) would argue that speaking of cognition in terms of bounded loci, *speaking of it in locative terms at all*, is a non-starter. This puzzle is also dealt with throughout the book.

1.10 No easy alternatives: The locative footprint of the embodied mind

In this closing section I will argue that abandoning the mind-*as*-a-place paradigm and replacing it with the mind-*in*-a-place approach will not be easy, or at least not as easy as it may seem to some of the philosophers proposing it. This is the case for at least two reasons which shall be developed in Chapter 4.

First, the locative framework used by the proponents of the paradigm shift is not precise, insofar as it is actually unclear whether the mind is involved in the notion of location or not. No effort has been made to explain notions such as *environment* (at a proper level of abstraction), *boundary*, *containment*, etc. Just as I stated above with respect to the so-called Cartesian cognitive science, these notions have to be defined in the newly emerging externalist context. This is required especially if we take into account that the mind-*in*-a-place approach is very much committed to the biological constraint, in a form similar to the one referred to above, and biological phenomena have a critical boundary-locative aspect to them. This conceptual muddle must, therefore, be clarified.

To illustrate this point, here is Francisco Varela's statement:

> If the mind is not in the head, where the hell is it? It's precisely the point here: it is in this non-place of the co-determination of inner and outer, so one cannot say that is outside or inside. The other consequence that follows, which is less commonly noted, is that the mind cannot be separated from the *entire* organism. [...] In other words, the organism as a meshwork of entirely co-determining elements makes it so that our minds are, literally, inseparable, not only from the external environment, but also from what Claude Bernard already called the *milieu intérieur*, the fact that we have not only a brain but an entire body.
>
> (Varela 2000: 73–74)

We are told on the one hand that the mind is *not a located phenomenon*, and therefore that it is somehow co-determined by the interplay between the inner and the outer, yet on the other hand, these very categories (inner and outer) are clearly meaningful, for otherwise they would not have been used to put this thesis forward. Are we then supposed to take them for granted as intuitively understandable? I suppose that Varela would not agree to the latter, given the fact that even on a purely biological level the issue of where and what organismic boundaries actually are is controversial (see Pradeu 2012; a point I shall return to in Chapter 6).

Moreover, however strange it may sound, Varela says that while the mind is not in any place, it is in a "non-place," therefore not only the locative preposition "in" remains in use, but we also obtain a new category of "non-place." Varela's move can be interpreted in at least three ways: first, as a kind of poetic expression without any literal sense. Of course, this is possible, but since "non-place" is supposed to be a notion that cuts through the inner-outer dichotomy, I would argue that it must be taken seriously. Second, one might argue that it is a way of saying that the notion of location simply does not apply to the embodied discourse of cognition. But this is also unconvincing, for the very same reasons. The situation we are dealing with is not – to use a famous illustration from Ryle (1949) – like asking: "all the players are on the pitch, but where is their team spirit?," where we have either a poetic way of speaking or a simple categorial mistake. In this case, if cutting through the inner/outer divide is supposed to be *a genuine conceptual breakthrough*, it must concern location, just like the categories of "inner" and "outer" do. I would therefore argue for a third option: that the somewhat puzzling "non-place" is a *specific kind* of location. The question therefore becomes – what kind? And the latter conundrum has not been answered systematically by any party within the enactive/embodied cognition movement due to their skepticism about traditional philosophy and about ontology and metaphysics in particular. Finally, note that Varela also uses the notion of *external environment*, and it is clear that this is a crucial technical notion within his entire philosophical project. Therefore, the next question becomes: what kind of locus is the said *environment*?

As we shall see in Chapter 4, proponents of embodied cognition declare that it is essential to the relation of *being-in-the-world*, that the relatum referred to as "the world" is not just a mere address, but a realm with salience and meaning. In other words, *being-in-the-world* is not a mere state of affairs, such as a toy being placed in a box, but an active pursuit of what they refer to as sense-making. However, as I shall argue, while the internal, or cognizer-related aspects of sense-making are explained convincingly by reference to what is known as autonomy conditions, integrity and the like (see Chapter 4), the world-related aspects, somewhat surprisingly – after all we are talking about an openly externalist position – beg many further questions and require more work. A clear suggestion is that *environment* means *a locus determined by sense-making*, but we do not learn much about what it means for a particular place to be delineated by sense-making; how sense-making is able to "alter" or "affect" specific places, so to speak.

According to the enactive/embodied cognition paradigm, what this *meaning* or *sense* stands for is determined by the needs of the agent or cognizer, which are in turn determined by the cognizer's conditions of autonomy, i.e., the conditions that govern the very existence of the cognizer as a closed-off, self-sustaining system. In other words, these conditions – to be characterized in greater detail in Chapter 4 – define the cognizer as a living creature, thereby determining its very integrity. And these conditions are also supposed to perform some function in the cognizer's environment. Richard Lewontin, who does not belong to the embodied cognition camp, yet somehow remains relevant to it, puts it perfectly:

> There is a confusion between the correct assertion that there is a physical world outside of an organism which would continue to exist in the absence of the species, and the incorrect claim that environments exist without species. Earth will continue to precess on its axis and produce periodic glacial and interglacial ages, volcanoes will erupt, evaporation from oceans will result in rain and snow, independently of any living beings. But glacial streams, volcanic ash deposits, and pools of water are not environments.
>
> (Lewontin 2000: 48)

In effect, accounting for what specific type of loci environments are is a non-trivial task, and referring to conditions of autonomy is a plausible way to begin. Yet, this is insufficient, especially if the alleged realm of sense is not only meaningful *at the moment* of a particular action, and not only *for the sake of* a particular action to be performed and a goal to be reached. Instead, at least in the case of more developed cognizers, it is a realm of relatively stable *structures* of sense (or *Umwelten*, as Jakob von Uexküll would say; see Uexküll 1926). This goes back to the issue elaborated upon in the preceding historical overview: we are not only doers but also understanders, and therefore any theory of human cognition needs to account for not only how the world momentarily gives us (or affords to us, as Gibson 1979 would say) meaningful cues, but also how this world *stays* meaningful and lends itself to human, and likely not only human, higher-level cognitive endeavors; how it *presents itself as* a relatively robust realm of salience and value.

To make the latter point clearer, let me now connect the preceding paragraphs with what I said at the beginning of the chapter, and thus sum things up. As already stated, even if we are necessarily embodied and placed in a certain environment, we are nonetheless not only doers, but also subjects engaged in a higher-level cognitive pursuit of "slackening the intentional threads," thus of taking distance from our interactions with the world in order to have an overview of them, to assess our own position with respect to them, etc. This must occur in a locus that makes room for it, in which achieving this specific momentum is possible and doable. Accounting for this capacity is, in my view, what fostered the mind-*as*-a-place view. Recall Augustine. The baseline there is that there must be a *safe refuge* from engagement with the world, from whose vantage point we can simply stand in front of a world that is already there, as if given to us. Before people developed a vocabulary to articulate the idea of a relatively stable, cognizer-specific *environment* which stands between the cognizer and external reality itself, and which Lewontin described so well, the most appealing solution to the problem of "slackening the intentional threads" was likely to postulate an internal realm, an *inner self* where this pursuit could be undertaken.

Since we now have the concept of environment, we can test possible alternatives or modifications of this traditional view while potentially maintaining some of its key elements. However, articulating the notion of environment as a concept that lends itself to general use requires us to elaborate upon it ontologically. Meanwhile, as stated in the beginning of this section, no one in the mind-*in*-a-place camp has yet undertaken this task. Instead, their use of locative terminology is loose and extremely unclear. Let me provide a few examples here.

In the previously cited passage, Noë claims that consciousness "is not something that happens inside us. It is something we do or make." It is, therefore, "more like dancing than it is like digestion" (Noë 2009: xii). He then adds the following:

> The locus of consciousness is the dynamic life of the whole, environmentally plugged-in person or animal.
>
> (Noë 2009: xiii)

On the one hand Noë states that consciousness *is not a located phenomenon*, but on the other hand it turns out that there is *a locus of consciousness* and that the *environmentally plugged-in* agent serves as that locus. There is, therefore, a lack of clarity which must be properly unpacked and elucidated.

We could read some of Noë's posits as conveying a strong assertion that the very idea of location does not apply to the conscious mind. This would be in line with the following statement from Di Paolo, who explicitly states that since "[c]ognition is sense-making in interaction," and it is "always a process that occurs in a relational domain," then "[a]s relational in this strict sense *cognition has no location* (original emphasis)" (Di Paolo 2009: 19). In the same vein, Thompson and Stapleton write that "[t]he spatial containment language of internal/external and inside/outside [...] is inappropriate and misleading for understanding the peculiar sort of relationality belonging to intentionality, the lived body, or being-in-the-world" (Thompson & Stapleteon 2009: 26).

Hence, in their view, enactivism does not appeal to location *at all*, the reason being its abandonment of the Cartesian *internal–external* dualism, a *specific* position regarding the boundaries of the cognitive system. However, they initially consider the Cartesian or (more accurately) empiricist version of this dichotomy as the only proposal on the table, seemingly unaware of the fact that there could be different ontologies of this crucial *in–out* boundary. It soon becomes clear why this is the case when we consider the concept of spatial containment invoked by Thompson and Stapleton as well as Di Paolo. We learn that "[i]t simply makes no sense to point to chunks of matter and space and speak of containment within a cognitive system" (Di Paolo 2009: 19).

So, this is the point of contention: it all depends on how we understand location and bounded loci. If *being located* only means occupying a certain portion of physical space, even more so if this space is supposed to serve as a container, then Di Paolo is likely right – referring to location, understood in this way, is misleading when it comes to the kind of interaction with the environment that cognition brings.

Note however that one can hardly bind cognition to *an environment* and at the same time believe that "cognition has no location." This is because "environment" *is* a locative term by definition. Clearly, "being-in-the-world," understood as being *placed in* an environment is *a* kind of location. As already shown, in the final analysis, the controversy over how the embodied cognition movement and enactivism address location boils down to the question of how the externalist movement (broadly understood) views the notion of environment and the bonds between the cognitive system and its system-specific surroundings.

The same considerations apply to Noë's "locus of consciousness." If this term is to be taken at face value, the conscious mind would turn out to be – in some refined sense – a *located* entity as well. What is this refined sense, and more generally, does the locative vocabulary eventually apply to the mind, consciousness and cognition, or not? This issue seems to have been left unresolved by proponents of the mind-*in*-a-place camp, as they have failed to provide satisfactory definitions of these locative concepts.

To expand this introductory critique of the somewhat loose use of various pregnant locative notions by members of the mind-*in*-a-place camp let us look at a different segment of the said position, namely the extended mind hypothesis of Clark and Chalmers (1998). While in the examples above the primary concern was the confusion regarding the notion of location, which clearly had to do with a presumed understanding of the *internal–external* boundary, here this very boundary emerges as the major issue, while the puzzle of location is left in the background. We read:

> Where does the mind stop and the rest of the world begin? The question invites two standard replies. Some accept the demarcation of skin and skull, and say that what is outside the body is outside the mind. Others are impressed by arguments suggesting that the meaning of our words 'just ain't in the head,' and hold that this externalism about meaning carries over into an externalism about mind.
>
> (Clark & Chalmers 1998: 27)

> [...] the human organism is linked with an external entity in a two-way interaction, creating a coupled system that can be seen as a cognitive system in its own right.
>
> (Clark & Chalmers 1998: 29)

> Some might think that the conclusion has been bought too cheaply. Perhaps some processing takes place in the environment, but what of mind? [...] In particular, we will argue that beliefs can be constituted partly by features of the environment, when those features play the right sort of role in driving cognitive processes. If so, the mind extends into the world.
>
> (Clark & Chalmers 1998: 33)

> What, finally, of the self? Does the extended mind imply an extended self? It seems so. Most of us already accept that the self outstrips the boundaries of consciousness; my dispositional beliefs, for example, constitute in some deep sense part of who I am. If so, then these boundaries may also fall beyond the skin
>
> (Clark & Chalmers 1998: 39)

Clark and Chalmers tell us that the mind *extends* the *boundaries* of the body and covers some portion of the environment, which suggests that, unlike in Noë's posit, it is not the case that nothing can be located *in* the mind, but rather that the boundaries of the mind are not the boundaries of the body. I agree, and this is basically the point I shall advance in due course.

On the other hand, Clark's and Chalmers's position can also be read as saying that the mind is stripped of boundaries, so it is not that the boundaries have been moved, but that the mind is topologically open. Further on, they stop referring to the boundaries of the body and start referring to the "boundaries of consciousness" without commenting on what the term "boundary" is supposed to mean in each case. Meanwhile, if taken seriously, the term in question cannot have the same meaning in both cases, since each is set up by different conditions – one referring to the functional closure of the organism, the other relying on some idea of a field of consciousness, as Aron Gurwitsch once put it (see Gurwitsch 2010), or something similar. Setting aside the issue of the boundaries of consciousness – an extremely subtle problem which we are not going to tackle here – let us consider the ongoing debate, already flagged above, in the philosophy of biology with regard to the criteria of biological individuality (see Pradeu 2012; Godfrey-Smith 2016; more in Chapter 6). It would suffice to prove that speaking of *the* boundaries of the body, as if this category simply referred to "skin and skull" (as Clark and Chalmers so illustratively put it) is simply wrong. Therefore, a more detailed ontological examination of the notion of boundary is required.

To my mind, all the puzzles relating to the way the mind-*in*-a-place paradigm understands location and boundaries stem from the fact that Clark and Chalmers, as well as Noë, Di Paolo, Varela and many others, seem to believe that such locative prepositions as "in," "inside" or "outside" have fixed, transparent and unproblematic meanings. But that is simply not the case, as we have already seen thanks to the cited linguists. Another line of defense might be that the term "environment" is sufficiently well defined in the biological sciences, and therefore there is no need for additional conceptual effort. I disagree for the following reasons: First, if we are going to talk about the environment that is specific to a creature's *cognitive* capacities (conceptually distinct from other aspects of its functioning), then we need a different set of *conditions*, because the ones usually referred to in biology are not designed to do the job we would expect them to do; second, if there is *a* concept of environment that connects biology, cognitive science, and perhaps some other fields of research, it needs to be defined at an appropriately abstract level. And that means a certain ontology of the environment. Meanwhile, although some proposals in this regard have been put on the table by Smith and Varzi (1999, 2002), none of them has been taken up by members of the mind-*in*-a-place movement.

We must ask, therefore, once again which sense of "in" fits best with "*x* is in the mind" or "the mind is in *x*." I hope we can see now that the puzzle of what "in" actually signifies in these contexts is by no means trivial. Given these imprecise remarks, I take it as at least provisionally proven that the conceptual links between mind (cognition), location and boundary are quite intricate, convoluted and, therefore, need to be elaborated upon in depth.

1.11 Conclusion

The time has now come to wrap up these introductory remarks and move on to more focused and detailed considerations. At the very least the following questions, which are themselves somewhat vast, must be answered if the ongoing paradigmatic struggle between mind-*as*-a-place and mind-*in*-a-place is to be ontologically clarified.

Q1 Is it possible (if so, is it still plausible) to conceive of the mind as *a locus*, i.e., as an entity or place in/at which some other entity can be located; and if so, what kind of locus might it be and for what kind of entities?

Q2 Is it possible (if so, is it also plausible) to conceive of the mind as *a located* entity, i.e., an entity that must be placed somewhere, and if so, what kind of located entity might the mind be and what kind of locus does it need?

Q3 Is it possible (if so, is it also necessary) for the mind to have boundaries, and if so, what kind of boundaries are they?

From the perspective provisionally assumed in this chapter, the fundamental tenet of the traditional mind-*as*-a-place view may not be any *particular* view on what constitutes the internal realm of the mind, but a much more abstract and general belief that the mind *is an entity that may serve as a locus*, as an address for certain beings. Usually, we tend to enlist percepts, sense-data, representations, thoughts, contents, meanings, beliefs and the like, but with a more general and abstract notion of bounded locus, this list could look different. It gives us an opportunity to approach the mind-*as*-a-place versus mind-*in*-a-place controversy in a new and more productive manner.

I believe – and I shall put this belief into practice in this book – that the fact that, unlike Augustine and Descartes, we now have the concept of environment, which originally comes from the biological sciences but proves much more general, opens up new prospects for dealing with the issues flagged in this chapter. If ontologically examined in detail – which is what I plan to do in this book – it may enable us to achieve a compromise position between the mind-*as*-a-place paradigm and its emerging mind-*in*-a-place alternative. The key notion in this effort shall be the concept of cognitive niche, which I shall elaborate on in Chapters 5 and 7.

Notes

1 Z. Herbert, "Kamyk", translated by Peter Dale Scott and Czesław Miłosz; available online e.g. here: https://allpoetry.com/poem/8507989-Pebble-by-Zbigniew-Herbert (retrieved last time on 2024.14.10). See also Z. Herbert, *The Collected Poems: 1956–1998*, Harper Collins 2010.

2 I have changed their original terminology not to cause confusion. They refer to a contained entity as the "trajector," and to the container as the "landmark." They provide reasons for this choice of terminology, but it would make little sense to bring it on board here.

3 I do not want to be misunderstood here; it was *a* concern, but not *the* primary concern, since the primary concern was the possibility of knowledge, ultimately grounded in the divinely inspired idea *of* God.

2 The Locative Commitments of Cartesian Cognitive Science

This chapter discusses the locative commitments of the tradition Rowlands (1999) dubs Cartesian cognitive science, whose contemporary renderings are known as the classical computational theory of cognition (in short – computationalism) and representational theory of mind (resp. representationalism). These are not necessarily the same things, yet both belong to Descartes' legacy. I will mostly be using the latter label.

The chapter lays the groundwork for the more extensive studies of representationalism to be undertaken in the next chapter. First, however, let us continue the historical sketch from Chapter 1 and examine what it is that makes this approach Cartesian and what strategies have been employed to date to deal with some of the problematic aspects of this legacy. My view differs somewhat from that of Rowlands, as I indicated in Chapter 1, and I will say more about this in a moment.

By "locative commitments" I mean the tacit assumptions and explicit claims made within a given theory about various locative relations such as *being-in*, *being-out*, or *being contained* as well as distinctions such as *internal* versus *external* or *proximal* versus *distal*, among others.

The central notion explored in this chapter is that of physical symbolic system, sometimes also referred to as a representational system (setting aside the differences between them for the time being). The debate I am going to wade into concerns the issue of whether or not, or perhaps to what extent, the representational system should be considered "environmentally plugged-in," to use Noë's (2009) phrase, thus whether or not it is fundamentally dependent in its functioning on the environment in which it operates. Since these are in large part empirical questions which must not be answered by theoretical fiats, my job here is strictly limited to providing a desirable degree of conceptual clarity with regard to the concept of environment. To do so, I will try to sketch out an ontology of *ecological* location as applied to creatures capable of cognition – thus an ontology of *ecological cognition*, to put it differently, as promised in the book title. This effort shall be undertaken and properly developed in Chapters 6 and 7.

DOI: 10.4324/9781003580997-2

This is, therefore, the beginning of a more detailed analysis of what I figuratively referred to as the *locative footprint* of representational systems in Chapter 1.

2.1 Introducing physical symbol systems

It is not an overstatement to say that cognitive science and a big part of the philosophy of mind as we know it today is based on Herbert Simon's and Allen Newell's *Physical Symbol System Hypothesis*, according to which a "physical symbol system has the necessary and sufficient means for general intelligent action" (Newell and Simon 1976: 116). This means, first, that "the intelligent machine is a symbol system" (Newell and Simon 1976), thus that what creatures capable of cognition do is manipulate tokens which are *processed as* symbols; second – that such mechanisms can be realized by physical complexes, natural or artificial. The hypothesis therefore makes "a specific architectural assertion about the nature of intelligent systems" (Newell and Simon 1976).

To begin, Simon and Newell emphasize that it is quite important to understand the wider historical context in which the concept of physical symbol system emerged. They reference Alan Turing, who made the "first step in this chain" (Newell and Simon 1976: 118), a group of logicians beginning with Bertrand Russell and Alfred North Whitehead, "putting the notion of proof and deduction on a secure footing" (Newell and Simon 1976: 117), and finally Emil Post and Alonzo Church, who aimed "to define the most general class of information processing systems" (Newell and Simon 1976). These developments in logic introduced an idea that may seem obvious to us these days but was in fact a pivotal innovation, namely that of purely syntactic symbol manipulation,

> a game played with meaningless tokens according to certain purely syntactic rules. All meaning had been purged. (…) Thus progress was first made by walking away from all that seemed relevant to meaning and human symbols. (…) This general attitude is well reflected in the development of information theory
>
> (Newell and Simon 1976)

It is worth adding to this brief summary that Church's and Turing's research agendas were developed in response to the *Entscheidungsproblem* formulated by David Hilbert and Wilhelm Ackermann in 1928 which problematized the possibility of an algorithm that could determine whether or not any statement in a fixed axiomatic system was universally valid. And speaking of Hilbert, I believe that Simon and Newell's hypothesis is based not only on a certain idea about intelligence, but also, tacitly, on a certain account of the rational *subject* which goes back to Hilbert's unpublished, rarely cited but highly significant "axiom of the existence of intelligence," which states:

> I have the ability to think things (or: of things) and designate them by simple symbols (...) in such a perfectly characteristic way, that I can always recognize them again unambiguously; my thought operates with these things under this symbolization in certain ways according to definite laws and I am able by introspection (*Selbsbeobachtung*) to know and completely describe these laws.
>
> (cited after Brożek & Olszewski 2014: 404; see Hallet 1994 and Brożek et al. 2014 for more on the philosophical context of Hilbert's ideas and Church's Thesis)

Therefore, there are certain assertions laid down as part of the very foundations of cognitive science as to the "architecture," as Simon and Newell dub it, of the rational subject or agent. Philosophically speaking, this means a certain ontology of the subject – the most general conceptualization of *what kind of a being* the subject/agent is.

That said, and adding even more to Newell and Simon's (1976) historical take, it is also worth noting that the idea of a universal means of solving rational problems, thus of an algorithm, is much older than Hilbert, Church and Turing, and goes back to Wilhelm Gottfried Leibniz, who already around the turn of the 17th century speculated about a machine capable of producing answers to all *solvable* problems (see Rescher 2013). Yet, it seems reasonable to ask: "solvable *by whom?*," which, again, directs our attention to the question of the rational subject or agent and the latter's basic "architecture."

Hilbert assumed the very *possibility* of a subject capable of "thinking (of) things" and solving problems, and so would Turing as well as Newell and Simon do following, consciously or not, Hilbert's axiom. However – as we saw in Chapter 1 – this assumption is by no means trivial philosophically. And Hilbert seemed to be perfectly aware of the shoulders of giants he was standing on.

Speaking of these giants, it may be illuminating for the story being told here to bring up the famous debate between Leibniz and Locke over the existence of innate ideas, which also constitutes the major difference between Descartes and empiricists who would employ the Cartesian "architecture" determined by the internal versus external chasm.

To put it in scholarly terms, Descartes, followed by Leibniz, argued that some ideas (at least one, according to Descartes – the idea *of* God) exist in the mind independently of any empirical data, while Locke argued to the contrary. However, what was really at stake, in the reading I propose for the purposes of this study, was in fact the question of what grounds the capacity of a *finite* subject to solve rational problems which seem to transcend the subject's finitude; thus, whether the finite individual mind takes part in some sort of bigger, more universal intellectual endeavor, or whether no such engagement is needed for it to be a problem solver. So, I believe that the debate was not so much about whether or not we are born with something planted in our minds – this is just a way of spelling out the issue in an intuitive way. The real concern was, and still is, whether our capacity for rational thought is anchored in something universal or not.

As already pointed out in Chapter 1, in the pre-modern era this connection with presumed universal standards of rationality was represented in terms of something like *participation* (participation in the intelligibility of the cosmos governed by a higher intelligence, whether considered a divine person or not). However, Locke and Leibniz were already laboring on a different playing field – the one established by modern science and Descartes' notion of the thinking substance. The unresolved question, for Descartes too, was how the thinking and the non-thinking (extended) substances are in contact with each other. Descartes' early works on optics, much in step with the spirit of his times, suggested a specific architecture of the mind-world connection: one determined by a barrier between the internal sphere of the thinking substance, and its external, spatially extended surroundings. In this context, the pre-modern notion of participation, thought of in a somewhat mereological fashion, thus in terms of the subject's *sharing a part* with something bigger, was no longer an option.

That said, keeping the issues of understanding and intelligibility of the world in mind, we must also realize that this little sightseeing tour through history could never be complete without mentioning Immanuel Kant. This is because while praising empiricism, Hume in particular, Kant famously accused the empiricists of positing impressions which are "blind" and as such cannot function as building blocks in our pursuit of *rationality* (see Kant 1999). Thus, like the pre-modern thinkers appealing to the authority of God – a view still held by Descartes – Kant claimed that there must be some higher rational authority governing empirical data. However, he did not follow the conservative path of returning to the idea of divine authority, and instead introduced a major innovation in the guise of transcendental subjectivity, which was a pivotal moment. Hence, Kant argued, in order to maintain the pursuit of rationality, we need a radically new conception of the role of mind. The higher rational authority is not God, and it is not an individual empirical subject either. In fact, it is not *a being* in the traditional metaphysical sense. Instead, when speaking of the transcendental subject, Kant referred to the *conditions of possibility* of any rational subject, of any rational grasp of the world.

Famously, Kant aimed at solving the problem posed by empiricism by making the case that – to put it in a somewhat simplistic manner – there are no internal ideas and all actual *contents* processed within the framework of cognition come from experience; nevertheless, there is a certain *structure* organizing these contents in the mind and making them intelligible. We see now perhaps the first clear-cut distinction between content and structure – arguably crucial to the future development of the notion of purely syntactic manipulation, stressed by Simon and Newell, and rightly so.

The latter move, together with the transition from the epistemic authority of God to the epistemic authority of a finite, constrained, even if somewhat unusual (since "transcendental") subject was momentous. Admittedly, insofar as the transcendental subject is thought of as constrained by *certain* cognitive structure or machinery, e.g., the transcendental categories of space and time or mechanisms of passive synthesis, Kant's theoretical shift arguably puts us on the path toward the contemporary notion of cognitive system. From that moment on, as Allison (2006) argues, our thinking about cognition definitely abandons "theocentric epistemology," invoking divine ideas that underpin the ideal standard of knowledge, in favor of investigating what a finite, constrained subject *can* do.

Since God was considered ideally rational, e.g., within Leibniz's system (see Leibniz 1969), there was no constraint imposed on the divine rationality, and it was therefore beyond the limits of inquiry. Meanwhile, Kant's posit created space for investigations into *an ideal, yet cognitively attainable* subject and cognitive mechanism. The notion of an ideally rational, yet constrained subject was quite unique. This specific combination of ideality and constraint proved crucial by laying the groundwork for abstract models of cognition (since speaking of ideals allows us to abstract from all things pertaining to the realizations of these models, and also to set aside all incidental "friction" having to do with our biologically limited cognitive capacities) which at the same time somehow fit together with limited rationality (since the transcendental subject is conditioned).

Historically, this particular coalition of ideas proved pivotal, especially with regard to the foundations of mathematics. Debates addressing the question of what an *ideal mathematician*, thus an *ideal subject constrained by specific formal and logical tools*, can do, and with what methods (e.g. finitistic or not; see e.g. Brożek et al. 2014 for more on the philosophical underpinnings of these debates) led to the idea of a computational machine, famously first formulated by Turing (see e.g. Turing 1950), which would then be translated into the notion of a physical computational system by Newell and Simon (1976). From that point on, as flagged in the beginning of this section, a whole new era begins.

Now, Rowlands claims that the "architecture" of cognitive systems posited by Newell and Simon was of a Cartesian type and this tacit presumption (the assumed Cartesian ontology, as I propose to put it) has been in operation until just recently. The question is, however, what makes this "architecture" genuinely Cartesian, and therefore also what (if anything) renders alternative views on the market non-Cartesian. I made some preliminary remarks on this in Chapter 1, expressing my doubts about Rowlands' view, and now I'd like to dig a little deeper.

2.2 The ecology of (non)Cartesianism: Descartes's notion(s) of location

Replacing the "participation" discourse of his predecessors, thus a somewhat mereological "architecture" of the subject-world bond, Descartes came up, although – as we saw in Chapter 1 – quite reluctantly, with *a locative architecture*. This was already anticipated, to a degree, by Augustine with his invention of the "inner self." In this new framing of cognition, both the subject and the external world become *loci* for entirely different kinds of entities – the latter for extended entities and the former for mental or intellectual entities. But if so, then the relationship between these two loci becomes a puzzle that returns in various forms, like the fundamental question of Cartesian epistemology, as to whether or not it is even possible to know the external world from the perspective of the internal, subjective sphere.

This locative aspect of Descartes' approach was elicited by Rowlands. It is crucial for a proper understanding of the drama which subsequently played out between Cartesian cognitive science and various non-Cartesian alternatives, thus also for a good grasp of what I aim at in this chapter. First, let me cite an extensive passage in which Rowlands makes his point:

> According to Descartes, the mind, like other things found inside the body, is defined by its function: and its function is to *think*. However, he argued that there is a crucial difference between the mind and all other organs found inside the body: the mind is a *nonphysical* substance. By this, he meant, fundamentally, that the mind is *nonspatial*. Physical things, Descartes claimed, have a single defining feature: *extension*. By this he meant that physical things *occupy space* or *take up room*. This, he thought, is precisely what makes them physical things. Therefore, the mind, being nonphysical, must also be nonspatial.
>
> However, there are actually two different aspects of the idea of space, and Descartes never clearly distinguished between them. On the one hand, there is spatial *extension* – taking up room. On the other hand, there is spatial *location* – existing *at* a particular place. If an object has spatial extension then it must also have spatial location. It is not possible for an object to occupy space without the space that it occupies being somewhere or other (...). But just because an object has spatial location, it does not necessarily follow that it has spatial extension.

> In effect, Descartes's view was that minds do not have spatial extension – this is what makes them nonphysical – but they do have spatial location. Every mind is located inside a (functioning) brain, and every (functioning) brain is located inside a body. Descartes was never exactly clear on the precise location of the mind; but somewhere in the vicinity of the brain' s pineal gland seemed to be his favored hypothesis.
>
> (Rowlands 1999: 11)

Long story short, according to Rowlands modern cognitive science rejects Descartes' dualism, thus the claim that there is a distinct thinking substance, yet it keeps Descartes' locative model in place. Mental entities, therefore, roughly put, are now considered physical, at least at base, contrary to what Descartes claimed. But, still, just as Descartes held, they must be *located somewhere*. Therefore, the most plausible option seems to be to place them within some kind of physically realized, thus extended system or machinery, like a computer (for those who find what is known as the "computer metaphor" compelling) or a brain (for those who believe that an actual nervous system is the only machinery capable of thinking).

This is the core belief of Cartesian cognitive science as Rowlands portrays it. Now, according to him, non-Cartesian theories within cognitive science want to get rid of this locative vocabulary. This means that

> non-Cartesian cognitive science also rejects, or is at least thought of as rejecting, Descartes's second idea, the idea inherited by the mind-brain identity/exclusive neural realization model. That is, it rejects the claim that mental states and processes occur purely inside the brains. Some of them do; but not all of them do. Mental states and processes are not just things that happen inside our brains; they are also things that happen, *partly*, in our bodies and even, *partly*, in the world outside of our bodies.
>
> (Rowlands 1999: 13)

One thing must be noted, however: non-Cartesianism, as spelled out by Rowlands, does not reject the internal versus external conceptualization of cognition; it only holds that cognition may also play out on the external side. Meanwhile, in my reading, the reform proposed by at least some members of the non-Cartesian church aims at a more fundamental reconfiguration. Some of them strive to *actually* get rid of the locative framework as such, but this move – as I will argue in this and in the next chapter – is not likely to succeed.

I view Descartes' locative schema and, therefore, also the alternatives to it in a different way and the remaining part of this section is devoted to rolling out this alternative reading. Namely, I believe that non-Cartesianism should aim at expanding the Cartesian locative framework by rendering it *ecological.* For the lack of an ecological framework is precisely the biggest hole looming in the Cartesian conceptualization – to be clear, a hole that Descartes himself could do nothing about, philosophizing two centuries before Darwin (so no blame game).

First, beginning with Descartes' own view, we have to acknowledge the fact that he purposefully employed two methods of analysis: the third-person analysis he adopted in his writings on optics and what we would today consider the psychology of perception, and the first-person analysis adopted in his *Meditations.* The first-person method harks back to St. Augustine, while the third-person method is obviously grounded in the scientific revolution of his times to which he himself contributed greatly. Adopting the two methods simultaneously but also separately must have seemed necessary to him, given the fact that he had no other way of conceptualizing the internal functioning of the mind (which is still an issue – more recently Husserl followed his path, and when it comes to the contemporary philosophy of mind, there is a debate on purely subjective aspects to cognitive functioning which cannot be captured from the third-person perspective; see Chalmers 1996).

Now, for the sake of this interpretation, I propose to conceptualize both kinds of analysis as taking place within specific abstract "spaces," as represented by the Cartesian system of coordinates. We have the third-person system of coordinates, which seems quite an intuitive tool for getting a "scientific" overview of spatially extended physical things, but we also have the first-person domain, represented as a different system of coordinates.

Now, since Descartes takes the mind as not extended, *res cogitans* must be introduced into the third-person system of coordinates as a specific point. As Rowlands puts it, this peculiar "point" has no extension, but it does have location in the physical world so represented, and it is this location that proves so problematic for the whole Cartesian model.

The first-person system of coordinates will be defined by a different set of variables, thus it will operate in different dimensions – for example, we can introduce here a certain measure of complexity or intensity of mental contents, as the British empiricists did; or a measure of their clarity and distinctness, which was dear do Descartes himself; or a measure of their semantic proximity/distance in something like what Gärdenfors (2004) calls conceptual spaces, etc. There are many options here. Either way, some kind of mental "space" is established. Sellars's (1956) notion of the "space of reasons" seems relevant here, too, and it also draws on the analogy between physical space and some kind of internal "space."

Aside from the details of each of these proposals, once we have this "mental" system of coordinates in place, perceptual inputs coming from the external world must now be represented as points – they are simple impressions, as Locke and Hume would put it, which means that they have no distinguishable parts within the *mental* domain. Note the parallel: the mind is a point lacking extension in physical space, and simple empirical data are points lacking "extension" in "mental" space – they are, so to speak, atoms of experience.

Given this simplified picture, a major problem for Descartes was, of course, how these two models, these two systems of coordinates (thus measures) – the one measuring the properties of physical entities, the other measuring the properties of mental entities – can be unified, which is what Rowlands likely meant by pointing to Descartes' failed attempts to localize the connection between the thinking substance and the physically extended substance.

However, though it somehow escaped Rowlands's attention, it is clear in the *Meditations* that a unified locative model of mind, which Descartes desired to elaborate, *cannot* simply place the mind somewhere in the body. Recall the fragment in which Descartes argues that the mind cannot be like a pilot "present in a ship" (Sixth Meditation 81; Descartes 2008: 57). Here Descartes makes his assessment of the location of the mind clear beyond all doubt – it must be *a different kind of location.*

Therefore, Descartes would not have appreciated the claim that "mental states and processes occur purely inside the brains," as Rowlands puts it, not only because of his dualist commitments, but because he recognized that the *kind of* location applicable to bodies (as analyzed from a third-person perspective) is not the same as that applicable to minds (as analyzed from the first-person perspective), and thus that neither of these is an appropriate characterization of the mind-body "fusion" he talks about. Recall that he says he is "closely conjoined to" his body and "fused with it, so as to form a single entity with it" (Descartes 2008).

So much for Descartes' dualism – "fusion" hardly sounds like one. Yet, it also suggests a certain helplessness, an acknowledgment of the lack of an appropriate conceptual framework, one that could facilitate even small progress in understanding cognition which somehow plays out in both of the above-mentioned "spaces." In other words, helplessness *not* with regard to how the mind should be placed within the third-person space, but rather about how to integrate the *two systems of coordinates*, the two measures, thus *two kinds of location* – the third-person and the first-person one.

2.3 Ecological location: A provisional account

What Descartes lacked (although, as mentioned several times, he was in no position to change this) was a genuine *ecological sense* of location, which boils down neither to the third-person "physical" space, nor the first-person "mental" one. I shall examine the ecological sense of location in Chapters 6 and 7, but this topic – as we shall see below – is quite significant for a proper grasp of the locative footprint of a representational/computational system and of the overall locative commitment of representationalism. Therefore, it needs to be provisionally addressed now.

To get a sense of what is going to be discussed, and what the said ecological location is about, consider an example that may at first seem completely random – a glass or mug that has the capacity to be *filled with* something; it can serve as a bounded locus *for* other things such as water or wine (recall some of the examples analyzed in 1.4 and 1.5). I propose to spell this idea out in terms of *locative capacity* which shall be defined formally in Chapter 6. The basic idea is that the kind of location attributable to the glass goes beyond the address occupied in physical space by the material that the glass is made of, since some portion of what we tend to call "empty" space counts as part of the glass's location, too, insofar as it can *accommodate* some portion of liquid. This "empty" space is exactly the place that is *filled*. The locative capacity of an entity, therefore, means that it not only has a particular location, but that it can also "provide" location to other things.

The location of the glass as a whole is therefore *ecological* in the sense that it is an amalgam of the location of the actual matter that the glass is made of, plus its locative capacity. In effect, a portion of wine, for example, not only occupy some unique address in the universe, as all things do independently of one another, but is also located *in relation to* the glass in a specific manner, namely it is *contained in* it.

Now, bearing in mind that this is just an illustrative analogy, we might ask whether or not cognitive (including representational) systems have any capacity to "accommodate" anything or, in some other unique way, to impact the locations of things around them. I will be arguing that we must assign some sort of locative capacity to cognitive systems if we are to fully understand their actual functioning.

The key point is that the flagged quality of being "ecological" does not just refer to a specific locative relation between two entities, like "being in," "standing on the right side of," etc., but to a certain *pattern* of locative relations. Think again of the glass filled with wine or water. The glass is an entity with an address, like any other thing in the world. The wine molecules also have exact locations which could perhaps be specified without even mentioning the glass they are in (some "liquid detector" may be able to ignore the glass and single out the wine itself). But what matters from the "ecological" angle is that the glass and the wine molecules maintain *the pattern* we articulate when we say that the glass is *filled with* wine or that wine *fills* the glass. The glass therefore not only has its own address in the world, but it also "offers" something to other entities in the form of what Gibson (1979) called "affordances." It affords a possible accommodation to some entities in its surroundings.

To sum up, a thing has locative capacity if it can intervene, as it were, in the setup of the locative relations surrounding it, as in the example just given. Simply put, if something has a locative capacity, it can "do" something with the locations of other things (see Chapter 6 for a more technical definition).

This enables us to provisionally characterize a *point of reference* within a fixed domain of locative relations (which is going to be unpacked in technical terms in Chapter 6, too). In everyday speech the concept in question can be referred to as a *viewpoint* or *point of view*. It seems quite intuitive and at the same time proves quite peculiar. For what does it actually mean to approach a thing *from a certain viewpoint*? Nothing changes about the thing itself. For example, a coin seen from above is the same coin as the one seen from the side. And yet there *is* a difference, since once we change the viewpoint, different features of the coin become accessible. And, crucially, points of view seem to be perfectly objective – some qualities of the thing are attributable to a fixed viewpoint, and others to a different one, regardless of who or what *stands at* these points and what cognitive apparatus this creature has. To use Aristotle's example, the road from Athens to Thebes is uphill when seen from the side of Athens, and downhill when approached from the side of Thebes. Whether we put a man, a bat, or a Martian there, being uphill and being downhill are two *matters of fact*, yet each is attached to the relevant viewpoint. All this means that it is crucial on some occasions to speak of features or qualities that are relative to cognizers *standing in a certain location*, but not created by the said cognizers.

The notion of ecological location can at least to some degree close the gap between the two "spaces" defined by Descartes. In the third-person space, we can define not only the locations of extended objects but also of fixed points of reference, thereby introducing a kind of "perspectiveness" there. Note that there is no room for "perspectiveness" in a physical space that lacks any points of reference: physical space is what it is, there is no special "valence," as it were, on top of any fragment of it. "Perspectiveness" in some sense adds a kind of valence. Hence, the subjective perspective is not introduced in its full-blown form, but it is *acknowledged*, and in some sense marked there, so to speak.

The "perspectiveness" obtained by the introduction of points of reference is pivotal if we are to understand, in a general sense, the notion of environment which in turn proves crucial in the mind-*as*-a-place versus mind-*in*-a-place dispute. This is because, as we learned from Lewontin (quoted in Chapter 1), the mere referencing of the physical stuff surrounding a given organism is not a plausible use of the term "environment." Of course, there is the physical space filled with the stuff that physics, chemistry, geology, seismology, etc. all talk about, yet this realm is *not* an environment. To put it differently – there is more to an environment than that.

Now, it is not particularly hard to provide a definition of environment in reference to the specific functions of an organism, for example, when speaking of a specific organism's metabolic conditions, such as how it gets oxygen (from air or water), what nutrients it needs, etc. However, once we begin to speak of "the environment" in a more abstract and generic sense, which is how the term is often used in numerous contexts, including in cognitive science and philosophy of mind, formulating a proper (sufficiently general) definition of it becomes quite challenging. In particular, it is not clear what it means for a given realm to be *the* environment relative to a specific organism's *cognitive* capacities. This shall be a major objective in Chapter 7.

Now, we must realize that the ecological sense of location was not available to Descartes for quite an obvious reason: we owe it to Darwin's work and the development of biology which came afterward. This realization sheds new light on what a non-Cartesian, but not necessarily anti-Cartesian project might be.

Rowlands claims that the key to a non-Cartesian cognitive science "is the extent to which we make use of things around us in order to solve problems and get things done" (Rowlands 1999: 13). He then says that human "cultural development is, in part, a process of creating external information-bearing structures: structures that could be used to enhance our ability to accomplish important tasks. One of the most significant of these structures is the development of written language" (Rowlands 1999: 15). While I agree with the general spirit behind this non-Cartesian hypothesis, it is not clear to me how we are supposed to understand the "around us" relation if the general locative vocabulary and the notions provisionally flagged in the previous paragraph, including the concept of point of reference, are abandoned or ignored. What are *external* information-bearing structures; more precisely – what does their being "external" and at the same time somehow relevant to the cognizer signify? Provided that "external" refers to the same domain as "around us," this domain cannot be *anything* around us, but rather a cognitively relevant surrounding. Therefore, we need a clearer conceptual grasp of what it means for this domain to be external, or rather to be "around" – to be precise: around a specific cognitive system, which is essentially an ecological relation.

To put it yet differently, my point is that non-Cartesian cognitive science should not pretend to abandon locative concepts, deeming them remnants of Descartes' preoccupations, while at the same time openly referring to "environment" and "being around." Instead, it should try to augment Descartes' *non-ecological* notion of location so as to make it ecological. Either our understanding of location is Cartesian or richer than that. If we see no option but to reject the Cartesian locative vocabulary we are still determined by these Cartesian limitations: the range of our options is still framed by Descartes, which is not a situation that non-Cartesians should welcome.

I, therefore, propose that what makes Cartesian cognitive science *Cartesian* is not the claim that cognition is located in the brain, as Rowlands and many others would have it, but a certain understanding of location itself. What would make non-Cartesian cognitive science more profoundly *non*-Cartesian is a new take on how the mind or a system capable of cognition is located and, perhaps, how something can be located in that system, too. Both of these relations should be attributed with a proper ecological sense. This, however, requires some conceptual effort, for while ecological notions are a well-established ingredient of the vocabulary of the empirical sciences, especially of the biological sciences, they are still somewhat loosely applied in cognitive science, not to mention philosophy of mind.

2.4 The default concept of representation and its tacit locative commitments

Even this highly simplified historical picture presented in previous sections gives reason to believe that philosophy did not join the computationalist camp when Jerry Fodor (1975) came up with his *Language of Thought* hypothesis. On the contrary, the notion of a computational system, or more precisely, of that system's basic architecture, already had some philosophical traction. The locative dichotomy *internal versus external* constitutes this architectural plan. It is this dichotomy that lies at the core of the debate between contemporary renderings of Cartesian cognitive science and a broad church of alternatives which I discuss in the next chapter.

This section begins with a more in-depth analysis of what Rowlands called Cartesian cognitive science, in particular the notion of representational system. However, someone might question whether there was a point to spilling so much ink about the historical evolution of abstract concepts such as location on the one hand, and intelligibility on the other.

Let me begin answering this concern with a reference to William Ramsey, who notes that:

> ... appealing to inner representations to explain mental phenomena has a very long and glorious history, going back at least as far as Aristotle. While our conception of mental representation has changed greatly over time, its assumed explanatory necessity has been a traditional assumption shared by a great number of thinkers. (...) Within cognitive science, the classical computational theory of mind is widely recognized as the traditional theoretical framework.
>
> (Ramsey 2017: 4202)

The key thing that Ramsey brings up is "explanatory necessity." Namely, postulating the existence of representations is supposed to be an indispensable part of the scientific endeavor to explain cognition. However, there is a risk, Ramsey says, having to do with the fact that:

> … representationalism is a core dimension of our ordinary, common-sense or 'folk' psychology. As various writers have noted, central folk posits like the propositional attitudes, images, memories, dreams, certain emotional attitudes and so on are all thoroughly representational in nature. So our tendency to define cognition in representational terms almost certainly stems, at least in part, from this folksy, common-sense conception of what is inside the mind.
>
> (Ramsey 2017)

Therefore, there is a risk of intermingling the properly scientific concept of representation, which has explanatory value, with the "folk" notion, and therefore of mistakenly expecting *a* science of representations to be a theory of propositional attitudes, imagination, emotion, etc.

On the other hand, there is also the risk, Ramsey claims, of making the scientific notion of representation a purely theoretical fiat, a prospective postulate, in the sense that any entity, mechanism or function is called representational in virtue of a scientist's decision, thereby bearing little or no resemblance to the "folk" notion. In the latter case the question of whether the notion of representation, so deeply ingrained in tradition, has explanatory value loses its ground – if anything can be referred to as a "representation" within a given theory, then certainly the term can be used to refer to something with explanatory power, too. But does this prescribed reference have anything to do with the reference and explanatory value of "representation" in a different context? Not necessarily, and therefore, if any particular scientist ends up with *their own* technical notion of representation, the general question of the utility of the concept of representation cannot even be properly posed.

We need to keep in mind that a general notion of representation laid the groundwork for cognitive science and constituted the explanandum that this whole cluster of disciplines was designed to tackle. Hence, it seemed to belong to a shared vocabulary enabling specialists from different disciplines to communicate. Given that, I would cautiously insist that we still need this general concept, intelligible to researchers coming from different places on the map of cognitive science. And Ramsey also makes this cautious suggestion.

His claim is that we need to adopt a notion of representation that will "overlap sufficiently with our pre-theoretical understanding" (Ramsey 2007: 13), drawing on "our intuitive understanding of what a representation is and does" (Ramsey 2007). Therefore, any technical notion postulated within a theory must be "recognizably representational in nature" (Ramsey 2007).

In Ramsey's view, there are three elements of the folk concept of representation that should be of some use to any technical rendering of the notion. The first is the quality of "aboutness" or intentionality, thus the fact that representations are about something else, usually something in the outside world. For Ramsey, as we shall see later on, this brings the key function of "standing for" which is constitutive of any state internal to the system if it is to function *as* a representation. The second element is causality: we assume that intentional states cause something, for example, my desire to drink beer causes me to move toward the fridge. Finally, there is a folksy class of non-mental applications of the concept of representing which also carries a lesson, namely when representational functions are ascribed to such entities as maps, drawings, traffic signs, etc. This is important, for in a sense it opens up a direct door from the folk notion to a more technical one. Namely, "it may be possible to gain some sort of insight into cognitive representation by exploring the representational character of things that are non-mental" (Ramsey 2007: 21). In particular, as we shall see, it is possible to construe a notion of *structural* representation by walking through this folk-to-technical door.

Now, what does all this have to do with my previous references to Descartes or Leibniz? Was this historical tour of any use? The point I would like to argue for here is that the Ramseyan folk-to-technical route is a sheer idealization of the more complex and looped dynamic that actually exists; to be precise (although it would require a separate historical study), I would risk the claim that there have been several "transfers" in both directions, from "technical" to "folk" and the other way around, and therefore it is by no means clear whether any distinctively "folk" understanding of the notion of representation actually exists. Rather, it seems that the notion emerged as a technical posit at some point (although it is not clear when) based on "folk" conceptual repositories (hardly elicitable now), and then returned to the folk vocabulary, thereby shaping the ways in which the general public began to understand what maps do, but also, to take an entirely different example, what attorneys do when they represent their clients. Shaped this way, the "folk" meaning likely reciprocally influenced the emerging cognitive science. Therefore, we should speak of an open-ended loop, not a linear transition from the folk to the technical (or vice versa).

If this latter hypothesis is true, we should not speak, in my opinion, of the "folk" notion of representation at all. Instead, although such terminological choices are not substantial, I propose to speak of the *default conception* of representation. What is more substantial, though, is the way in which we attribute meaning to the said default conception. Since appealing to what "ordinary people" (whoever they are) think would hardly be informative due to the open-ended loop invoked above, what we can do is refer to specific philosophical traditions in which this concept appeared. And *this* is the reason why the reference to Leibniz, Locke, Descartes, Hume, Kant, but even to Plato is relevant (Ramsey mentions Aristotle in the fragments cited above). It tells us about the evolving meaning of the concept we are about to provide with a technical, operationalized sense as part of cognitive science, and with an up-to-date ontological scaffolding. Crucially, this applies not only to the concept of representation, but to any presumably *non*-Cartesian posit as well, which – again – justifies the need for at least some level of historical self-consciousness.

Given all the considerations made so far, I propose that *the default conception of representation* satisfy the following conditions:

- Representations are located inside the mind or subject and as such cannot be located outside the mind.
- Representations do not and cannot overlap with external entities (i.e. share any parts with whatever is outside the subject).
- Representations, nevertheless, have the function of *standing* inside *for* something located outside, thus they maintain intentional relations with external entities.
- Representations, in virtue of this intentional relation, can in various ways resemble external entities, e.g. structurally, or provide information about external phenomena.
- Representations, insofar as they provide information about external entities, can cause the subject they are located in to act in a particular way.

To conclude, before going into more detail with regard to representational systems, let me single out what the *locative commitments of the default concept of representation* are. This part also summarizes the sketchy and scattered historical remarks made in the above segment of this chapter as well as in Chapter 1.

First, Descartes introduced a locative vocabulary into our thinking about cognition by drawing a sharp line between the internal sphere of the subject and what began to be called the "external world." This vocabulary had previously been tried out by Plato, among others, with his "Trojan Horse" model, and by Augustine, who laid the groundwork for Descartes with his idea of the "inner self," although neither ultimately adopted it. One commitment of the default concept of representation, as seen from this Cartesian angle, is quite straightforward, namely that the locative relations of being-*in* and being-*out* play a constitutive role in cognition: being-*in-the-mind* is constitutive of entities such as impressions, sense-data or, in the modern vocabulary, representations, whereas being-*out-of-the-mind* plays a constitutive role in entities conceived of as real and objective, those traditionally referred to as "mind-independent." These locative relations are, however, assumed as given and are never actually examined and scrutinized. This work is going to be done in the next chapters.

Second, the idea of intentionality, also included in the default concept of representation, refers to a peculiar relation whose purpose is to bridge the gap between "in-the-mind" and "out-of-the-mind." Assuming that such a bridge is *possible* in the first place is another, somewhat tacit, locative commitment of the default conception. It is tacit in the sense that those working with the default concept make no effort to unpack this aspect of intentionality, and in most cases are not even aware of how problematic and peculiar it is. Nicholas Shea (2014) says that thoughts, for example,

> ... can be about objects and properties that are not present to the thinker, that are distant in time and space, that are hypothetical or may only be actualised far in the future, or that are entirely imaginary. If thinking is a physical process realised by or within people, how then can thoughts reach out and be about such things?
>
> (Shea 2014: 496)

The key phrase here is "reach out." This should really make us stop and reflect for a moment. Shea's articulation depicts intentionality as a somewhat revolutionary capacity to traverse spatial and temporal distance without actually physically doing so. This is a certain "move" within the first-person "space" defined by Descartes, but there is no parallel move in the third-person space. How is this possible? Shea does not explore this conceptually – he is interested solely in the underlying mechanism.

Moreover, think of more primitive cognizers that do not have this peculiar capacity for "as-if-moving" attributed to intentionality (e.g. the most primitive cognizer van Duijn et al. 2006 talk about – the unicellular organism): such a simple cognizer can only be "concerned" with entities and happenings occurring on its surface. If it has any first-person "space" to speak of, there can be no movement in this space, thus no cognitive connection to anything, without actual sensorimotor activity and without movement within the third-person physical space. Meanwhile, intentionality "reaches out," thus transcends the bounds of the physical *here* without there being any concomitant physical move. What this whole book attempts to do, in some sense, is to spell out an ontology of this "reaching out." The latter involves, as I will argue, a genuinely ecological bond which requires real conceptual effort to unpack.

We are so used to intentionality's puzzling locative dynamic of "reaching out" as if it were obvious that nature supports this kind of effort at all. But upon reflection, I believe, we should come to the conclusion that it must have been a significant "innovation" in our cognitive evolution and an "achievement" of great adaptive value. Therefore, it is a plausible intellectual exercise to problematize this locative or – as I prefer to say for reasons to be outlined – *ecological* aspect of representations and their built-in intentionality.

2.5 The architecture of representing: The physical symbol system

With a long intellectual history behind it, including Turing, Church, Hilbert, but also Descartes, Locke, Leibniz and Kant, the notion of *physical symbol system* (hereafter PSS) introduced by Newell and Simon (1976) is the cornerstone of cognitive science. Newell is quite emphatic about it when he writes:

> The physical symbol system is to our enterprise what the theory of evolution is to all biology, the cell doctrine to cellular biology, the notion of germs to the scientific concept of disease, the notion of tectonic plates to structural geology.
>
> (Newell 1980 p. 136)

Here is what this concept stands for:

> A physical symbol system consists of a set of entities, called symbols, which are physical patterns that can occur as components of another type of entity called an expression (or symbol structure). Thus, a symbol structure is composed of a number of instances (or tokens) of symbols related in some physical way (such as one token being next to another). At any instant of time the system will contain a collection of these symbol structures. Besides these structures, the system also contains a collection of processes that operate on expressions to produce other expressions: processes of creation, modification, reproduction and destruction. A physical symbol system is a machine that produces through time an evolving collection of symbol structures. Such a system exists in a world of objects wider than just these symbolic expressions themselves.
>
> (Newell & Simon 1976: 116)

The term "physical" stands for the fact that the said systems "clearly obey the laws of physics – they are realizable by engineered systems made of engineered components" (Newell & Simon 1976).

Newell (1980) gives a parallel explication of PSS. He talks about symbols and symbol manipulation, yet he begins by pointing to the locative architecture of PSS, which is of great importance given our goals here:

> [PSS] consists of a memory, a set of operators, a control, an input, and an output. Its inputs are the objects in certain locations; its outputs are

> the modification or creation of the objects in certain (usually different) locations. Its external behavior, then, consists of the outputs it produces as a function of its inputs. The larger system of environment plus [PSS] forms a closed system, since the output objects either become or affect later input objects. [PSS]'s internal state consists of the state of its memory and the state of the control; and its internal behavior consists of the variation in this internal state over time.
>
> (Newell 1980: 142)

Note that Newell explicitly uses the terms "location" and "environment," assuming, I submit, that we already know what they refer to. This fragment is crucial if we are to assess what the locative footprint of PSS is. On the one hand, in a somewhat obvious and straightforward way, PSS exemplifies the Cartesian internal-external divide, since what drives its functioning is referred to as "input," while its products are referred to as "output." The Cartesian underpinnings of PSS also manifest themselves when Newell declares:

> Although little can be said about exact boundaries, some interior milieu must exist within which the symbol system can freely and successfully interpret expressions.
>
> (Newell 1980: 158)

There seems to be nothing particularly interesting here, just the standard language of Cartesian cognitive science. And yet we learn that "inputs" are "objects in certain locations" (Newell 1980: 142). What does this mean though?

To start with a trivial observation, the "objects in certain locations" which serve as "inputs" cannot be external objects such as chairs and tables because the latter clearly are not the kind of entities to be accommodated by the "interior milieu" of the symbol system. However, this triviality leads us to an interesting possibility – which, as it turns out, Newell might even be quite open to – that of extending the system, its milieu, in (more or less) the way proposed by Clark and Chalmers (1998). I will come back to this.

For now, however, setting aside this somewhat unorthodox option, if the system is thought of in the standard manner, everyday objects in the system's surroundings cannot enter the system. On the other hand, calling them "objects" suggests that by "input" Newell does not mean something like sense-data or mere receptor stimulation. He seems to have a richer concept of "input" in mind. If so, then the "locations" he alludes to also become quite mysterious, for the very same reason – the term cannot refer to the addresses of things in the Cartesian "third-person" space, i.e. within the purely physical domain of evaporation and volcanic eruptions, to cite Lewontin (2000) again. This is because insofar as physical space proper is concerned, the only objects that can reach a physical system are energy-carrying particles. Meanwhile, Newell really seems to be speaking of distant chairs and tables, thus everyday mesoscopic entities. This means that Newell's "location" must refer to a thicker concept, and the candidate that comes to mind first, given the fact that Newell also speaks of "environment," is ecological location, characterized by certain *patterns of locative relations* around a system conceived of as a fixed "point of reference." This is also suggested by Newell's reference to "larger systems" composed of PSS *and* its surroundings.

All of these puzzles necessitate a better conceptual grasp of the conceptual ingredients involved here: of the location of PSS, the location of the objects it deals with, what kind of locus PSS' environment is, etc.

Meanwhile, to continue the introduction of PSS, the concept originally proposed by Newell and Simon is linked to two other notions: designation and representation. While PSS processes physical tokens, these are thought of as symbols, while their being symbols is possible only if they designate something external to the system. We read:

> An expression designates an object if, given the expression, the system can either affect the object itself or behave in ways dependent on the object. In either case, access to the object via the expression has been obtained, which is the essence of designation.
>
> (Newell & Simon 1976: 116)

There are several interesting things here. First, designation is *not* about what is going in the system's "interior milieu." The invoked "access" to the object, which Newell and Simon dub the "essence of designation," refers to the possibility of doing something *directly with the object*. Therefore, "access" in its most fundamental sense, if I am correct, is grounded in the possibility of the system behaving in a specific way in its environment. The crucial question is this: what constitutes this possibility? To be more precise – what kind of arrangement in the system's surroundings makes the *access* bond possible? Newell and Simon, quite rightly, avoid starting from heavily loaded concepts such as knowledge or information, and begin with something thinner, as it were, likely more intuitive. Yet, even an "intuitive" concept like access, spelled out in terms of behavior, cannot be taken for granted if the Cartesian internal versus external dichotomy and therefore the distinction between the "interior milieu" and the rest of the world is assumed upfront. Given Newell & Simon's clear adoption of the Cartesian architecture of cognition, even the most "intuitive" sense of cognitive access, grounded in the notion of behavior, cannot come cheap – we need to say what happens with these two domains, the system and its surroundings, that *makes room for* behavior and allows behavior to account for *cognitive access*.

The idea that I will be articulating stepwise throughout this book is that cognitive access in this most fundamental sense is made possible by a certain arrangement of locative relations between the system and selected ingredients of its physical surroundings – by chains and patterns of locative relations between the system and the things around it which make the physical surroundings *an environment*.

Now, as for the concept of representation, it is almost identical to the notion of designation, yet with two subtleties that make a difference, in my reading. We read:

> Representation is simply another term to refer to a structure that designates:
>
> X represents Y if X designates aspects of Y, i.e., if there exist symbol processes that can take X as input and behave as if they had access to some aspects of Y. (…).
>
> (Newell 1980: 176)

First, Newell speaks here of "a structure" that designates, which was not there in the definition of designation itself. The suggestion here is that speaking of representations refers uniquely to certain *internal structures* within the system; structures that work as "images":

> The term representation focuses attention on the image of the distal object in the symbolic structure which represents it.
>
> (Newell 1980)

It is not clear what this "image" is, but some grasp of if shall be possible once we tackle the notion of structural representation later on.

Second, we have a reference to *aspects*. Newell explains:

> The qualification to aspects of Y, rather than just Y, simply reflects language usage in which X can be said to represent a complex object Y without being faithful (i.e., designating) to all aspects of Y. Representation is sometimes formulated in terms of a mapping from aspects of Y to aspects of X. Implicit in this formulation is that something can be done with X, i.e., that processes exist that can detect the aspects of X that are images of aspects of Y. Hence the whole forms a designatory chain.
>
> (Newell 1980)

The problem is that what we have here, at least at first glance, is a kind of circularity: *aspects* are referenced as part of the above definition of representation, but when Newell explains "the qualification to aspects," we are supposed to already know what the relation of representing stands for. Yet, a simple way out of the circularity is suggested by Newell himself when he refers to the relation of designation, which he already defined earlier. Let us then try to replace the word "representation" with "designation" in the latter quote and say this: "X can be said to designate a complex object Y without designating all aspects of Y." This sounds plausible. If the previously given definition of designation holds, this should mean that X can either affect some aspects of the object or, in a different way, behave in relation to these aspects. Newell does not explain what he means by "aspect," although he suggests that it has to do with selection: PSS is selective in the sense that it cannot designate all the properties of an object. Therefore "aspects" may stand for selected properties.

Now, understood this way, aspects are just like Gibson's (1979) affordances. They are opportunities "offered" to the system to act thus and so. I shall discuss the latter in greater detail later on, but here the following remark should suffice: if aspects are properties selected out of the whole array of an object's properties that the PSS can effectively designate, they must be thought of as properties that are *relative to the system* thought of as a point of reference in the sense proposed above; therefore – they must be taken as located not only in the system's physical surroundings, but also in the *ecological* space constituted by the system.

Therefore, although drawing any final conclusions at this point would be premature, a provisional take is that the concept of PSS involves two locative commitments:

- the explicit locative commitment of the concept of PSS embraces the Cartesian *internal* – *external* divide and the idea of the system's "internal milieu."
- the implicit or tacit locative commitment of the concept of PSS is that the system operates not only in a physical space but *in an environment*. Moreover, there is a suggestion that PSS makes up a higher-level system together with entities in its surroundings and with selected aspects of them (which are its cues for action, thus something like Gibsonian affordances). This tacit locative commitment needs to be made explicit, in my view, and articulated properly.

2.6 Embedding the physical symbol system

Although PSS is an abstract model which could in principle be realized by a variety of physical complexes, the intention to implement it primarily to capture actual cognition is clear in the works of Simon and Newell. They first formulate a hypothesis according to which PSS "has the necessary and sufficient means for general intelligent action" (Newell and Simon 1976: 116). In a similar vein John Haugeland says that "[r]easoning (on the computational model) is the manipulation of meaningful symbols according to rational rules (in an integrated system)" (Haugeland 1985, p. 39). The reference to reasoning is supposed to direct our attention to what humans *actually* do. This is also clear when Newell comments that according to the hypothesis he and Simon put forward

> these symbols [the symbols inside PSS – KW] are in fact the same symbols that we humans have and use every day of our lives. Stated another way, the hypothesis is that humans are instances of physical symbol systems, and, by virtue of this, mind enters into the physical universe.
>
> (Newell 1980: p. 136)

Jerry Fodor with Zenon Pylyshyn go further and say that

> it's the architecture of representational states and processes that discussions of *cognitive architecture* are about. Put differently, the architecture of the cognitive system consists of the set of basic operations, resources, functions, principles, etc., whose domain and range are the *representational states* of the organism.
>
> (Fodor & Pylyshyn 1988: 10)

I said that Fodor and Pylyshyn go further than others since by explicitly referring to "organisms" they seem to be targeting not only higher-order or more advanced human cognitive functions such as reasoning, but cognition as such. Therefore, Fodor and Pylyshyn certainly, but others as well, at least to an extent, adopt the biological constraint referred to in Chapter 1.

Now, the question is how these strategies of embedding PSS in real-world cases, thus the different realizations of the biological constraint within Cartesian cognitive science, relate to the problem of the locative footprint of PSS, especially the latter's ecological location. In other words, the concern is whether at least some of these strategies provide us with a plausible account of the locative relations between living creatures, considered as exemplification of PSS, and their environments.

To begin with, if PSS is to serve as a model of what real-world cognizers do, then more needs to be done to explain how PSS performs its function. For it is one thing to say that PSS operates on symbols designating external objects, and another thing to say how it actually "reaches out" to these objects. We, therefore, need a more substantial account of what is going on *between* the system *and* its surroundings.

Fred Dretske famously articulates this system-surroundings bond in terms of information, the "flow" of information, strictly speaking, and indication, which is basically the same thing for him. A system represents an object possessing a property if it "has the function of indicating" (Dretske 1995: 2) that property "by occupying different states" (Dretske 1995). These states are "the expressive elements" (Dretske 1988: 52) of the system: "*what they represent* (about the object – KW)" is *that* it has one property or another. Then comes his example of a speedometer, where pointer positions such as 55, 80, 123, correspond to different car speeds (55 km/h, etc.).

The phrase "expressive elements" used by Dretske is far from clear though. Dretske's use of the propositional form when he claims that the system represents *that* the object is in a given state suggests some sort of linguistic machinery internal to the system. This is explicitly proposed by Fodor (1975), who holds that "computation presupposes a medium of computation – a representational system in which computations are carried out," and then proceeds to hypothesize that there is an internal tool at the system's disposal called the *language of thought* (hereafter LOT). He claims that LOT is the best hypothesis at the moment (strictly speaking at that moment, in the 1970s) regarding how this system operates. According to the LOT hypothesis, the representational system operates by employing an internal language-like medium. This does not mean, however, that this internal language is identical to any spoken language, to the effect that English speakers differ in their LOTs from German speakers. Instead, LOT is a species-specific internal structure or format enabling the system to represent concepts in the form of symbols.

The key thing about LOT is, on the one hand, the analogy with linguistic structures, and on the other hand, its contribution to a broader view that Fodor calls *representational theory of mind* (hereafter RTM). The reason why certain brain operations are like a language is that there are rules of making complex symbol tokens out of simpler symbol tokens; these rules are sensitive to the tokens' physical properties only, not to what these symbols *stand for*, while at the same time maintaining the function of "standing for." This means that the manipulation of tokens ignores the semantic component of "standing for" while preserving it at the same time, thus it does not allow the whole complex structure to lose its function of representing. These purely syntactic rules boil down to specific algorithms run by the brain. In the case of formal languages, it translates roughly into the notion of deduction, i.e. a series of operations on formal structures which nonetheless – and this was a discovery of paramount significance in the wake of mathematical logic as we know it today – preserves the structures' semantic properties.

However, it is one thing to say that the algorithmic, deduction-like reconfigurations of token/physical symbols in LOT "secure" the semantic properties of these symbols, and another thing to explain how it comes about that they *have* any semantic properties in the first place. We learn very little about this from Fodor, while the only thing Dretske does is introduce the somewhat metaphorical concept of the "flow of information" (the very concept of information is taken for granted). In other words, information itself seems to be something already available and understandable by the time we try to grasp what it means for it to "flow" between the world and the system. As we shall see later on, however, this is not necessarily the case, and a theory of *what* information is (not of the amount of information, as in the classic posit by Shannon & Weaver 1949), especially in the proper ecological context, is still very much needed.

I will be arguing in Chapters 3 and 5 – and this is the reason why I bring up this issue here as a kind of preparation – that semantics, thus both "informing" and "standing for," require a certain *ecological* framework. In other words – and this goes back to the provisional remarks on intentionality made above – *designating*, *referring*, *indicating* and finally *standing for something else* are all relations made possible by the relation of ecological location which is neglected in virtually all theories of representation.

To be clear, the accusation raised by the embodied cognition camp, that representationalism generally ignores the notion of environment, is somewhat over the top, yet what is indeed lacking is a *general* theory of what *makes* physical surroundings *an environment* in which meaning or information *can* emerge.

Another idea about the functioning of PSS comes from a different tradition, and at the same time it brings along a different heuristic. This time we are not supposed to think of the internal functioning of PSS as a kind of language system, but rather as a mechanism. In a stronger rendering, PSS *is* a mechanism according to this view. This is actually suggested by Newell and Simon when they explicitly write, without unpacking it in greater detail, that "[a] physical symbol system is a machine" (Newell and Simon 1976: 116).

An apt articulation of this idea has come recently from Miłkowski (2013) and Gładziejewski and Miłkowski (2017), building especially on Bechtel (2008) and Craver (2007). Namely, a mechanism is characterized as a set of components and operations which jointly enable the system as a whole to exhibit a certain capacity.

We need to pause for a moment though. The "capacity" they talk about is an *observable* instance of cognitive functioning, for example, the use of vision, decision-making, or memorization. This is the *explanandum* belonging to the manifest image of the world, as Sellars (1956) would put it, whereas mechanistic *explanations* provide a certain model of the observable explanandum. As part of the pursuit of *explanation*, the system is theoretically decomposed into various components and their operations. Therefore, mechanisms as well as components are individuated by reference to their function within the larger system (Gładziejewski & Miłkowski 2017). This means that the distinctions between the mechanism's various functions or operations, or various mechanisms within a larger mechanism, are somewhat contextual: there is no single pre-given set of mechanisms attributable to a given system, such that the cognitive scientist's only job is to discover them. The cognitive scientist must, as it were, distil the mechanism they are willing to, and properly equipped to conceptually capture and explain. At the same time, *once* a certain mechanism has been distinguished, there are criteria that allow the cognitive scientist to determine its true or genuine function. At least this is the way I read the proposal at stake.

This interpretation brings certain consequences with it, and I am not sure whether Miłkowski and Gładziejewski would accept them. My reading is that a complex mechanism such as a real-world living creature can be divided into subsystems (component systems) in various ways, and one of such subsystems satisfies the conditions of PSS, thus the organism in question can count as an exemplification of PSS, but there is no predetermined, ready-made recipe for that subsystem decomposition. However, once it is done, one way or another, there *are* objective truths about the functions of these subsystems. Analogously, Frege once stressed that the North Sea is a geographical fiat drawn by man, but *once* it is conceptually distinguished it *is* objectively true that, for example, Norway has access to the North Sea and Poland doesn't.

Why is this important from the locative perspective? First, as already stressed in Chapter 1, some subsystems have specific locative footprints, meaning that a given subsystem *s* not only occupies some portion of physical space, but that *s* is characterized by a setup of *s*-specific locative relations: those occurring within *s* itself as well as those between *s* and selected elements of its surroundings. In this context, for each subsystem distinguished in mechanistic terms there emerges the question of whether or not it defines its own specific locative footprint, thus its own specific setup of locative relations, or just makes use, so to speak, of some other subsystem's locative setup.

My claim is that PSS *does* have its own unique locative footprint. This is exactly the fact that comes out in all these mysterious concepts such as "standing for," "indication," or "flow of information." They all indicate that *something quite specific* happens between the cognitive system (the cognitive subsystem of a larger systemic whole) and its system-specific surroundings. However, the available theories of PSS, including the mechanistic approach, do not say anything explicit about this locative feature and do not even problematize the issue properly. To be clear – they say a lot about *how* cognition has to do with the system's environment, as we shall see, but not about what makes such and such area around the system *an environment* appropriate specifically for the system's *cognitive* functioning.

Second, the question of how subsystems are singled out is important because the answer can bear on whether or not it is possible to speak of larger systems, mechanistically thought of, composed of organisms capable of cognition *and* selected ingredients of their surroundings. A full theory of this sort goes far beyond the limits of ontology, but a general architecture of such higher-level cognitive systems shall be tried out in the final stage of these investigations, in Chapter 7.

Now, going back to the issue of the embedding of PSS, behind all the embedding strategies mentioned above, whether it is the strategy adopted by Newell and Simon, or LOT, Dretske, or mechanicism, there is the idea of taking the brain if not as the sole realizer of PSS, then at least as the central part of any embedding story. Meanwhile, there is a relevant debate concerned with the question of whether neuronal representations, as the neuroscientific literature calls them, are real entities localized in the brain or just a useful theoretical fiction.

Roskies (2021) notes that neuroimaging "has largely shifted away from identifying the primary changes in regional brain activation for cognitive tasks (…), to looking at complex patterns of signal changes and the ways in which they relate to one another and to task demands" (Roskies 2021: 2 – preprint). This shift "has been characterized as a change from a focus on activation to a focus on information" (Roskies 2021), and herein lies the core reason, according to Roskies, why some notion of representation might be in order. What this shift stands for is in fact a certain evolution of research objectives parallel to the development of brain scanning technologies. More recent studies "utilize the *pattern* of responses across multiple voxels rather than focusing on localized regions of greatest change" (Roskies 2021: 3). This means that subsystems within the brain are differentiated differently now. For example, the technique called Similarity Analysis (RSA) "takes as input activation levels in an array of voxels, but instead of using this information for classification, it looks for internal similarity relations (…)" (Roskies 2021: 4–5) between patterns of activation. Therefore, what RSA does is "the calculation of pairwise similarities between patterns of response," instead of aiming at a one-to-one mapping between regions of the brain on the one hand, and kinds of stimulation on the other. This creates a new need for the concept of representation which is supposed to spell out the relation between these multi-voxel patterns of brain activation and behavior.

Now, one might argue that moving to neuroscience makes it possible to speak of representations without any locative commitment, thus without necessarily provoking all the puzzles mentioned above. This is not the case, however. As Roskies notes, "[a]ll philosophical theories of mental content rely on the idea that the brain must allow the organism to track and respond in adaptive ways to the environment" (Roskies 2021: 8). This means that representations must have a specific function *inside* the system, but the specification of this function relies on referring to what is *beyond* the boundaries of that system. Otherwise one might argue that the whole story could be told in purely causal terms, in terms of brain "gymnastics," as it were (echoing Chemero's 2010 critique of "mental gymnastics"), and without any reference to the world outside. It seems, therefore, that the two concepts – representation and environment – come on stage together even when we build our philosophical theory of cognition on the foundation of neuroscience. For if it is a neuroscience-based story spelled out in terms of involving, for example, such notions as agency and success or failure, then room is opened for a non-redundant notion of representation and at the same time a non-trivial concept of environment. As Roskies puts it, "representations must be *used, consumed* or *interpreted* by the system, and they must play a role in explaining intelligent behaviour" (Roskies 2021), a claim in which she follows Millikan (1984), among others. Meanwhile, behavior is obviously an environmentally plugged-in phenomenon.

Therefore, grounding our philosophical theory of cognition solely in neuroscience won't work since, to cite Roskies once more, despite

> the unsettled nature of theories of content, there is little doubt that there are causal processes that relate brain activity to external stimuli, and that play a role in transformation of early perceptual representations to more articulated representations higher in the processing stream.
>
> (Roskies 2021: 9)

Yet, even if there is, indeed, "little doubt" that there are causal processes relating the brain to external stimuli, what we mean by "external" here is more puzzling.

Clearly, if the concept of representation is to be used in this context, "external" must refer to something more than just stimuli emerging on the system's surface that happens *not* to be caused by the system itself. Instead, the term "external" is expected to have a thicker sense linking the brain to objects or states of affairs in the system's environment. However, "environment" cannot refer to physical space filled with physical stuff, as Lewontin (2000) pointed out, but rather to a realm in which it *makes sense* in the first place to speak of whether a particular behavior has succeeded or failed in achieving *a purpose*. There is no purpose in a chunk of physical space alone; purposes emerge in relation to the organism. But how does it come about that what is happening on the system's surface, stimulating the reaction of receptors, is connected with worldly states of affairs in *a* manner that isn't merely causal? By "not merely causal" I mean something informing behavior, perhaps affordances, however they are articulated – something setting up *conditions* of the behavior's success or failure.

My point, already reiterated many times, is that part of the answer to this puzzle must be to get our environmental talk straight and to confront the ontological puzzle inherent in it upfront and explicitly. So, neuroscience (just like the "flow of information" talk, LOT, or mechanicism discussed earlier), as informative as it is for any comprehensive philosophical theory of cognition, cannot be a refuge for those who would prefer not to deal with the need for a general account of the ecological location of cognitive systems.

2.7 Conclusion

While Chapter 1 unpacked some deep historical roots of the traditional mind-*as*-a-place approach to cognition and made it clear that the locative terminology was supposed to serve a greater purpose – i.e., to understand how the pursuit of intelligibility or understanding is possible – this chapter focused specifically on the conceptual backbones of Cartesian cognitive science, as it was dubbed by Rowlands, and elaborated in greater detail what it means for this paradigm to be, indeed, Cartesian. Key concept, including Physical Symbol System and representation (or the relation/mechanism of representing) have been analyzed and their implicit ecological commitments or requirements have been elicited. The next chapter dwells more on the latter.

3 The Ecology of Representational Systems

Faced with the problems outlined in Chapter 2, one might want to adopt one of the following two strategies: first, to argue that all the troubles having to do with the unresolved locative commitments of Cartesian cognitive science and PSS stem from a lack of clarity as to the kind of job the notion of representation is really supposed to do in cognitive science. Therefore, if we clarify representation's role, the locative commitment turns out to be unproblematic.

Second, someone might make the opposite case, namely that these problems come up together with the notion of representation, and if we manage to get rid of it while keeping the core of the PSS model in place, the locative commitments become, again, unproblematic.

What I will be doing in this chapter is as follows: I shall examine the idea put forward by Ramsey (2007) that there is a very specific task that the concept of representation is expected to perform in cognitive science. On this basis, I shall examine whether any of the two strategies invoked above are accurate. First, I will argue that once we clarify the function of representation, the problem of locative commitment gets clarified, too, which is beneficial in and of itself, but does not make the problem disappear. Second, I will make the case that if we follow Ramsey and interpret, for example, the informational account of cognition as essentially non-representational, we shall also obtain a clearer overview of the extent to which an account of ecological location is needed. There is no way for the latter to disappear.

3.1 A challenging job: What we want representations to do

Ramsey (2007) is concerned with the question of when exactly the notion of representation plays an explanatory role in cognitive science, as distinguished from mere representationalist jargon. He claims that while representation does play that role in the classical computational approach devised by Newell and Simon, thus with the PSS architecture in place, it is

DOI: 10.4324/9781003580997-3

no longer the case in many other approaches, such as connectionism or the informational theory of cognition advocated by Dretske.

To begin with, Ramsey acknowledges that *representation* is a cluster concept. As already discussed earlier, researchers in cognitive science either rely on something they take to be a general pre-theoretical notion or they come up with proscriptive, technical definitions which may posit relations that are not *recognizably* representational but are nonetheless posited as representational within a particular theory. Sometimes they do both.

To make his point about recognizability clearer, Ramsey refers to Charles S. Peirce and his notion of the interpretant. The key point is that if something is supposed to serve as a representation, it must be *interpreted as* such; therefore, if a given theory provides no account of this specific interpretive function, its posits are not recognizably representational. Yet, the goal here is not to postulate a homunculus, a disembodied interpretant hidden in our brains (to be clear – Peirce did not talk about any such creature either), but to emphasize that representations are entities or states that are *used in a certain way*. Something qualifies *as* a representation by playing a certain kind of *role*. Ramsey's approach is therefore pragmatist, meaning that "to be a representation is to be something that does a certain job" (Ramsey 2007: 23).

This, indeed, is a key issue. The explicit attribution of a function or role is a shield against naïve reification that would make representations out to be specific entities planted in the brain. A similar point can be made about the notion of information. Ramsey aptly points out elsewhere that "information is not some sort of substance that can be 'processed'" (Ramsey 2017: 4203). There is no such *thing*, *entity* or *substance* as information, and the same holds true for representation. Being a representation is *a role*, and – the crucial next step – that role, given the PSS model, plays out *inside* the system. Thus, the system itself is organized and can be mechanistically broken down into different subsystems, so that one subsystem takes something delivered by a different subsystem *as* a representation. The interpretant is therefore, in a sense, internalized, but also broken down. In effect, the proper task of theoretical analysis is "to understand how something can play a representational role *inside* a given cognitive system" (Ramsey 2007: 23).

The pragmatist reference to roles and functions brings out something that I provisionally call the *functional description challenge* which is a generalization of what Ramsey originally refers to as the *job description challenge* for the notion of representation. The idea is this: a theory must provide a description of what exactly a given concept is supposed to do within that theory, such that no other concept can replace it. With regard to representation, the challenge means a call directed to all those who use the concept, urging them to actually point out what specific function it serves within their theory of cognition. If a theory of cognition "invokes internal representations" (Ramsey 2007: 34) in its account of a certain process, there must be "some unique role or set of causal relations that warrants our saying some structure or state serves a representational function" (Ramsey 2007: 26). There needs to be some "explanatory benefit in describing an internal element of a physical or computational process in representational terms" (Ramsey 2007). Therefore, the said theory "should provide us with conditions that delineate the sort of job representations perform, *qua* representations, in a physical system" (Ramsey 2007: 27).

Why does the job description challenge matter? The key observation Ramsey makes is that the term "representation" has become part of a certain jargon in cognitive science, therefore, it is used in many theories in which, in his view, it has no genuine function, no explanatory role to play. I shall not analyze here if he is right or wrong with regard to each specific case. The question I am asking is whether or not (and if so, how?) Ramsey's pragmatist strategy of clarifying the concept of representation contributes to the puzzle of the locative commitments of representationism.

In my reading, the crux of Ramsey's proposal can be spelled out by means of a simple thought experiment: imagine a Martian or another "little green man" with a very good grasp of causal relations but no sense at all of symbols or representations – no concept of representation. Now, the Martian is observing a certain system on Earth which performs certain tasks. It seems that all of the system's actions have rather simple causal explanations in purely physical terms. For example, there is a part of the system that looks like claws on top of a steel arm, which grabs little balls from a flat platform and then throws them into two baskets. The claw grabs a ball, then goes up, and this is caused by a steel arm pulling it up – no mystery here, the Martian thinks. Furthermore, the steel arm does what it does because of a certain hydraulic mechanism; this hydraulic mechanism does what it does because it is pushed by a string of moving parts channeling the energy generated by the controlled burning of a fuel, e.g. gasoline. No mystery here either. Yet the steel arm is also attached to a light source labeled as a "scanner" which throws light on the flat platform delivering the balls, and it turns out that when the ball is green it is pulled up by the arm and the claw and then thrown into the basket on the left, and when the ball is red it travels almost the identical way, yet lands in the basket on the right. And here a mystery is looming for the Martian: there must be some connection between what the scanner does, the color of the balls, and the direction in which the arm goes. But what kind of connection? It must be causal, of course, for what else can it be? Perhaps causal+, the Martian speculates, since there must be something there in addition to causality.

The helpless Martian will or will not figure out that what he is lacking is interpretation, as defined by Newell and Simon, who write that the system

> can interpret an expression if the expression designates a process and if, given the expression, the system can carry out the process. Interpretation implies a special form of dependent action: given an expression the system can perform the indicated process, which is to say, it can evoke and execute its own processes from expressions that designate them.
>
> (Newell and Simon 1976: 116)

When speaking of "expressions," they mean symbols inside a PSS operating like a Turing machine. In the example just given what is interpreted is a certain property of the balls, what we call "color," but what the scanner measures is in fact a certain cluster of properties of light reflected by each ball. However, there is no simple causal connection between the light and the machine doing what it does. For there are two processes that the machine can execute, and which one is executed depends on the detected properties of each single ball. The machine therefore "interprets" a certain input by adjusting its task to that input. It takes this input in a way that crucially differs from the way it takes gasoline input and this difference is something that our Martian struggles to conceptualize because he lacks the concept of representation. So here the concept in question does a real explanatory job, or rather it would do the job, had the Martian been able to grasp the concept.

Therefore, the core of Ramsey's message is clear: the concept of representation must be able to provide answers to questions like "why is the system doing *a* and not *b*?" when purely causal explanations are not sufficient.

3.2 The input-output concept of representation

Ramsey's claim is that the classical computational theory of cognition is the paradigmatic exemplification of genuine representational theory, thus a theory in which representations actually do something. He singles out two concepts of representation that satisfy the job description challenge. As we shall see, both of these involve certain commitments and, therefore, call for a more elaborate theory of location.

The first concept refers to the *input-output* distinction. The general idea is quite straightforward: there are causal "bridges" between the input provided to the system and the output produced by it that would be impossible without some tokens functioning inside the system not only as causes of specific actions, but also *as representations* of states that are external to the machinery at stake. Recall the ball machine and the Martian grappling with it. The input was what the scanner reads, the output was the action of putting the balls into one of two baskets. There is a causal bridge from the input to the output, and yet for this bridge to stand there must be elements whose functioning as representations glues certain segments of it together.

The question Ramsey asks is this: "why are internal representations necessary for functional analysis when we are dealing with cognitive systems?" (Ramsey 2007: 72). His answer "stems from the way the sub-systems and sub-routines in computational processes are typically understood" (Ramsey 2007: 72). Namely, usually it is assumed

> that many of the tasks performed by the inner sub-systems should be seen as natural 'parts' of the main computations that form the overall explanandum. That is, they should be defined as procedures or sub-routines that are natural steps in a process that instantiates the more sophisticated capacity that is ultimately being explained.
>
> (Ramsey 2007)

Now, crucially, if a sub-process is thought of "as a sort of internal mini-computation" (Ramsey 2007), its inputs and outputs *must also* be regarded as representations.

Thus, we get a model that includes more than just input and output; something like a "bridge" between the two. Using this metaphor, Ramsey depicts the structure of subsystems as a series of intermediate "pylons" bridging input and output. In doing so, he modifies the so-called "Tower Bridge" model of the representational system proposed by Cummins (1989). Whereas the original model included only two "pylons" – one for input and one for output – Ramsey adds the intermediate structures that represent, we might say, a certain division of cognitive labor. His key point is that in order to understand what the function of representation is for the whole system, that is, between the "input pylon" and the final "output pylon," we must be able to trace what is going on, how the role of "standing for" is realized within this complex structure – between the "pylons" that make up its internal structure.

Hence, Ramsey summarizes:

> Data structures serve as representations because that is how the internal sub-systems treat them, given their job descriptions (e.g., performing addition, assessing chess moves, etc.). Serving as a representation of some feature of a target domain here amounts to serving as the sort of input or output required by a sub-processor solving a problem related to that domain. The content of the representation is critical for this role because unless the symbol stands for the relevant computational argument or value, it is impossible to make sense of the sub-system as a computational sub-system doing its job.
>
> (Ramsey 2007: 74)

The decomposition of the system into subsystems turns out to be crucial in accounting for how the system does the job of representing things *inside* itself. Otherwise, it's just another black box postulated as a representational system, with no explanation of what makes it representational. Meanwhile, the crucial part is happening inside, between different components of the system; between its subsystems.

There is another concept of representation within the computational approach that satisfies, in Ramsey's take, the job description challenge, but I shall bring it up in due course. Meanwhile, here is what I would like to do. Before I proceed, a key question must be posed: does Ramsey's Tower Bridge model of the Input-Output theory of representation help us to solve the problem of the locative footprint of PSS and thus answer the question of what kind of locative commitment representationalism makes? My answer is yes, and the next section makes it explicit.

3.3 Where does the "embankment" end and the "bridge" begin?

Ramsey's version of the Input-Output theory of representation takes an interesting and plausible step by transplanting the Cartesian internal versus external architecture to the internal realm of the PSS. In other words, while keeping the Cartesian distinction intact, Ramsey makes it much more fine-grained; he increases its resolution and uses it not only to model the default low-resolution distinction between the cognitive system as a whole and the rest of the world, but also the internal dynamic of the system. So, the Cartesian internal versus external dichotomy morphs into something like *[the internal versus external] versus external* dichotomy, where the left side stands for a complex string of many internal versus external distinctions drawn within the system as a whole.

This decision, however, comes at a price, which is noticeable from a more dogmatic Cartesian perspective. Namely, the default internal versus external dichotomy, the foundation of Cartesianism, becomes somewhat less dichotomous. This is because once we obtain a higher-resolution model of the internal side, the original dichotomous line fades and becomes less clear, more context-dependent. Think of the following example which does not pertain to cognition but serves as a useful heuristic (I shall come back to it in Chapter 6). Imagine the boundary between the interior of a complex organism such as an animal or a plant and its exterior. Actually, there is a big debate in the philosophy of biology (briefly mentioned in Chapter 1; to be referred to in Chapter 6), about biological individuals and the criteria of biological individuality. For if we zoom in we discover that, to take the most striking case, the animal cannot thrive without millions of symbiotic bacteria which, *strictly* speaking (i.e. speaking in terms of genes and reproduction), are *not* parts of the organism. However, some scholars argue (e.g. Pradeu 2012) that we need to adopt a different criterion of individuality, thus a different criterion for drawing the line(s) between what is inside and what is outside the individual, e.g., a criterion determined by the immune system, not by the physical barriers (to be discussed in greater detail in due course).

Whether Pradeu is right or not, the point that I would like to elicit here is that *once* we zoom in on the interior of a complex system, obtaining a higher-resolution picture of it, the boundary between the system *as a whole* and its surroundings may become more granular and turn out to be itself a complex structure, not a simple clear-cut barrier. Of course, this does not entail the boundary's decomposition, and some boundaries may stay clean and clear even as parts of a more fine-tuned model, yet the example prompts certain questions regarding PSS. Namely, once we zoom in and distinguish a plurality of input-output structures inside the system, how is it possible to distinguish the "frontier input," i.e., one that is *not* an output of another internal subsystem, but comes from the domain that is genuinely external to the system as a whole? In other words, what criteria enable us to draw such a frontier line?

I spill so much ink on this puzzle because, in addition to Ramsey's own intended goals, this is a plausible way of problematizing the issue of the locative commitments of representationalism. To demonstrate this, let me start from what an advocate of the extended mind hypothesis might bring up when confronted with the Tower Bridge model.

Here is a question that Clark and Chalmers (1998) might ask: is everything that happens beyond the standard low-resolution boundary of the system – the boundary determined by the system's "skin and skull" – actually distinct from the internal representational "Tower Bridge"? Think, for example, of a magnifier used by a 17th-century researcher. The magnifier clearly alters the inputs on the researcher's retina, thereby "mediating" between details of the external world that the researcher would otherwise be unable to see, and the researcher's nervous system. But if so, why not include the magnifier as another pylon of the "Tower Bridge" that the researcher's cognitive machinery is composed of? One might reply that if something happens on the surface of the magnifier, it plays no representational function within the system simply because the magnifier is not part of the researcher's body. Yet, the latter statement is exactly the sticking point here: it *assumes* that the conditions determining what is part of the body are *also* the conditions determining what is part of the *cognitive* "Tower Bridge." Meanwhile, the key idea behind the extended mind hypothesis is that this latter assumption may be false.

The point that the extended mind advocate could make is this: the "decision" as to what counts as a "pylon" of the cognitive "Tower Bridge" is not made by the factors determining the physical integrity of a cognitive system.

Instead, the relevant "decision-making" competence is "decentralized" so that one "pylon" of the cognitive structure "decides" what counts as another "pylon," just like in the case of the function of representation attributed to a "pylon" by the one standing next to it. Therefore, if the relevant "decision-making" competence as to what is *inside* and what stays *outside* the cognitive "Tower Bridge" is dispersed throughout the system, then the retinal image does not play the role it does just because it is part of the body, but because of the "decision" of the subsequent "pylon" in the visual system or higher up the neural "chain of command." If so, why shouldn't it be "decided" somewhere *inside* the system that what happens on the surface of the magnifier also plays a representational role?

To be clear, the question about the magnifier could not be answered by referring to a theoretical fiat. Eventually it would have to be an empirically informed decision. My point, however, is that the example, as part of the conceptual analysis being performed here, suffices to make the case for a certain further augmentation of Ramsey's metaphor. Namely, staying within the same metaphorical realm, I propose to introduce the notion of an "embankment" of the representational "Tower Bridge." My claim is that once we endorse a more fine-grained picture of the representational system, e.g., modeled as the Ramsayan many-pylons "Bridge," there is no ready-made, universally applicable answer to the question of where the system's "embankment" ends and the system itself begins. For example, the visual representational system may differ in terms of its boundaries and the boundaries of its "embankment" from the olfactory representational system (see e.g., Skrzypulec 2019 for more on the ontology of olfactory objecthood). Metaphorically speaking, the relationship between actual cognizers and their surroundings hardly resembles clear-cut, engineered river basins. It may be much more like a natural river with sandbanks and backwaters. This shows that the problem of the locative commitments of representationalism, at least as portrayed by Ramsey, is unresolved, thus calling for a more elaborate conceptual analysis.

All that being said, the weak point of Ramsey's model is that it takes the surroundings of the representational system as "plain." Here is what I mean: there is a complexity of pylons within the "bridge," replacing the too simple two-pylon structure proposed by Cummins, and yet the "embankment" on the sides of this new complex bridge is not modeled in any way. Thus, in a sense, the Tower Bridge model takes the surroundings as having no complex structure whatsoever, and especially no structure that might "partner up" with the complexity of the operations composing the Bridge. If we imagine a bridge, the area around it is simply blank.

My point is that if the decision as to where a particular representational "bridge machinery" begins is going to be made on an empirical basis in each case, then the model, if it is to stand, cannot leave the "embankment" blank.

This is because there may be a certain dynamic playing out between a particular subsystem of the representational machinery and the latter's local surroundings which decides on what is included as a vehicle of representation and what is not (see Chapters 7 and 8). Just like the particular dynamics between the metabolism and the immunity of an organism, coupled with the organism's local microbial surroundings, determine which bacteria are functional parts of the biological individual and which are not. Note however that it would be impossible to tell the latter story if biology made use of a model in which the surrounding microbial complexity was represented as a blank slate. The takeaway is that we need a model of cognitive systems, perhaps a version of PSS (perhaps even a version of the Tower Bridge model), that somehow does justice to the complexity of the system's surroundings. And this is the job to be done by a certain theory of *the location* of representational systems – a theory of their system-specific environments.

But what is it exactly that *counts as* an environment relative to the representational "Tower Bridge" and not to other subsystems of the organism? In other words, the zooming-in proposed by Ramsey must have a *fixed* resolution, for it would make little sense to provide a model of PSS in which we take atoms and electrons jumping from one orbit to another as "pylons" in the representational "bridge." Here the job description challenge plays a crucial role, for it is the factor that decides how fine-grained the model can be, thus how far we can go when it comes to distinguishing subsystems within the PSS. At some point there will be nothing recognizably representational, and this is the signal to stop.

Now, I argue that the same applies to the PSS's surroundings: simply put, not everything that is going on in the physical surroundings of a cognitive system counts *as* its environment; only entities, states of affairs or processes that are somehow relevant to the system, distinguished with the system-specific resolution. Think again of the analogous case of biological identity. The immune system decides which bacteria are allowed to functionally partake in the living body, but electromagnetic waves going back and forth through the microbial layers are irrelevant, and the immune system is not even sensible to them; they are simply *not* part of the *immune-specific environment*. On the other hand, these same waves, unlike microbes, are crucial building blocks of the environment defined by the subsystem responsible for vision (also with a limited resolution determined by the system's fixed sensibility).

3.4 In search for a proper "embankment" for cognitive systems

The question is, therefore, what actually counts as a potential "partner" specifically for the representational system, not other subsystems of the living creature and what decided on the resolution of its "embankment."

This question is not only about the selection of inputs on the surface of the system; it is rather about how some parts, fragments or aspects of the living creature's surroundings play *the role of the environment* for its representational (sub)system.

To get a sense of what I mean here, let us go back to the somewhat out-of-the blue example of the glass (recall Chapter 1). Suppose the question is what counts as an entity that *may* potentially be located in the glass. Air is not a good candidate, since it is always there, so to speak, and allowing air to function as a proper "partner" (a "filler" in this case) for the glass would trivialize the being-in relation. Further on, say, X-rays are not entities that could be *in* the glass, simply because the glass is no barrier to them. Noteworthily, this has little to do with the causal relations between the glass and its surroundings. Most likely there are unnoticeable chemical processes going on between the material that the glass is made of and the air. Yet they are completely irrelevant to the relation of being-in. In contrast, think of a fly that got inside the glass – it makes sense to say that the fly is *in* the glass despite the fact that there is no actual physical or chemical bond between the fly and the material bulk of the glass. Therefore, being-in is in principle about something else, as I provisionally explained in Chapter 2 (to be characterized more technically in Chapter 6). Namely, there is some sense in which the glass "offers" an accommodation to the fly, in a more or less Gibsonian sense, but not to the air or the X-rays. Now, if we think of a more specific locative relation such as the relation of *filling* the glass, the fly becomes irrelevant, too, for the glass makes this kind of "offer" to wine, water or even blueberries, but not to flies (a swarm of flies would make the example more complicated, but let us put this aside).

The takeaway for us is that what counts as an input to the *representational* system depends on what the *proper environment of* a representational system is, as distinct from the environments of different kinds of systems. This latter issue is left unresolved by Ramsey.

Note that for a minimal cognitive system such as an *E-coli* which van Duijn et al. (2006) build an argument upon, the environment boils down to the chemicals *in its proximity*, but certainly this is not the case for creatures capable of vision or auditory perception. Therefore, what *counts as* an environment for a system capable of audition is not (or not only) the proximal mechanical wave carried by the air, but a distal entity that can *be heard* by the system. This means that there emerges a certain bond between the location of the system and the location of the entity.

Note what Newell writes in this context in relation to his understanding of designation:

> There are two keys to this definition [of designation – KW]. First, the concept is grounded in the behavior of a process. Thus, the implications

> of designation will depend on the nature of this process. Second, there is action at a distance: The process behaves as if inputs, remote from those in it in fact has, effect it. This is the symbolic aspect, that having X (the symbol) is tantamount to having Y (the thing designated) for the purposes of process P.
>
> (Newell 1980: 156)

The "symbolic aspect," as he calls it, consists of the peculiar fact that the system takes some inputs *not* for what they "in fact" are, thus certain physico-chemical reactions on the surface of the retina, for example, but "as if" some remote entities were able to affect the process. The phrases "as if" and "in fact" are crucial here, since they show that Newell's theory of designation must assume that the *de facto* inputs do somehow put the system "in touch" with remote entities. In other words, the "symbolic aspect," i.e., the very phenomenon of symbolicity, is taken for granted here while its crucial locative aspect remains untackled. And yet it is quite a mysterious phenomenon. For assuming that the world may exist without symbolicity and the peculiar locative architecture behind it, and likely did for a quite long time, answering the question of how symbolicity is even *possible* and what its basic conditions are becomes of paramount significance.

These are extremely broad questions and there are some theories on the market that try to tackle them from various angles, for example, biosemiotics (see Favareau 2010; Emmeche & Kull 2011). And yet my point – one I hark back to all the time – is that there is a certain locative/ecological architecture and a certain locative/ecological dynamic underlying what Newell calls the "symbolic aspect," which must be elicited and articulated if we are to understand cognition as something environmentally plugged-in.

To get a sense of what's being problematized here, think of a seemingly trivial question, which nonetheless proves quite troubling, namely how are we supposed to understand the *distance* cited by Newell? This cannot be a purely physical distance, thus a distance in physical space. For from a purely physicalist perspective, there is no way to get in touch with a distant thing without either moving from one place to another or emitting some kind of energy. But nothing like this happens in the case of cognition understood in terms of designation. Cognition is forceless here; it has no power to move anything in physical space; it has no capacity to exercise physical power. Therefore, the "distance" involved in cognition must be something else.

Newell seems to suggest that what determines the distance relevant to cognition – we may call it *cognitive distance* – is in fact not physical distance as such, but the possibility (or impossibility, let us add) of some specific *access*. The point is not that physical distance does not matter, but rather that some other, cognition-specific *measure* must be imposed upon the physical domain if cognition is to be able to deal with distance. What matters is *access* to a thing, not how far the thing is from the system, as measured in meters, miles, etc. A different measure is needed. We read:

> In [PSS], the second aspect of the definition is provided by the mechanism of access, which is part of the primitive structure of [PSS]. It provides remote connections of specific character, as spelled out in describing assign. This specification is generated by enumerating for each of the ten operators plus the control the precise access needed to carry out their specified operations. Exactly these and no other forms of access are needed. This access is needed to exactly three types of entities: symbol structures, operators, and roles in symbol structures.
>
> (Newell 1980: 156)

It is quite striking that Newell speaks of "remote connections of specific character." For this is exactly the most intriguing issue. What is the nature of this "remote connection" and what kind of theory could help us unpack it? Cognition somehow *deals* with distance, Newell says, thus it sets up "remote connections" with distanced entities, but the latter must be located in a different, *not-only*-physical kind of "space" *if cognition is to have any power over this realm*. This must be a "space of access," so to speak. But what kind of space is it? It cannot be the Sellarsian "space of reasons" inside our minds, for when approached from the Cartesian standpoint the sought realm is clearly external. And yet it must be somehow determined by cognition.

This is another point when a somewhat more elaborate examination of locative relations becomes crucial. The purpose is not to nail down what cognition is from the vantage point of a philosopher's armchair, for at the end of the day localizing actual cases of cognition and cognition's underlying machinery is an empirical matter. However, what needs to be done, I hold, is to clarify the most fundamental conceptual architecture pertaining to various kinds of locative bonds between things and cognitive systems; a conceptual architecture that frames the empirical research.

Now, Newell gives an interesting hint as to how the "remote connection" he has posited could work from a logical perspective. Namely, it could be based on the quality of transitivity; in his view – the transitivity of the relation of designation:

> An important transitive law is illustrated in this, in which if X designates Y and Y designates Z, then X designates Z. In the case in point, there is first the acquisition which, through access to the actual external structure, creates a structure in the memory of the system that depends on this external entity; then the preservation of that memory structure through time yields a memory structure at some later time that still depends on the object.
>
> (Newell 1980: 157)

This gives us some initial idea of how it may be possible to go outside the system with this *string* of designations, but if so, we would have to agree that the relationship of designation determined by a given computational process actually goes beyond the boundaries of the system conceived of in a standard way, so that, e.g., a state in the receptor designates not the bird singing in the outside world, but another state, this time one at the very surface of the system, one that caused a certain receptor response; then the latter state designates another, this time happening in the system's immediate physical surroundings; and so on. We, therefore, have a long string of microstates, states designating one another in a row – and the row finally reaches the singing bird which is considered to be the distant target that cognition *remotely connects the system with*. But perhaps not with the bird, but with its vocal organs; therefore, the objecthood of the target must also somehow be "construed" or "decided" as part of the computational/designation process (which is going to be briefly discussed in Chapter 6).

Newell's idea of a string of designations seems promising, but it requires that the cognitive process encompass states outside the biological vehicle of the representational system. And if the latter is to be the case, we need to have a certain road-map, so to speak, of how to assign subsequent designators in the row – the world is after all full of intermixed causal connections, and the question is what distinguishes *the pattern* of hearing the bird as opposed to the pattern of hearing the wind that blows and moves the leaves around the bird. These patterns single out *specific* chains of causal connections; from a different perspective – the patterns are "filled" with specific causal chains as when water fills a particular riverbed or stream. If so, we need to be able to define a *specific space* in which this is played out, a distinctly "cognitive space" around the system; a space in which talk of "remote connections" makes sense. This shall be done in Chapters 6 and 7.

3.5 Where the "bridge" stands: The "pontoon bridge" argument against PSS

Given that the Tower Bridge model takes the system's environment for granted while at the same time not paying enough attention to it, i.e., to what makes it *the* environment of *this* particular system, one might build an argument against the whole model based on that negligence. And, indeed, as we shall see in Chapter 4, this is a frequent argument in the embodied cognition and enactivist literature. Varela, Thompson and Rosch set the tone by writing:

> (…) species brings forth and specifies it own domain of problems to be solved (…); this domain does not exist "out there" in an environment

> that acts as a landing pad for organisms that somehow drop or parachute into the world.
>
> (Varela et al. 1991.: 198)

If we translate the "parachutist" metaphor into something more in line with the Tower Bridge metaphor of Cummins and Ramsey, we might say that the argument advanced by the philosophers just cited, and many others in their camp, says something like this: what representationalism describes is not like a bridge actually built in a specific location, spanning a specific river or valley, and therefore rooted in specific ground. For those who erect such a bridge must take into account the local ground conditions (is it rock or soil, what kind, etc.), the local properties of the terrain that is supposed to be bridged; the whole system of roads to which the bridge is designed to contribute as a new efficient part of the system, etc. This all means that the environment of the bridge, when considered by architects and engineers, cannot be blank. Now, carrying on the metaphor, what representationalism proposes therefore is something like a pontoon bridge which is in principle erectable anywhere, but for that reason also hardly efficient in the long run.

The "pontoon bridge" argument, as I propose to call it for the sake of this discussion, says that while the cognitive system is placed in real-world surroundings, and while a majority if not all representationalists would stress that placement, the system is nonetheless *not constituted* by this location, it simply *happens to be* placed somewhere and receive some inputs from its whereabouts. In other words, the argument makes the case that representationalism has no conceptual tools permitting to articulate a unique and, in a sense, intimate relationship between a particular cognitive system and *its* system-specific local environment. Therefore, the term "environment" is merely a *façon de parler*, just like, according to Ramsey, the term "representation" in many cognitive science theories, where it is used quite frequently but has no real job to do.

In response, members of the representationalist camp may reply that there is enough textual evidence to show that the pontoon bridge argument is not fair. For example, Miłkowski defends Newell, claiming that his views are much more "nuanced" and "his arguments about the explanatory role of the external environment were not sufficiently analyzed in the debate on situatedness and embodiment" (Miłkowski 2017: p. 2 preprint).

I think that Miłkowski is largely right. The anti-representationalist literature does not always engage what theories of representations or other approaches within the computationalist tradition actually say (there are exceptions, of course, including, quite tellingly, Varela et al. 1991, where computationalism and connectionism is tackled in depth). This may be due, I suppose, to the fact that referring to "representations" and "representational content" has become ubiquitous and, if Ramsey (2007) is right, in many cases there is no substance to these references. Therefore, if a particular use of the term "representation" carries no substance, there is no substance to opposing it either. Hence both representationalism and anti-representationalism end up with opposing jargons.

That said, I propose to take what I referred to earlier as the *functional description challenge*, a generalization of Ramsey's (2007) job description challenge, and come up with an analogous task in reference to the concept of environment. This is the challenge of providing a job description for the concept of environment. The task is designed not only for representationalists, since, in principle, it may also be the case that some embodied cognition proponents use "environment" as a mere *façon de parler*. So the quest for fairness which Miłkowski invokes becomes somewhat operationalized in the form of a call issued to everybody, to both sides of the debate, to provide a job description for the concept of environment.

Before we move on, however, a certain problem with the newly introduced job description challenge should be elicited and briefly addressed. Ramsey (2007) originally referred to what he regarded as the "folk" notion of representation, which I have replaced with what I prefer to call the *default concept* of representation, thus an open-ended string of folk and more technical senses which trickled down from one vocabulary to the other over the centuries. The intention behind Ramsey's posit and mine was that we need at least a loose, yet sufficiently useful sense of something that plays a *recognizably* representational role. Based on the relevant literature, I outlined certain conditions for the latter. Now, recalling again the seminal quotation from Lewontin (2000), the problem is that we would have to make an analogous move here and characterize a *recognizably environmental* function for some entities. What does this stand for, however?

I propose the following two conditions. First, relevance to the capacities and needs of the inhabitant system. This means that the concept of environment as employed in a given theory must stand for how it is that certain segments or aspects of the physical surroundings are related, in a positive or negative way, to the system's maintenance of its integrity, its survival, the achievement of its goals, etc. In other words, how they contribute to the system's performance or endanger it.

The second condition I propose is that the concept must elicit *specific* locative relations between the above-mentioned aspects of the physical surroundings and the system. Physical space filled with physical stuff is always there. Therefore, using the concept of environment to refer to *that* would trivialize it. When it comes to *an* environment, the locative relations must provide information about what is going on between the system and its surroundings. For example, if a mouse hiding in its burrow cannot be attacked by a buzzard hovering in the sky, this means that there is a certain relation – *containment* – played out between the mouse, the buzzard, and the burrow. The very same relation would occur between another rodent, say a degu, and a hawk *if* they were placed in the very same *locations* the next day. This means that there is a certain abstract relation between *these locations* which constitute specific environmental conditions for all the creatures placed there.

These two conditions, I propose, set the *minimal* job description challenge for the concept of environment. In sum, each theory using the term "environment" should be able to say, first, how the term applies to specific locative relations occurring between a system and the parts of its surroundings cast in the *role* of its environment. Second, the theory should be able to say how these parts of the surroundings are *relevant* to the system's needs and capacities.

To be clear, these conditions cannot be understood to mean that only a theory belonging to the embodied cognition camp can satisfy them. In principle, even a theory advocating the strict cut-off between the system and its environment could use the term "environment" in a non-trivial way if it says something about what makes the walled-off realm an environment of this particular walled-off system. Therefore, Cartesian cognitive science cannot *a priori* be banned from proper use of the concept at stake; the latter is not the exclusive property of a particular faction or movement.

The pontoon bridge argument can now be reformulated so that it splits into two possible arguments: a simple version would make the point that representationalism in either form does not even see the need to satisfy the job description challenge for the concept of environment. Therefore, it obviously cannot satisfy it, which means that the concept at stake is just part of environmental jargon. The other version of the argument would say something more substantial: it would refer to theories existing within the representationalist paradigm that can be seen as making an effort to satisfy the challenge, somehow aware of its significance, and it would try to make the point that a given theory under consideration fails in this effort. These are arguably two different things: to not even see a challenge and to see it, but fail to tackle it.

3.6 Representationalism hires the concept of environment

I will now investigate whether the pontoon bridge argument in any of its two versions applies to representationalism at all. Let me begin, again, with a classic. Newell writes the following about a PSS's location:

> It [a PSS] is a machine which exists in an environment consisting of objects, distributed in a space of locations. We can imagine the objects having some sort of structure and dynamics, and doing their individual and interactive thing in this space.
>
> (Newell 1980: 142)

And he also writes:

> Behave and input have played a muted role in the exposition of [PSS], only because the emphasis has been on the basic functional requirements for symbolization and for universality. These capabilities must exist in some interior system, and thus can be illustrated there, without involving the interaction with the external world. (…) But without some reliable transduction from external structure to symbols, the symbol system will not be able to produce reliable functional dependence on the external environment.
>
> (Newell 1980: 167)

Someone might argue that this already puts the pontoon bridge argument to bed since Newell could not be clearer here about the importance of the system's placement in an environment of some kind. And yet this fragment is somewhat more of a mixed bag. Indeed, the simple version of the pontoon bridge argument does not apply – PSS's environment is not something that Newell forgot about or ignored. Going into more detail, it is also worth noticing that he uses the term "space of locations." This can be interpreted as an indication that environments are not just physical surroundings, but that they can be modeled as sets of specific locative relations built upon the physical layer. However, Newell does not develop this point, so it may also be the case that this was just a rhetorical move on his part, of no theoretical significance. Somewhere in between these two readings would be a position that I am quite prone to take, namely that Newell did have an unspecified intuition that the relation of *being in an environment* could not boil down to PSS' placement in the physical space, but he did not formally and explicitly spelled out this intuition as a proper part of his theory.

In the second quotation Newell admits that PSS was indeed theorized about in disregard of its environmental conditions, while a real system always maintains an "interaction with the external world." But on the other hand he seems to be thinking that this disregard was justified, at least to an extent. This is because, in my reading of his point, symbolization is something that can only be properly grasped as a process "in some interior" of the system. This means that for symbolization *as such* it is not relevant in what *specific* environment the system is placed, provided that it is placed somewhere. On the other hand, he speaks of the symbols' "functional dependence on the external environment," which suggests a non-trivial notion of the environment's *relevance* to the system.

A proper assessment of Newell and of classic computationalism with respect to its locative commitments would require much more than these few paragraphs, but my provisional take is this. First – as already pointed out – the simple pontoon bridge argument does not apply. However, taking symbolization as in principle something that takes place in the "interior" of the system makes Newell's theory vulnerable to the other rendering of the argument. This is because it seems at least possible that a system's environment is completely eliminated if we somehow secure inputs, thus certain causal happenings at the system's surface, so that, e.g., specific receptor firings are identical to the input usually delivered by the environment (which is what philosophers have been exploring for some time in the Cartesian tradition, beginning with Descartes' demon, up to the movie *Matrix* and most recent proposal by Hoffman 2019). For if the environment is just a source of surface perturbations *made into symbols solely by an internal machinery* (and not, at least in part, by action within this environment, as, for example, Hutto & Myin 2013 would argue) it may not be there at all. Therefore, assuming that the real-life systems *are* in fact located in natural environments, and therefore that real-life symbols *are* tied to these environments, it turns out that computationalism is unable to say anything substantial about this specific *tie*. Causation is not enough, for even the "fake" inputs *are* causal factors. Going back to my metaphor, the internal complexity of PSS that Ramsey so convincingly elicited is like a pontoon bridge pumped here or there, thereby entering into causal bonds, yet without any genuine bond with its surroundings – a bond that would make a difference in terms of what a particular system is and how it performs symbolization.

One could even make the point that Newell's view trivializes the concept of environment, for if symbolization is based exclusively on internal mechanisms, then Newell's reference to the functional connections between the system and its environment is empty. I would not go that far, however, for it seems clear to me that Newell does not consider his theory a complete model of cognition and, therefore, leaves certain issues open to further specification. The question of environmental placement is, I believe, one of these issues. Therefore, there is no *a priori* reason to assume that a more substantial conception could not be built on computational grounds. Actually, it has been built, and I shall refer to it later on – I am thinking of the idea of structural representations which clearly makes the relation between the system and its environment non-trivial.

Meanwhile, let me bring up another important issue here, which someone might also refer to in support of the pontoon bridge argument. Namely, it is said explicitly that PSS behaves "as an (almost) arbitrary function of the environment" (Newell 1980: 139) which is referred to as the *universality* of PPS and has to do with symbolization. Specifically, a machine is universal if it "can produce any dependence of output on input. Such a property is desirable for an adaptive, intelligent system which must cope with environments whose demands are not known at the time the system is designed" (Newell 1980: 147).

Universality means that PSS cannot be overly bonded to any particular environment, for if it was, it would hardly be flexible, thus unable to respond to novel circumstances. An even stronger version says this: if the input-output function is mediated by symbolization, then it is necessarily able to "produce any output behavior," for otherwise symbols *would not be symbols* but something like a natural indicator or signal, e.g., when smoke indicates/signals fire. Symbols are by definition free to symbolize anything the system wants them to symbolize.

This is a significant moment, for on the one hand a proponent of embodied cognition, as I mentioned, could invoke this property to make the case that PSS is like a "pontoon bridge," merely pumped here and there and maintaining no connection with local environments, yet at the other extreme, a proponent of computationalism could make the same thing into a virtue, so to speak. The PSS researcher could, therefore, say something like this: you want cognition to be constituted by local environments, and perhaps that is the case with regard to many "primitive" systems capable of minimal cognition (e.g. van Duijn et al. 2006), but the ability do decouple from a local environment is a cognitive *achievement*, and the ability to do so by means of symbolization is a uniquely human capacity. So, yes, cognition articulated in terms of symbolic computation *is* decoupled, and that is in fact a great feat. In this context, we may recall Chapter 1 discussing the rationale behind the mind-*as*-a-place paradigm and Merleau-Ponty's (1962/2005) notion of "slackening the intentional threads."

The issue is quite delicate. On the one hand, insisting on universality leads, at least ideally, to an account of cognition that is completely independent of the specifics of what is going on around the system, and perhaps also independent of the specific bodily (and evolutionary) system hardware. Surprisingly or not, the latter means going back to some sort of Cartesian dualism (note that classical functionalism was accused of dualist commitments). On the other hand, however, some level of universality does seem a reasonable postulate and, indeed, such specifically human cognitive tools as language do enable us to abstract from a large number of qualities uniquely attributed to this or that local milieu (for how language is accounted for in the embodied cognition literature see Di Paolo et al. 2018).

In my reading, the issue is another manifestation of the need for a general theory of locative relations between the system capable of cognition and its surroundings; a theory that would enable us to speak of relations between real entities, yet defined solely *in terms of their location(s)*. Such a theory would equip us sufficiently, I believe, to tackle philosophically the puzzle of what being-in-an-environment stands for at a very abstract level, thus without reducing the relation in question to any specific, empirically observed habitat. To put it differently, we need a more elaborate elicitation of the general principles determining a cognition-specific location and thus cognition-specific environments. This means a general ontology of the kind of environment that cognition is supposed to be coupled with, and at the same time *one* that cognition is able *to abstract from*. Such a conceptual framework would enable us to point to qualities of real-life environments that cognition is decoupled from while at the same time eliciting the qualities – I will figuratively call them "architectural" features of cognitive environments (cognitive niches as I put it later on) – that cognition not only does not abstract from, but indeed relies on in its pursuit of abstraction.

In this spirit, I will argue that cognition imposes a certain *structure of locative relations* on things in the system's surroundings, providing a blueprint for how both abstraction *and* environmental placement operate at the same time. So the defense line brought by the proponent of computationalism stating that abstracting from environmental bonds is exactly what symbolization achieves, shall be addressed in due course.

3.7 A first look at structural representations: How (not) to make PSS more embodied

Computationalism built upon the notion of PSS is by no means doomed to fail under pressure from the embodied cognition movement. As we shall see, it can have a more serious, more substantial approach to environment. In other words, there are tools in the computationalist toolbox to make PSS more embodied or more embedded in an environment. Two strategies are possible here: one keeps the concept of representation, refines it so that it involves a non-trivial relation with the system's surroundings, thereby satisfying the job description challenge presented above. This strategy is realized by the concept of structural representation.

The other strategy abandons the concept of representation, but at least in some fundamental respects stays within the boundaries of Cartesian cognitive science and computationalism. Here I see the classic proposal by Gibson, which shall be addressed later on, or the most recent theory of biological information proposed by Terrence Deacon (2021).

This section will be concerned with structural representations. To begin, let us briefly analyze the following statement by Dretske:

> What determines the reference for a *de re* mode of representation (the object it is a representation of) is not *how* it is represented, but a certain external causal or contextual relation I will designate as C. There is nothing in the content of the representation, nothing the representation *says*, which makes it about this object rather than that object or no object at all. *De re* modes of representation have their reference determined contextually, by the relation I am here calling C. Since the

> veridicality of an experience depends on it reference on what object (if any) it is an experience of – the veridicality of experience is determined, in part, by context (C).
>
> (Dretske 1995: 24–25)

In my reading, the contextual relation C is exactly thought of as a factor supposed to embed PSS in its environment, in the local circumstances, with the specific states of affairs found there. Relation C makes a particular representational content *de re*, which means that it is about specific things in the real world. Now, there are many possible answers to the question of what C actually is. Dretske himself articulates C in terms of information ("flow of information," as he dubs it elsewhere; see Dretske 1981).

But there seems to be a different option on the table, namely to consider C as a *structural* bond between the system and some states of affairs or objects in its surroundings. This is the route I shall analyze below. My main claim will be that C, however understood, must also be a locative relation; it must have a locative aspect to it, making it so that the system plays the role of a point of reference for a certain broader arrangement of locations. I believe that, insofar as this locative aspect is not unpacked properly, relation C does not shield representationalism from the pontoon bridge argument. Yet, when unpacked – it does the job well, as we shall see.

I begin with the very idea of structural representation (S-representation hereafter). First, let us go back to Ramsey, as he considers the notion in question to be one of the two non-redundant uses of the concept of representation; thus, one of the uses that successfully answer his job description challenge. The first one – the concept of input-output representation – has already been discussed.

According to Ramsey's reading of the allegedly folk concept of representation, the notion of S-representation draws especially on our intuitions regarding artifacts such as maps or pictures. The key idea behind the concept of S-representation is quite simple: an S-representation somehow resembles or maps *within* the system the structure of an object or a state of affairs *outside* the system. Just like a map which structurally resembles a given town or region.

Ramsey clarifies one crucial thing however. It is one thing when an *entity* playing the representational role structurally resembles an external *object*, and a different thing when the resemblance is between

> the system in which the representation is embedded and the conditions or state of affairs surrounding what is represented. A map illustrates this type of representation. The individual features on a map stand for parts of the landscape not by resembling the things they stand for, but rather by participating in a model that has a broader structural symmetry with

> the environment the map describes. (…) Given this structural isomorphism between the map and the environment, the map can answer a large number of questions about the environment without the latter being directly investigated.
>
> (Ramsey 2007: 78)

It is, therefore, of crucial importance to a proper understanding of the concept of S-representation that we should not think of specific objects within the system that are supposed to resemble their external targets. Instead, the relation of structural resemblance, spelled out in terms of isomorphism or, in a weaker version, homomorphism, is supposed to occur between the system, or perhaps one of its functionally distinguished subsystems, and a fixed external state of affairs. Therefore, there is a particular *functional pattern* composed of relations within the system, for example, a pattern of neuronal firings (recall Roskies 2021), and a fixed external state which is also composed of relations. Structural resemblance occurs between these two relational structures, and not between some internal *thing* and an external *thing*.

The concept of S-representation comes from Swoyer (1991). We read:

> [T]he pattern of relations among the constituents of the represented phenomenon is mirrored by the pattern of relations among the constituents of the representation itself. And because the arrangement of things in the representation are like shadows cast by the things they portray, we can encode information about the original situation as information about the representation. Much of this information is preserved in inferences about the constituents of the representation, so it can be transformed back into information about the original situation.
>
> (Swoyer 1991: 452)

Cummins (1989) calls S-representation "simulation representation." The key intuition here refers to models of various kinds, for example, technical drawings of a machine. Ramsey gives the example of a family whose relational structure, with relations such as "parent of," "married to," etc., can be nicely represented by a graph and – crucially – someone can learn something about the family from the graph itself, even without knowing any of its members. One can "simulate" family relations, Ramsey says, even not knowing who is who, thus to whom a particular node in the graph refers. For it is "irrelevant that there are no components of the system that consciously interpret the symbols; that doesn't prevent the system from using some of its components as symbolic surrogates while running its simulations" (Ramsey 2007: 86). So, according to computationalism spelled out in terms of S-representations, "cognition should be understood as a process in which brains run simulations, and consequently employ representations of aspects of whatever domain is simulated" (Ramsey 2007).

However, when it comes to the family example, abstracting from who is who, which is supposed to characterize simulation, proves quite problematic. Clearly, the intention is not to say that standard cognitive tasks are like this, thus the blind family simulation is not supposed to work as an illustration of the human epistemic situation. The point that Ramsey makes is that computation itself, standing at the core of our cognitive functioning, is *in principle* independent of the specifics of a particular situation; thus, it is universal in the sense invoked earlier. We can, therefore, imagine someone, e.g., a person Ramsey names Bob, who performs simulations in his head, thus operates on S-representations of the said family, without knowing the names of the individuals belonging to it. I can image that I am a historian of European aristocracy and Bob may be my assistant. I can give him two mixed family trees with blinded names, say with numbers instead of names, tell him to figure out the intricate bonds between persons 345 and 12, and not inform him that the families he is about to work on are the Habsburgs and the Jagiellons. The point is that he can still come up with results and identify structures of interconnected nodes that only I can decode and relate to actual people.

Now, this view of S-representations is problematic insofar as it adds to a more widely formulated charge that structural resemblance is cheap: anything can be structurally homomorphic or isomorphic with anything else. Yet, Ramsey calls this kind of worry a "red herring," and replies that it

> doesn't really matter that the drawing is isomorphic with dozens of other family trees or, for that matter, dozens of other states of affairs. It is used as a model of this family, and not some other, because this is the family that is the subject of Bob's problem solving efforts.
>
> (Ramsey 2007: 94)

This means that the fixed problem domain itself "is what makes determinate the target" of Bob's model.

In this context Ramsey emphasizes that "representational systems do not operate in a vacuum; they are embedded in the world in various ways, and this embedding helps determine the actual tasks they are attempting to perform" (Ramsey 2007: 95).

However, this leaves the problem of *embeddedness* unresolved. Ramsey simply takes this concept for granted. At the end of the day, Ramsey suggests, Bob may always become familiar with the specifics of the families he simulates. Bob's situational or environmental "plug-in" is, therefore, a brute fact, period, and there is nothing to theorize about, Ramsey seems to be saying. Therefore, unfortunately it seems that his account of S-representations does not satisfy the job description challenge for the concept of environment (admittedly, this is only a provisional assessment).

Shea also stresses that "representations interact causally in virtue of non-semantic properties." He then adds:

> If so, a complete causal description of the behavior of the system is available that doesn't mention semantic properties at all. We can describe how proximal stimulation at input will cause the system to undergo various internal transitions that eventuate in movements at output.
>
> (Shea 2014: 498)

At the same time he holds that:

> [W]hat adverting to content does achieve, however, is to show how the system connects with its environment: with the real-world objects and properties with which it is interacting, and with the problem space in which it is embedded. The non-semantic description of the system's internal organisation is true of the system irrespective of its external environment. Content ascriptions help explain how it interacts with that environment.
>
> (Shea 2014)

This is because

> When a system is embedded in a particular environment, entities within the system thereby acquire a suite of new, relational properties. The 'information' of information theory is a matter of covariation, so embedding a system in an environment gives rise to a host of new informational properties. An input register that could in principle carry information about very many different things now carries information about a much narrower class of conditions.
>
> (Shea 2014)

All this means that, according to Shea, there is nothing philosophically troubling about environmental embeddedness as such, full stop. For if one had any doubts regarding these content-involving "explanations," one is reminded that all these things "are all perfectly un-mysterious natural facts about the embedded system" (Shea 2014). So, if I got the message right, there is nothing to philosophize about.

Meanwhile, if we recall all the great thinkers listed in the previous two chapters and what they aimed at, the "semantic" phenomena Shea talks about turn out to be precisely *the most* mysterious facts that philosophy has been pondering for the last couple of hundred years. At least from the point when Descartes, driven by his first-person meditational method and inspired by his own scientific work in optics and analytical geometry, came up with the dichotomous internal–external architecture of cognition (see also Putnam 1987 about the "invention of the external world"). For, given this architecture, maintained and clarified by the concept of PSS, there is *no* straightforward way of connecting the interior of the system with an external domain. Theorists working on sense-data such as Russell and Moore, and phenomenologists led by Husserl struggled to define such a connection; Russell, Frege and Wittgenstein undertook the same effort in the domain of the philosophy of language (Frege's notion of *Sinn*, Russell's descriptivism, Wittgenstein's notion of logical form, all aiming at linking the internal, thus the "intellectual," "the meaningful," with the external, the "physical," or what have you). Of course this connection or "access," as Newell (1980) calls it, may simply be proclaimed, assumed upfront, and while it is quite understandable a proclamation in cognitive *science*, it can hardly be a plausible strategy in the philosophy of mind given its own history, invoked above.

Shea speaks of relational properties acquired by internal states thanks to environmental placement, but we hardly learn anything about what a relational property is in this context, or about its relata outside the system. Of course we can, again, proclaim that there is an environment already waiting to partner up with the system's internal states. Yet, in keeping with what we learned from Lewontin (2000), let me stick with the conviction that evaporation and volcanic eruptions are *not* environments, which means that we have some more philosophical work to do in order to understand *what general conditions* must be satisfied by an environment as a specific locus. In other words, we must understand how environments are brought forth by living *and* cognizing creatures, which is the aim of the embodied cognition movement, especially of followers of Varela.

To put it differently yet, given the job description challenge for the notion of environment, we might say that the way Ramsey and Shea use the term "environment" does not stand up to the challenge. This is not the end of the story, however.

3.8 A second look at S-representations: Getting more serious about embeddedness

Gładziejewski and Miłkowski (2017) can also be read as answering the pontoon bridge argument as well as the cheapness argument dismissed by Ramsey. The main point they make is that the similarities between fixed states of the system and selected states of affairs in the world must be *exploitable*. In a key fragment, they make a bold move, as if reaching out to the embodied cognition camp, writing that "S-representations do not have to be construed in terms of passive, pragmatically detached 'mirrors of nature'" (Gładziejewski & Miłkowski 2017: 338). Instead, they should be thought of as tools at the disposal of an active agent, a living creature – thus as a causally relevant factor fueling the success of the organism in "getting things done" in its surroundings. This notion of exploitable S-representations, they claim,

> can prove useful in resolving problems that seemingly plague similarity-based theories of representation. For example, one might claim that because of the ubiquity and 'cheapness' of structural similarity, similarity-based theories imply a problematic panrepresentationalism. But this can be avoided if we cut down the class of representation relevant similarities to exploitable similarities (...).
>
> (Gładziejewski & Miłkowski 2017)

Clearly, referring to the actual *use* that organisms make of their representations disarms the accusation of cheapness, for the only similarity that matters is the one needed to succeed at a particular task, and if the relevant setup of the representational system's internal states happens to be identical to other structures in the universe, be it an arrangement of rocks in some part of the surface of Mars, *it doesn't matter*.

I agree with Gładziejewski and Miłkowski at this point and shall not dig deeper into the cheapness argument. However, the question is whether referring to the exploitation of structural similarities as "fuel for success" can also fuel answers to the pontoon bridge argument. It seems that it could, given that sensorimotor coordination, responsible at the most fundamental level for the capacity to act, must be a capacity that is well-tuned and adaptable to local circumstances. However, once we look at the issue in a bit more depth, it turns out that the pontoon bridge argument has a deeper level still that needs to be addressed. But let me proceed stepwise.

The idea of exploitable representations and "fuel for success" enabling organisms to "get things done" in the world comes from Peter Godfrey-Smith (1996) who works within the information-processing paradigm and strives to make it more biologically embedded, following the path championed by Ruth Millikan (1984). The mechanistic approach to representational systems sketched out in the previous chapter and well-grounded in Newell and Simon's (1976) original PSS proposal is also adopted. Gładziejewski and Miłkowski think of the system as a cluster of mechanisms, i.e., operations whose aim is to produce specific outcomes. That said, the crucial idea is that "structural similarity between the representation and what it represents is what contributes toward the mechanism's proper functioning" (Gładziejewski and Miłkowski 2017: 341).

They also adopt Woodward's (2003) interventionist account of causation according to which X causes Y when there are circumstances B such that if an intervention changes X in B, then Y would change, too. This enables them to define the success of S-representations as follows:

> [T]o cause success, interventions into the value of X (which corresponds to the degree of structural similarity between the representational vehicle and what it represents) should result in systematic changes in the value of Y (which corresponds to the degree of success of the mechanism that makes use of an S-representation in performing its mechanistic function or capacity).
>
> (Gładziejewski & Miłkowski 2017: 343)

The authors stress that S-representations are of course simplified and the resemblance relation is partial only.

Building on this theoretical base, Miłkowski (2017) admits that the role of environment "is crucial in biologically plausible accounts of rationality, developed already by Simon in his theory of bounded rationality" (Miłkowski 2017: 2). The key to "rationality," as it is understood here, is (limited) behavioral flexibility. In this context Miłkowski brings up Simon's example of ants and their navigation capacity. To succeed in the task of navigation "the ant uses simple rules which may be seen as rational – not ideally rational but rational enough to fulfill its goals. In other words, the ant may be said to display bounded rationality (...)" (Miłkowski 2017: 4). Because according to Miłkowski, "sensitivity to information about the environment and the organism itself is usually presupposed to underlie flexible behavioral strategies" (Miłkowski 2017: 3), and "flexible behavior is adapted to the current niche" (Miłkowski 2017), it seems that to succeed at its task, the ant must be able to map its environment in some way, and use this map, thus an S-representation, as a causally relevant factor. And "as long as the function of such mechanisms is to process information, they should qualify as computational mechanisms" (Miłkowski 2017). Therefore, *structuring the internal mechanisms* in relation to the structure of the niche is in essence a representational relation.

It seems clear that the notion of environment is used here in a non-trivial way, thus as something that really has a role to play within the theory. I believe this makes the concept put forward by Miłkowski (2017) as well as Gładziejewski and Miłkowski (2017) fit to satisfy the job description challenge for the notion of environment. On these grounds, the representational system cannot be thought of as a pontoon bridge merely pumped up here or there.

All that being said, there is another problem. Beginning at a meta-theoretical level, it is not clear – and I would argue that this is a more general issue in cognitive science – which "image of the world" Gładziejewski, Miłkowski and other proponents of S-representations refer to when speaking of *objects in the system's environment*, thus also when speaking of the structural similarity of relational structures, etc. Is it the "manifest image," as Sellars (1956) called it, or the "scientific image"? Arguably, these categories are not well defined. The "scientific image" depends on what we take as the prototype of science, and whether we believe that there is just one such prototype, usually physics, or many possible ones. However, there seems to be a consensus that the "scientific image" makes us re-consider many of the mesoscopic phenomena we take for granted as parts of the "manifest" layout. This is because at least some important features of the manifest image turn out to be products of certain underlying cognitive mechanisms, as cognitive psychologists have convincingly proven.

Most obviously, when we adopt physicalism and take reality to be composed solely of clouds of elementary particles dancing in space and transmitting energy, everything else becomes a fiat, a result of "worldmaking," as Nelson Goodman (1978) would say. But even aside from such a radically reductionist and/or constructivist approach, the problem remains. For structural representationalists seem to be assuming that *there is* such a thing as *a fixed set-up of structures* in the outside world which can potentially be represented and exploited; that there are boundaries cutting up our surroundings into discrete objects, processes, relations, etc. to be mapped by the cognitive system. For example, all the cues that the ant has to represent and exploit to successfully navigate are already *there*, in the world, as if waiting for the ant to come and map them. In other words, however large and convoluted this nexus of structures might be, they *are there*, awaiting the arrival of a cognitive system. Meanwhile, if we look at what the scientific image of the world actually offers, there may be no such ready-made realm, and in effect, the ways in which we "draw boundaries across the board," as Varzi (2016) put it, depends on what kind of sensorimotor and cognitive capacities we have (see Chapter 6 for more on that). Take the famous bat illustration proposed by Nagel (1974). Although we can hardly *imagine* what it is like to be a bat, we can nevertheless *think* that it is likely that the boundaries between objects drawn by the bat's cognitive system are different from ours. This makes it hardly meaningful to refer to *the same* environment which the said bat is supposed to share with, say, a mouse living in the same cave, or with us.

Therefore, one might argue that representational systems are not only intentionally selective; they must intervene, so to speak, in their surroundings at a more fundamental level *if any* arrangement of structures *is to show up*. Aside from Nagel who made this issue famous in Anglo-American philosophy of mind and within the debate on purely subjective qualities (qualia), this is also the crux of the observation made by Jakob von Uexküll a hundred years ago, which gave rise to his influential notion of *Umwelt* (see von Uexküll 1926, 1934/2010). Each organism capable of interacting with its surroundings thanks to specific cognitive tools lives in *a* world, something akin to a bubble, determined by these very tools, he says. This line of thought, as we shall see in Chapter 4, is now being carried on by embodied cognition/enactivism.

This, of course, causes a lot of theoretical problems, beginning with the question of the metaphysical status of these *Umwelten*, how they are brought forth, etc. Some of these concerns shall be addressed in this book. Yet, this general reference to the plurality of possible *Umwelten* is sufficient to problematize the assumption that seems to underlie the concept of S-representations, namely that the structures to be represented are assumed as given. And this assumption is by no means obvious.

Going back to structure talk, the problem is what *specifies* the external structure *to be mapped* before it is mapped, which eventually boils down to the metaphysical question of what a *perceived object* as such is. Should objecthood be assumed as given? This is quite problematic because different senses may impose different conditions on what *being a perceived object* means, thus, among other things, different boundaries (see Chapters 6 and 7).

Someone might argue that this problem is solved by the theory of exploitable representations. For example, Miłkowski claims that causally relevant regularities in the environment can be parts of explanations of cognitive phenomena. The key here is the distinction between causally relevant properties or regularities and noise. In response to my remarks one might say that the distinction is drawn by specific cognitive capacities, and that what we refer to as "environment" is all that is *not* noise to these capacities.

However, according to Gładziejewski and Miłkowski (2017), for cognition to come on stage there must *already be* an environment that lends itself to tasks; there must be a problem domain. This is because cognition *is what it is* insofar as it allows the system to solve problems. Therefore, if cognition had also taken part in bringing forth these task-loaded environments, as von Uexküll might have argued, there must be *some still unelicited aspect of cognition*, a missing feature of the cognitive bond between the organism and its physical surroundings; one that is *not representational* in the proposed sense, i.e., one that does not boil down to the exploitation of structural similarities in order to solve problems.

This missing aspect of cognition is instead somehow responsible for "drawing lines across the board," to use Varzi's (2016) nice phrase again, thus for the coming into being of these *structures-to-be-represented*. Varela et al. (1991) speak of *enactment* in this context, which causes a lot of friction within the embodied cognition movement. The idea, therefore, might be that cognition is Janus-faced, as it were: one of its functions is to structurally represent, but the other and more fundamental function is to enact what is then supposed to *be represented.*

The problem that is left unsolved can, therefore, be put this way: if we take the environment to be a reservoir of information, we must realize that there are different such reservoirs for different creatures: the ant discussed by Miłkowski (2017) makes use of a reservoir of information that differs from the environment/reservoir of, say, a mouse; the latter's differs from the one attributable to a hawk; the latter differs from that of a human, etc. So, if similarity is a two-argument relation between an internal state of the system and an external state of affairs, and the latter is somehow also conditioned by what kind of system we are looking at, we need to say more about what this latter conditioning is and thus what the external *structure-to-be-represented* actually is. For in addition to representing and information flows, there must be some other relation between the system and its surroundings; one that *makes* the physical surroundings *an environment* by, possibly among other things, "distilling" certain structures out of a huge variety of them. And we still don't know much about the latter process. This is the deeper level of the pontoon bridge argument which S-representations do not address.

3.9 Conclusion

This chapter dug deeper into the problem of the locative commitments of representationalism and computationalism more broadly (thus Cartesian cognitive science, to use Rowlands'1999 term again). Drawing on analyses of Ramsey (2007), his Tower Bridge model of the representational system, and his job description challenge of the concept of representation, I discussed a much needed extension of the Bridge model so that it includes the system's environment (illustrated as the "embankment" where the "bridge" is supposed to be anchored), and came up with an analogous job description challenge for the concept of environment. All this enabled me to articulate an argument (the "pontoon bridge" argument) against representationalism, making the case that representationalism either ignores of fails to provide a job description for the concept of environment.

One worry, quite successfully answered by a line of arguments going from Millikan, through Godfrey-Smith to Shea, Miłkowski, Gładziejewski and others, was that PSS thought of as a "pontoon bridge" maintains no genuine bond with the place where it is set up. However, if we think of S-representations as "fuel for success" and diligently unpack this relation in terms of mechanisms and interventionist causation, it can no longer be maintained that the cognitive system is not sensible to the local specifics of its environment. On the contrary, the system seems to be strongly coupled with its surroundings.

Yet, the deeper issue we found ourselves faced with at the end of the chapter refers to the fact that the cognitive system may not be a bridge at all. This means that it is not something just *added* to the environment, however sensitive to the latter's details it may be, but rather something that transforms or even constitutes the environment. Perhaps we should think of the cognitive system as something like a dam rather than a bridge, thus something that brings about a significant change in worldly goings-on. But instead of thinking of the Hoover Dam or some equally spectacular construction, think rather of dams built by beavers – they *use* the local material and necessarily, in a sense, *represent* the local arrangement of things, for otherwise they could hardly survive, but at the same time they *alter* these local arrangements by seriously intervening in water flows. Does something similar happen in the case of cognition?

At this point, we have no answer to that question, but some partial answers shall be provided over the course of subsequent chapters, since, in my reading, embodied cognition addresses precisely this deeper level of the system–environment *constitutive* dynamic. This leads up to a general account of *cognitive niche* construction, to be given in Chapter 7.

4 Introducing 4E and Its Locative Commitments

This chapter introduces the emerging non-Cartesian approach to cognition which comes under many names including embodied cognition, enactive theory, enactivism, situated cognition, etc. This is a coalition of views in the philosophy of cognitive science maintaining some internal diversity but united at least in the realization of what I provisionally dub the mind-*in*-a-place approach in Chapter 1. Its main objective is to show that cognition, mind, or consciousness, are phenomena that not only happen to be placed in an environment, but are *constituted* by this location – by direct bonds between the subject capable of cognition and their surroundings.

Investigating the locative commitments of the non-Cartesian paradigm, as in the case of computationalism/representationalism, means unveiling tacit assumptions as well as explicit claims about what kind of location is attributable to a system capable of cognition and the entities that the system connects with thanks to perception, action, or reflection.

While Cartesian cognitive science, as Rowlands (1999) calls it, was a tent so big as to necessitate setting aside many details and referring mostly to the conceptual foundations laid by Newell and Simon (and their direct offshoots), the tent that we are about to enter now is no less crowded. And no less internally diverse, as illustrated, for example, by the controversy between so-called radical enactive cognition, a position taken by Daniel Hutto and Erik Myin (2013), and autopoietic enactivism, which can be (as understood, e.g., by De Jesus 2015) attributed to Francisco Varela, Evan Thompson and Eleonor Rosch (1991). I, therefore, need to make some upfront selection here and focus on the most fundamental concepts. The concept of autopoietic/autonomous system which can be seen as PSS' counterpart on the other side of the barricade shall be the focus of my effort, which admittedly reveals some preference toward the autopoietic tradition. Yet, the result to be obtained, I believe, will facilitate the much broader task of placing the non-Cartesian paradigm on firm philosophical footing.

DOI: 10.4324/9781003580997-4

4.1 An introductory encounter with 4E

The tent that we are entering is so internally complex that even naming it can be a matter of controversy; to be clear – a controversy that I want to avoid. Rowlands (1999) crediting it to Shuan Gallagher, has proposed the label "4E," where the capital letter "E" stands for embedded, embodied, enactive and extended (but, e.g., Feiten 2020 speaks of "4EA," adding "affective" to the list, so even here we have a certain plurality).

Briefly unpacking each of the "Es" should give us some idea of what the purported paradigm shift in the philosophy of cognitive science is about, and what elements of it, if any, make it revolutionary. What is worth emphasizing again, I will be focused solely on themes having to do with location and boundaries, which nonetheless happens to be – in my reading – quite crucial to 4E as such.

The term "embedded" means that 4E breaks with the Cartesian conceptual architecture constituted by the *internal–external* dichotomy which left no room for any closer tie or middle ground between the subject and its surroundings. However, as we shall see, this break does not provide a clear conceptual alternative, thus an explicit conceptual architecture that could actually replace the one set up by Descartes. Articulating such an architecture is one of the key goals of this book.

The term "embodied" means that the cognitive system must be thought of as a real-world living creature. At this point 4E puts emphasis on the so-called life-mind continuity thesis, drawing on the ideas that Varela developed in tandem with Humberto Maturana (Maturana & Varela 1980), first of all the notion of autopoiesis. In short, this is the idea that cognitive capacities are continuous with other processes defining a living creature. Thus even if cognition is not identical with life (as Maturana & Varela suggested; van Duijn et al. 2006 think similarly; see Moreno et al. 1997 for a different view), it is nevertheless much older in evolutionary terms than the Cartesian tradition (traditionally rather anthropocentric) would have it (also see, e.g., Thompson 2007; Di Paolo 2005; Di Paolo et al. 2017). As Andy Clark puts it,

> the thesis of strong continuity would be true if, for example, the basic concepts needed to understand the organization of life turned out to be self-organization, collective dynamics, circular causal processes, autopoiesis, etc., and if those very same concepts and constructs turned out to be central to a proper scientific understanding of mind.
>
> (Clark 2001, p. 118)

And this is exactly what autopoietic enactivism argues for (see De Jesus 2015; Cummins & De Jesus 2016; Kirchhoff 2016 from a different standpoint; also Stewart et al. 2010 for an overview).

As for the term "enactive," it is worth emphasizing that it may have at least two senses. The less controversial one is that cognition is in principle an activity or is grounded in activity; that it is constituted by actions undertaken by subjects in their surroundings (see O'Regan & Noë 2001; Noë 2004, 2009). This means that the subject is not a passive recipient of the environment's "deliveries" in the form of sense data, impressions, or mere physical stimuli. Rather, the subject interacts with various "aspects of the environment," as Hutto and Myin (2013) put it, which means, in my understanding, something more than causal perturbations. Instead, the cognizer is a dynamic "sampler" of what its environment has to "offer."

The more controversial reading, as we shall see below, speaks of the environment of a living and cognizing creature as being "brought forth," thus in a sense constructed, co-determined or co-constituted, by the acting cognizer (see e.g., Rolla & Figueiredo 2023). This is the view famously articulated by Francisco Varela, Evan Thompson and Eleonor Rosch in their groundbreaking (1991) book *The Embodied Mind*. The work smuggles in a sort of "idealistic" commitment according to some, e.g., Pascal and O'Regan (2008). This interpretation, however, is a gross misunderstanding, as I will try to show in due course.

Finally, "extended" is the most reluctant member of the group, already cited in Chapter 1. It derives from the so-called extended mind hypothesis put forth by Clark in collaboration with David Chalmers (Clark & Chalmers 1998). Actually, there is no agreement as to the extent to which this idea fits in with some of the other ideas laid out above (see Menary 2007, 2010). Clark, for example, quite openly adheres to the computational tradition, which is not what some other members of the 4E movement would accept (e.g., Varela et al. 1991 openly reject it). In short, the idea is that the range of vehicles of cognition – thus the material stuff responsible for running the cognitive machinery in the real world – is not limited to, or closed up within the boundaries of the living individual. Cognition is not limited to the nervous system. Instead, some entities in the subject's surroundings can help (or impede) it along, too. I shall not discuss this hypothesis here. Clark and Chalmers's argument concludes with the claim that there is in principle no difference between information stored in the brain and information written in a notebook, insofar as the *vehicle function* is concerned (Clark develops this view in various other publications, e.g., Clark 2008, while Chalmers, according to a footnote added to their 1998 paper, is more skeptical). Let me stress the "insofar" part – there are lots of differences otherwise, but *from the perspective of the vehicle-of-content function*, there is no difference, they say. Controversial as it is, I decided to include the "extended" strand here due to the fact that it alludes to the issue of the boundaries of cognitive systems, which shall prove crucial later on.

Rowlands stresses the fact that the term "non-Cartesian science of mind" is more aspirational than descriptive. This is because "as yet" (which refers to the late 1990s, and may or may not be the case now) it "has no clear conceptual foundation" (Rowlands 1999: 26). Meanwhile Cartesian cognitive science proposes "a framework whose foundational principles are explicit and well understood" (Rowlands 1999: 25–26).

In response to Rowlands's diagnosis, the task I undertake in this book by clarifying the locative vocabulary used within the 4E movement contributes to the conceptual foundations of non-Cartesian science of mind, whatever form this future science might eventually take (see Baggs & Chemero 2021 or Miłkowski & Nowakowski 2021 for more on the prospects for 4E).

4.2 The conceptual backbone of 4E: The autopoietic system

In Chapter 3 I tried to make the case that Cartesian cognitive science nowadays is not as ignorant of or indifferent toward the issues of embodiment and environment as some parties within the 4E movement suggest. On the contrary, there have been serious theoretical developments inside this paradigm that seek proper conceptual tools to capture the fact that PSS is an abstract model *realized by actual living creatures* and that all such realizations take place in a specific environment. In other words, accusing contemporary Cartesianism of neglecting embodiment is simply unfair.

Therefore, my strategy is not to show that 4E discovers the importance of environment and embodiment, as if no other theorists were aware of it, but rather to make the case that 4E takes these notions "more seriously," as I put it here. This is, of course, just a rough and ready rhetorical device articulating, on the one hand, the key idea of the system's co-determination or co-constitution, and of the system's cognition-specific locus on the other. For this is something that, indeed, cannot line up with the Cartesian paradigm. Along with this "seriousness" about embodiment and environment, 4E is much more "serious" about experience, too, which has been shown to be quite problematic inside the computationalist or representationalist camp (see e.g., the debate about qualia: Nagel 1974; Dennett 1988; Chalmers 1996; here, quite surprisingly, however, Descartes himself would side more with 4E).

The question is what makes 4E's commitment to embodiment stronger or more fundamental. An initial answer could be that 4E does not start by creating an account of cognition as realized by actual living creatures whose nature and functioning is assumed as given. Instead, 4E starts from a certain model of the living system and aims at finding a place for cognition there. The difference, therefore, is in the overall framing of the problem. In 4E the question is how the functioning of organisms gives rise – how it *gave* rise, if evolution is our concern – to cognition as a proper part or an emergent product of the very processes of living.

That said, we must not lose sight of how entangled 4E and computationalism actually are, basically as two chapters of one broader story. As already indicated, the emergence of information science was one of the things that gave rise to notions such as the Turing machine and finally PSS. Yet, another branch of this "tree of knowledge," to use Maturana and Varela's (1992) apt title, comes from developments in theoretical biology which gave rise to the concept of a system (e.g., the pioneering works of Ludwig von Bertalanffy 1968) and what is now called system science (see Thurner et al. 2018). This enabled researchers to approach a wide variety of problems in biology, psychology, social science, engineering and economics *in terms of systems*. And both of the paradigms under investigation here, i.e., computationalism and 4E, share this innovation as their root. While the former's conceptual keystone is the concept of a *computational* system, the keystone of the latter is the concept of an *autopoietic* system. The mechanistic approach, briefly sketched out as part of my recapitulation of representationalism, is another thing they have in common. For, in principle, both kinds of systems are said to be specific *machines*. Maturana and Varela (1980) speak explicitly of autopoietic machines, too.

The autopoietic system stands out as the fundamental conceptual root of 4E. This is the reason why I shall bring extensive quotes from Maturana and Varela (1980). My introduction of basic problems having to do with the locative footprint of the cognitive system thought of in the autopoietic-enactivist manner gravitates around their seminal book. Further on I shall focus more on Varela's collaborative work with Thompson and Rosch.

Here is a definition to begin with:

> An autopoietic machine is a machine organized (defined as a unity) as a network of processes of production (transformation and destruction) of components that produces the components which: (i) through their interactions and transformations continuously regenerate and realize the network of processes (relations) that produced them; and (ii) constitute it (the machine) as a concrete unity in the space in which they (the components) exists by specifying the topological domain of its realization as such a network.
>
> (Maturana & Varela 1980: 78–79)

Autopoietic systems/machines are distinguished from allopoietic ones which produce something different from themselves (think of any human-made machine). What is specific to the former and impossible for the latter is that what the autopoietic machine produces is *its own components* – simply put it (re)produces itself (which is what the term "autopoiesis," coming from ancient Greek, means).

Organisms are physical autopoietic machines or "autopoietic systems in the physical space." Note the parallel to the notion of PSS. In both cases we have a certain abstract model of the functioning of actual living creatures. Therefore, the difference between computationalism and 4E is not about abstractness, with the former allegedly too detached from how real organisms operate. Both approaches are very abstract, and both put stress on the cognitive system's physical realization. So what is it that makes the conceptual foundations of 4E more "serious" about embodiment? The answer is: cognition does *not* just *happen to* the autopoietic system; instead, it is considered to be part of *the very fabric of thatsystem*. We read:

> A cognitive system is a system whose organization defines a domain of interactions in which it can act with relevance to the maintenance of itself, and the process of cognition is the actual (…) acting or behaving in this domain. Living system are cognitive systems, and living as a process is a process of cognition. This statement is valid for all organisms, with and without a nervous system.
>
> (Maturana & Varela 1980: 13)

This initial answer, however, needs some additional clarification if we are to understand its implications for 4E's locative commitments. For note that based on what we have just read, if a system interacts with its surroundings in any manner, this equals cognition. This is why it used to be said that Maturana and Varela endorse not only life-mind continuity, but life-mind identity. The risk, however, is that this step trivializes the concept at stake, i.e., mind or cognition. Some thinkers argue that if cognition is everywhere, there is no point in searching for its unique features and origins, and eventually we learn nothing from the identity claim (see e.g., Godfrey-Smith 2016).

I am not going to defend (or criticize) the identity claim, since searching for the "mark of the cognitive," as the literature sometimes dubs this pursuit, is not the goal of this investigation (see van Duijn et al. 2006; Barandiaran & Moreno 2006; Arnellos & Moreno 2015; Keijzer 2015; Allen 2017). However, I shall argue that there is a certain dynamic having to do with location which makes the *continuity* thesis non-trivial.

In other words, my claim is that identifying the locative footprint of an autopoietic system is not an additional theoretical effort but a key part of understanding how autopoiesis *becomes* cognition and how cognition contributes to that system-specific footprint (see 4.4 where the issue is introduced).

4.3 The locative footprint of autopoietic systems

To begin with, a possible justification of the claim that 4E's concentration on embodiment and environment is more profound than computationalism's might be that while PSS is said to be a closed structure whose mechanism is fully defined in terms of linear chains of internal symbol manipulation, 4E defines the cognitive system as an open-ended loop of system–environment interaction. Daniel Hutto and Erik Myin provide an excellent articulation of this idea by referring to how "[v]ariables in the environment influence and are influenced by variables in the brain and the non-neural body in a recurrent manner, making it impossible to conceive of these as linear relations holding between inputs and outputs" (Hutto & Myin 2013: 6). Therefore, which is crucial from the perspective of this study, "there is no way to isolate properly mentality constituting 'inner' organismic responses from 'outer' ones that allegedly stand over and against the former as mere causal contributions from the environment" (Hutto & Myin 2013). Then they conclude that insofar as the enactivist model is concerned, "there is no prospect of making any such principled division" (Hutto & Myin 2013). I shall address this latter issue in due course and come up with a more nuanced approach.

Meanwhile, it may come as a surprise that the backbone of 4E, the concept of autopoietic system, seems to be, at least at first glimpse, very internalist. We are told that the organization of the autopoietic machine "must be such as to define the process as occurring completely within the boundaries of the machine which the very same organization specifies" (Maturana & Varela 1980: 79). The system is, therefore, a functionally closed "concrete unity in space," and its functioning seems quite idiosyncratic – contrary to what Hutto and Myin would endorse.

There is a tension here, and a puzzle: how is it that a coalition of views aiming at reforming our conceptions of cognition so as to get rid of the Cartesian *internal versus external* dichotomy and anchor cognitive functioning in living creatures' actual dealings with their surroundings, starts from a concept that may seem to be a faithful exemplification of that dichotomy.

To resolve this tension, let us start by defining the *space* in which autopoietic systems operate. The following fragment suggests a possible answer from Maturana and Varela:

> In a natural physical unity like a crystal, the spatial relations among the components specify a lattice organization which defines it as a member of a class (a crystal of a particular kind), (…). This is not so with an autopoietic machine. In fact, although we find spatial relations among its components whenever we actually or conceptually freeze it for an observation, the observed spatial relations do not (and cannot) define it

> as autopoietic. This is so because the spatial relations between the components of an autopoietic machine are specified by the network of processes of production of components (...). A crystal organization then lies in a different domain than the autopoietic organization: a domain of relations between components, not of relations between processes of production of components; (...) We normally acknowledge this by saying that crystals are static."
>
> (Maturana & Varela 1980: 79–80)

The term "spatial relations" most likely refers to *physical space* in this fragment. The first point to notice is that according to Maturana and Varela relations in physical space cannot specify an autopoietic system because the direction of specification is exactly the opposite, so to speak. This means that the relations in physical space that characterize a given system are themselves determined by the internal processes responsible for the system's autopoiesis. Autopoiesis is not defined by space, but all actual spatial relations within the system are defined by its autopoiesis.

Hence, in a sense, there is nothing interesting to be said about the autopoietic system in terms of its footprint in physical space – it has a spatial dimension, obviously, but analyzing it says nothing significant about the core of what makes the system what it is. And yet, this does not mean that there is nothing important about its *locative* footprint, if we keep in mind that location may not refer to physical space only. On the contrary, I believe that unpacking the autopoietic system's specific *locative* footprint resolves some of the tension between the focus on the interactions highlighted above as one of the key features of 4E, and the movement's roots in Maturana and Varela's works on autopoiesis.

First, Maturana and Varela distinguish physical space from what they call the *phenomenological* domain. The latter is "defined by the properties of the unity or unities that constitute it," meaning that "whenever a unity is defined or a class of unities is established which can undergo transformations or interactions, a phenomenological domain is defined" (Maturana & Varela 1980: 137). This sense of the term "phenomenology" is by no means standard and unfortunately remains somewhat unclear. Aside from the term itself, the point seems to be that there is a domain generated by interactions *within* the autopoietic machine; a domain that needs to be distinguished from the physical space in which the machine is realized. The physical space, Maturana and Varela claim, is "the space within which the phenomenology of autopoiesis of living systems takes place" (Maturana & Varela 1980: 137). Thus, the physical serves as the base for the phenomenological.

To get at least a provisional grasp of this "phenomenological domain," let us go back to the example given by Maturana and Varela. The key difference between the crystal and the autopoietic system is supposed to be that in addition to its location in physical space, the system is located in a domain that *it itself internally creates*, while crystals are "only" placed in physical space. I propose to read this as follows: first, in the case of the crystal, specifying the locative relations between the components requires assuming the position of an external observer. This does not mean that there needs to *be* an observer for these relations to occur; rather, an observer is needed to single them out. This is because every such singling out, every specification, requires a vantage point or a point of reference from which it can be said that, for example, the crystal component *x* is located 5 mm to the left of component *y*. In other words, some system of measurement has to be *imposed on* the crystal or any other such complex but static object, and it must be done from the outside, by an observer. Where else could such a measurement come from? The notion of the observer proves crucial here. Crystals themselves, quite obviously, cannot define and impose a measurement on themselves.

Meanwhile – and this is the key – autopoietic systems *can* take stock of themselves, so to speak. They can be self-directed, which results, as I see it, exactly in the emergence of phenomenological domains. In short, therefore, relations within the phenomenological domain are specified by the autopoietic system itself functioning as the observer *of its own internal dynamics*.

Yet this view is still strongly internalist, and we still do not know how to ground Hutto and Myin's (2013) insistence on cognition as "dynamic interactions" which are "loopy, not linear." Let us then take a further step which unveils the fact that this somewhat idiosyncratic "phenomenological domain" of a system is possible precisely *due to interactions* with other systems, and moreover – that the said domain is constituted by certain locative relations.

Maturana and Varela stress that although every change that an autopoietic system undergoes is caused solely by its internal process of autopoiesis, systems can interact with one another in the sense that

> the autopoietic conduct of an organism A becomes a source of deformation for an organism B, and the compensatory behavior of organism B acts, in turn, as a source of deformation of organism A, whose compensatory behavior acts again as a source of deformation of B, and so on recursively until the coupling is interrupted.
>
> (Maturana & Varela 1980: 120)

This is referred to as *behavioral coupling*. To be clear: one system cannot determine the behavior of other systems directly, but there is an indirect bond insofar as A causes perturbations to B and B changes its autopoietic processes accordingly.

This indirect connection between two internal processes of autopoiesis gives rise to a consensual *linguistic domain*, as Maturana and Varela call it, which is defined as "a consensual domain in which the coupled organisms orient each other in their internally determined behavior through interactions that have been specified during their coupled ontogenesis" (Maturana & Varela 1980: 136).

The term "linguistic," just like "phenomenological," is employed here in a very non-standard way, which we must keep in mind. The phenomenon of a linguistic connection between two systems is defined in terms of their internal pursuits of autopoiesis. This linguistic domain has hardly anything to do with what we would intuitively call "language." It plays out at a much more "primitive" level than Fodor's LOT, for example.

Once we have the linguistic domain in place, we can define the observer as an autopoietic system "capable of interacting with its own states (as an organism with a nervous system can do), and capable of developing with others a linguistic consensual domain," meaning a system that "can treat its own linguistic states as a source of deformation and thus interact linguistically in a closed linguistic domain" (Maturana & Varela 1980: 120–121).

The key thing here is that the observer, as defined by Maturana and Varela, is not a mysterious creature that does not belong in the model they develop. Instead, the observer is *also* an autopoietic system. The idea they put forward is that some systems are capable not only of interacting with other systems in the linguistic domain, i.e., of connecting their processes of autopoiesis in such a way so that the perturbations caused by one system modify the respective processes of another system, but they can also cause certain perturbations *to themselves* and react accordingly. This means that such a system is capable of *tracking its own states* in the linguistic domain.

We have here an interesting case when a capacity developed as a result of co-evolution with other systems, and primarily devoted to tracking others, gives the individual autopoietic system an extra capacity with respect to itself. So the phenomenological domain, internally determined by the system, *is possible only if the system interacts with other systems* in the way just described. This is because, as I proposed above, the phenomenological domain is constituted by the system's ability to specify relations within its own internal structure, thus to act as an observer of its own functioning. Meanwhile, being an observer is made possible by the system's engagement in the interactional linguistic domain.

I propose the following reading: the autopoietic system is capable of determining *points of reference for its own internal functioning*, thus of imposing, in a sense, a system of measurement *on itself*, unlike the crystal which is not able to do so. The notion of a point of reference can be nicely illustrated – which is what I did in Chapter 2 – by entities that can afford, in the Gibsonian sense, an accommodation to other things, like in the example of the glass filled with wine. Provisionally put (see Chapter 6 for a more technical characterization), for an entity *x*, to be a point of reference means that *x* is able to establish a *pattern* of locative relations binding some of the entities surrounding *x* with one another *and with x*. Therefore, insofar as the functioning of the autopoietic system is composed of some internal elements standing in locative relations to one another, specified by the system itself, it can be said that the autopoietic system defines its *own system-specific* locus *from within*, without needing an external observer. This "internal" determination is what makes the autopoietic system crucially different from crystals and other complex spatially extended entities when it comes to its locative footprint.

Therefore, the internal phenomenological domain is grounded in the interactional linguistic domain. This means that although the functioning of autopoietic systems is still somewhat idiosyncratic, it is only possible in a domain whose emergence is due to these interactions. By contrast, the latter feature does *not* apply to PSS which is supposed to be merely placed in a pre-given physical domain waiting to be structurally represented within the PSS. Therefore, one might say that the functioning of the autopoietic system is at least less idiosyncratic than the internal functioning of PSS.

4.4 On becoming more serious about embodiment and prospects for more seriousness about environment

All the things just said have two consequences – we might say two *serious* consequences in the sense that they make the conceptual backbone of 4E *more serious* about two things: about embodiment and about environment.

The important point here is that a shared domain established by interacting autopoietic systems can itself be considered, in my reading, as *a higher-level autopoietic system*. Maturana and Varela hold that autopoietic systems

> can couple and constitute a new unity while their individual paths of autopoiesis become reciprocal sources of specification of each other's ambience, if their reciprocal deformations do not overstep their corresponding ranges of tolerance for variation without loss of autopoiesis.
> (Maturana & Varela 1980: 108)

In this manner an autopoietic system "can become a component of another system (...)" (Maturana & Varela 1980: 110).

This is the sense in which, I propose, the autopoietic system is *embodied*. Namely, the said embodiment does not boil down to the mere fact that organisms are considered physical autopoietic systems, realizations of a more abstract schema, just like PSS is the physical realization of the computational system. The crux of the autopoietic system's embodiment is the fact that *autopoiesis scales up*, as it were, meaning that the system co-determines a "larger body," one might say, higher-level autonomous systems, together with some of its partner systems. This gives rise to what Maturana and Varela call the linguistic domain. And this shared domain is the proper embodiment of the autopoietic system, not just physical space. It is a richer, thus more "serious" notion of embodiment than the one available to computationalism or representationalism which take the space in which cognitive systems operate as existing "out there," independently of what cognitive systems are doing.

Now, 4E's conceptual backbone's being more serious about embodiment makes room for a debate on whether or not – if so, in what sense – it is also more serious about the notion of environment, thus about the fact that the cognitive system is environmentally plugged-in. In my reading, the crux of this latter "seriousness" is the already highlighted fact that representationalism takes the environment as given, waiting to be represented, whereas 4E wants to say something about *how* the physical surroundings of a cognitive system *become* its environment.

To get a better sense of why the latter is critically important, note that from the perspective of a single autopoietic system *alone* nothing can be considered *external* in the proper sense; it simply *is not internal*, as it were. This means that the system maintains its boundary and is capable of registering and reacting to perturbations occurring on that boundary, but what happens on this boundary is the whole "worldview" that the system can get. "What's at my surface is at my surface, and that's *all I can tell*," we can imagine it saying. So it is not *external* in the proper sense, since the system does not yet have any "notion" of "exterior" that would refer to realms beyond its boundary.

This is worth emphasizing because – as I pointed out in several places in the previous two chapters – philosophers and cognitive scientists frequently talk about a cognitive system's bonds with its environment, its dealings with the environment and distant things in this environment as if it were obvious that the system itself, alone, is capable of seeing itself *as placed in some broader domain*; as if it were able to take a glimpse from above and see *itself and the surrounding realms*. But how so? From the perspective of the system alone, strictly speaking, there is *no environment*, *no exterior* of any sort. There is *no distal object* seen in virtue of the light it reflects; this is all a *description from the perspective of the observer* who is capable of seeing the object *and* the system from its own perspective. From the system's own standpoint there is something happening on its surface; that's *all* there is.

So, if an external domain is not assumed, then its emergence has to be explained. Therefore, it cannot be part of the story of autopoietic systems from the start. That said, the story told by Maturana and Varela can also hardly be dubbed internalist insofar as internalism puts stress on internal or interior-oriented processes and *neglects* exterior-oriented ones. For it is impossible to actually neglect the external and highlight the internal if there is *no* concept of "external" in operation. Therefore, what seems to be internally oriented is not quite so, strictly speaking, given that the very concept of something's *being internal* assumes that the counterpart notion of another thing's *being external* is already understandable. If this is not the case, internality is not, strictly speaking, part of the conceptualization.

We are at a level of conceptualization where the idea of an exterior does not apply, nor, therefore, does the idea of an interior. This means that the conceptualization proposed by Maturana and Varela is not internalist, strictly speaking; it goes deeper than the *internalism–externalism* debate and is supposed to provide the *internal–external* divide as such with a meaning.

Yet, in this context, Maturana and Varela emphasize a point that may seem trivial otherwise: that observers are also autopoietic systems. Thus, we can speak of groups of systems playing the role of observers to one another, and therefore we can also speak of *a domain established by them playing that role*. And this conceptual move lays the foundation for a non-trivial, thus more serious, as I decided to put it here, concept of environment.

To unpack this idea, suppose we have three systems A, B, C. The relation of observing between systems A, B and C unfolds a new domain of location in which A and B are placed *as observed* by C, and the same applies to A and C *as observed* by B, and B and C *as observed* by A.

I propose that if they serve as observers to one another, a certain new network of locative relations emerges with *observers playing the role of points of reference* in the network. This means that *the relation of observing*, when A serves as the observer of B and C, creates a pattern of locative relations between B and C on the one hand, and A as the point of reference. The same applies to A and C from the reference point of B, and to A and B from the reference point of C.

Therefore, *the locative footprint* of autopoietic systems does not only differ from the footprint of crystals and other such entities, which is what I argued for in the previous section; moreover, their locative footprint is of the *ecological kind* in the sense that autopoietic systems together establish a specific *shared* locus defined by their functioning as observers to one another and to themselves. Let me stress this point: unlike in the case of PSS, here we are provided by Maturana and Varela with a certain description of how it happens that this genuinely *ecological* location of the autopoietic system *begins* to emerge. It is not assumed upfront, pre-given, and simply awaiting the arrival of autopoietic systems. Instead, it is a location established by the systems themselves as they interact.

However, I hold that we still lack a more detailed description of *how this emergence of the ecological location develops*; how it gives rise to the specific locative footprint of more complex systems and their – as it will be dubbed later on – cognitive niches. Maturana and Varela do not give sufficient answers. Here is why.

It is generally agreed that the notion of autopoietic system applies primarily to something like the "atom" of life, thus the simplest living creature. Insofar as known forms of life are concerned, it is the model of a single cell. Therefore, a more general concept may be needed if more complex forms of life are to be captured, and especially if cognition in a more recognizable form, e.g., perception, problem solving, is to come on stage.

Moreover, while *acting* in a certain fixed environment is not a definitional feature of the autopoietic system, more complex systems capable of flexible sensorimotor coordination may be in part constituted by what they *do*, which is what 4E as a whole strongly emphasizes.

For that reason, among others, the 4E literature does not speak of autopoietic systems very often but instead comes up with the more general notion of an *autonomous system* which satisfies the following conditions:

Considered abstractly, for a system to be autonomous, its constituent processes must meet the following conditions:

(a) recursively depend on each other for their generation and their realization as a network;
(b) constitute the system as a unity in whatever domain they exist; and
(c) determine a domain of possible interactions with the world.

(Thompson & Stapleteon, 2009, p. 24, original punctuation changed)

The last point is pivotal, insofar as it refers *not* just to the fact that one system is a source of perturbation to another, thereby giving rise to a domain in which systems are observers for one another – as in the case of autopoietic systems – but to genuine *activities* undertaken by systems.

The main idea, as I see it, is that as the complexity of inter-system relations increases, there also emerge different ways in which the systems are relevant to one another as well as different ways in which other things in the world are relevant to them. Here I focus only on how this new level of complexity manifests itself in locative structures, while many philosophers in the 4E tradition substantiate this notion in step with their research agendas, coming up with such influential notions as, for example, participatory sense-making (De Jaegher & Di Paolo 2007).

This scaling-up of complexity applies not only to the realms in which the systems operate, it also applies to the systems themselves. I therefore understand the relation between the concept of autopoietic system and the concept of autonomous system somewhat similarly to the relation between the concept of computational system and the concept of representational system. The latter is a specification of the former, namely it consists of computational mechanisms working on representations, thus on symbols *standing for entities external to the system*. It is believed that virtually all real-world, biological computational machines are representational, and yet the concept of computation is more general in the sense that it *does not have to* take anything that *actually stands for something external* as its input. Here it might be said that autopoiesis provides the most general characterization of what a living creature is as a complex network of processes, but insofar as complex real-world organisms (especially animals) are concerned, they, in a sense, do more than that, and their internal processes are tied in a non-incidental manner to their *actions*. The concept of autonomous system, therefore, captures these real-world exemplifications of autopoietic systems whose functioning is constituted by active interactions – by doing things in the shared world.

This key interactional or agential aspect attributable to autonomous systems is captured by another notion which is fundamental to the 4E movement, namely the concept of structural coupling. I propose (see also Werner & Kiełkowicz-Werner 2022) that an autonomous system is *structurally coupled* with its surroundings if the system selects and sometimes also transforms some segments of its surrounding, which includes other autonomous systems. These entities are exploited by the system in the process of maintaining its autonomy. Further on, the selected and/or transformed entities determine future states of the system. This means that structural coupling is not a linear process, but rather a looped co-determination of the autonomous system and its surroundings (see Varela et al. 1991, p. 150).

Metaphorically put, structural coupling means that a living creature "establishes a *perspective on the world* with its own normativity" (Di Paolo et al. 2010, p. 39). This is usually referred to as *sense-making*, i.e., making the world relevant to the system's capacities and needs.

Cummins and De Jesus are more concrete in their characterization. Namely, if we think of two systems – they write – O and M, and,

> for example, in the process of phylogenesis, O were to acquire the capacity to make a novel discrimination, for example, detecting a specific chemical, this will necessarily lead to a congruent change in the structure of M. O and M are said to be structurally coupled.
>
> (Cummins & De Jesus, 2016, p. 7)

Crucially, structural coupling is not a definitional quality of autopoiesis alone. For it is in principle an *externally* oriented feature. The concept, therefore, captures the next step in the evolution of complexity. Grounded in the structures that build up the autonomous system as a creature capable of action, thus of active interactions with other systems and a broader set of things, here we have emerging *structures of active interactions* – certain *paths* and also *patterns* of interactions.

So, it seems that according to 4E, environments arise on the basis of shared phenomenological domains, as Maturana and Varela (1980) called it, as next steps in the evolution of complex and thus somehow *organized* interactions; that they are more complex spaces which, crucially, include more complex *autonomous* systems, and also a variety of other things. Going back to Lewontin's (2000) remark, even if evaporation and volcanic ashes are not environments, they *do* contribute to the creation of environments; they are material that goes into the making of environments. In simple terms, we can provisionally characterize an environment as a shared domain of the interactions of various autonomous systems together with *selected* fragments of the underlying physical medium in which they operate.

All that being said, there is a gap in the conceptual backbones of 4E, I'd say, between the level of autopoietic systems and their first, as if reluctant and superficial interactions on the one side, and the level of full-blown shared environments on the other. This is because we would need some additional concepts to grasp structural coupling and sense making *not* as *already existing* pursuits, but *how they came about* in the first place. For suddenly we are informed that autonomous systems have their normativity, their own perspective; that they distinguish things in their surroundings from that specific perspective, etc., which suggests a highly complex structure of locative relations, with the autonomous system clearly playing the role of the point of reference with respect to a rich variety of entities. All this does not apply to the autopoietic system. Yet, we learn nothing about *how the system managed to become the point of reference* as we look through the conceptual roots of 4E, and we learn nothing about how its interactive partners, so to speak, are singled out – *how the relevant boundaries are drawn* and how the relevant locative relationships are set up.

To fill the gap, I propose, we need to give a real job to the concept of cognition (as flagged in the closing remarks of 4.2). It turns out that cognition is responsible for an environment's stepwise coming into being on the basis of systems' interactions – for its *enactment*, as Varela et al. (1991) call it. I will articulate this fundamental idea in terms of *cognitive niche construction* which, rolled out in Chapter 7, constitutes the crux of this book.

Needless to say, I will be focusing on cognition as a factor that brings something new to the *locative* architecture of environments, obviously without any pretense to provide a full theory of cognition (which is predominantly an empirical business). As emphasized at the very beginning, this is *a locative-ontological study of cognition*, which is by no means supposed to transgress its proper limits.

To sum up this part, 4E is *at least potentially* more serious about the environment in the sense that, first, it aims at understanding *how environments as such emerge* instead of taking them for granted. Second, it develops the initial core notion of the autopoietic system and defines a more general and complex concept of a system whose functioning is constituted by active interactions in this emerged environment. The latter posit is spelled out in terms of autonomous systems and their structural coupling. In effect, the "seriousness" here boils down to the fact that an environment attributable to a given system is not just a locus where the system *happens to be placed*, as if "parachuted" there, to use Varela's et al. (1991) figure of speech; instead, it is a locus that *emerges in step with the system's capacities, needs and actions*, while at the same time contributing to the emergence of the system itself. This means a loopy relation of *system–environment* co-constitution or co-determination.

4.5 Becoming serious about experience: 4E's phenomenological roots

Varela, Thompson and Rosch (1991) begin their groundbreaking book by invoking what they call *fundamental circularity*.

> A phenomenologically inclined cognitive scientist reflecting on the origins of cognition might reason thus: Minds awaken in a world. (...) We reflect on a world that is not made, but found, and yet it is also our structure that enables us to reflect upon this world. Thus in reflection we find ourselves in a circle: we are in a world that seems to be there before reflection begins, but that world is not separate from us.
>
> (Varela et al. 1991: 3)

They say that we find ourselves in the world which is not of our making, and yet at the same time this world manifests itself to us in a specific way – a way that does in some manner depend on our cognitive apparatus and thus, in a sense, fits our cognitive measure. This recognition situates 4E as a paradigm that cannot ignore *experience*. One might be tempted to say *subjective* experience, but this would situate us in the tradition that sees the subjective and the objective as opposites, which is not something that 4E endorses.

By referring to experience, 4E stresses the fact that the reality under our feet always manifests itself to us a certain way; that it is *a presentation* (Noë 2012 talks of *presence* in this context, but I take it to be a different conceptualization of the same phenomenon).

That being said, at least two points need to be stressed. First, the environment in which the autonomous system is located and with which it is structurally coupled not only provides meaningful perturbations, i.e., perturbations that the system can use to act successfully and maintain its integrity. In addition, the environment also *shows up* in a certain manner; it has a layout that fits the cognitive capacities of the system. Therefore, it must be possible for roughly the same segment of the assumed physical surroundings not only to constitute various system-specific environments in the sense provisionally spelled out earlier, thus system-specific patterns of interactions or structural coupling, but also to manifest itself in the form of system-specific presentations. So, we end up with the genuinely metaphysical question of why and how it is the case that anything presents itself in the first place. *Why there presents something rather than nothing*, one might ask in Leibnizian fashion (see Werner 2022).

Second, it is also important to realize that these presentations, whatever makes them possible, are all that we have access to; that this is what cognition always begins from and makes use of, even the most abstract and technically advanced scientific models. For what these models strive to explain is *this* world around us, thus *a* certain presentation. So while Sellars (1956) famously distinguished the manifest image of the world from the scientific image, 4E opposes the distinction, at least insofar as the latter is considered to be free of all the limitations of the former. Reality *as we cognize it*, thus the manifest image, constitutes the explanandum of any scientific endeavor, and at the end of the day all the "devices" that science makes use of – its concepts, formal models, empirical verification methods, and various other tools – are also produced within the boundaries of the manifest image, making this manifest world intelligible. As Ludwig Wittgenstein put it in his unique enigmatic style, (*Tractatus*, 5.621) "[t]he world and life are one" and (*Tractatus* 5.63) "I am my world. (The microcosm.)" (Wittgenstein 1922/1999: 89).

Maurice Merleau-Ponty is also clear at this point, writing that the world

> is inseparable from the subject, but from a subject which is nothing but a project of the world, and the subject is inseparable from the world, but from a world which the subject itself projects. The subject is a being-in-the-world.
>
> (Merleau-Ponty 1962/2005: 499–500)

Given the significance of the fundamental circularity, in addition to its "seriousness" about embodiment and environment 4E is arguably also more "serious" than representationalism about *experience*. And yet, this again brings up the issue of internalism and whether or not 4E succumbs to what it was supposed to oppose, namely the *internal vs. external* dichotomy. I have been trying to explain how the distinction itself is born *of* the autonomous system's self-maintenance and interactions, and therefore cannot be used *a priori* as an interpretative tool, and now the same needs to be demonstrated with regard to experience. As before, there is a certain locative dynamic underlying experience, having to do with how autonomous systems manage and establish specific loci. Unfortunately, 4E has not developed sufficient locative vocabulary to articulate the specificity of these experienced or experiential loci. As before, I shall unpack the topic provisionally, referring the reader to further chapters for a more technical treatment.

At the beginning of the 20th century, two scholars in particular attempted to examine and formulate a precise description of this presentational aspect of what we usually simply consider *the* world. I am thinking of Edmund Husserl and Jakob von Uexküll. The 4E movement draws on both of them – on Husserl via Merleau-Ponty (especially Varela) and Gibson (especially Chemero), and on von Uexkull, less often but more directly (see Feiten 2020, for example).

Beginning with Husserl, the accusation of internalism directed at 4E stems from the hundred-year-old controversy over whether the project of so-called phenomenological reduction, which is the cornerstone of Husserl's method of analysis, should be seen as an inward-directed move.

Phenomenological reduction is a form of "intellectual gymnastics," as Chemero (2009) might say, whose aim is to take in the whole variety of phenomena that we are faced with solely *qua phenomena*, thus only as something *given to the conscious mind* and therefore without any assumption as to whether it refers to or stands for something "real," "external," "objective," etc. In other words, the first step is to recognize that the manifest world we are dealing with *is* a manifestation or presentation. Then, in the second step, phenomenological reduction consists in the decision to consider this manifestation or presentation exactly as it manifests itself, thus *solely qua presentation*, without any presumption as to what is it a presentation *of* and what kind of relation occurs between it and what it presents.

I abstain from any judgment as to whether or not phenomenological reduction can succeed in its task, and whether the contents it yields are indeed what should be philosophically analyzed. The only thing I am concerned with now is the locative dynamic behind this "intellectual gymnastics." Is it actually, as the familiar accusation has it, a radical *inward* move in the sense that what we are supposedly advised to do by Husserl is to fathom our inner self. Or perhaps we should follow Dan Zahavi (2003) who argues that to perform the reduction "is not to abstain from an investigation of the real world in order to focus on mental content and representations, as it has occasionally been claimed (…)"; it does not involve "an exclusive turn toward inwardness," and therefore does not "imply any loss. On the contrary, the fundamental change of attitude makes possible a decisive discovery and should consequently be understood as an *expansion* of our field of research." Zahavi points out that Husserl compares phenomenological reduction with "the transition from a two-dimensional to a three-dimensional life" so that "the perpetually functioning, but so far hidden, transcendental subjectivity is disclosed as the subjective condition of possibility for manifestation" (Zahavi 2003: 46).[1]

I follow Zahavi's reading. Phenomenological reduction is *not* about going *inside* the mind. On the contrary, recognizing the familiar world *as* something given to consciousness could be read the other way around, thus as, in a sense, an *outward* move or – which seems a much better conceptualization given that the *internal versus external* division is not in operation, not even established at this level of analysis – as an *extension* of the boundaries of the self. This results from discovering that "I am my world," as Wittgenstein (1922) emphatically put it.

Let me stress that insofar as this expansion of the boundaries of the self encompasses the entire realm of phenomena, thus the whole world that we have access to, the very distinction between internal and external becomes inadequate and needs to be established first, before it can play any role. This is because at the level of phenomenological reduction there is nothing that we can refer to as external, thus as not belonging to the presentation, which in effect makes the locution "internal" redundant, too (which was also true for the autopoietic system, as we saw above in 4.4, yet in a different context).

This is the crux of Husserl's proposal, followed at least by the autopoietic current within 4E. What Husserl aims at is an *in principle a recategorization* of the mind-world relation, to the effect that the Cartesian internal–external scaffolding is no longer the most fundamental ontological distinction determining our thinking about cognition.

Merleau-Ponty comes up with a similar idea and articulates it in a way that explicitly refers to perception as a factor constituting a special *locus*. First, he criticizes empiricism for sharply distinguishing "the physical and chemical properties of the stimuli" (Merleau-Ponty 1962/2005: 28) from subjective "projections." Second, he proposes that if "we admit that all these 'projections', all these 'associations'" (Merleau-Ponty 1962/2005) that empiricism postulates are "based on some intrinsic characteristic" of the perceived object, then "the 'human world' ceases to be a metaphor and becomes once more what it really is, the seat and as it were the *homeland* of our thoughts" (Merleau-Ponty 1962/2005). In this "human world" as a "homeland" perception and action are "ways of positing an object (…)" (Merleau-Ponty 1962/2005).

Therefore, insofar as 4E follows Husserl and Merleau-Ponty, experience is taken there as something *beyond the internal–external dichotomy*. But – crucially – this does not mean abandoning locative conceptualizations.

Note that the conscious mind, which is no longer thought of as a container cut off from its surroundings but rather as something expanding its boundaries into the surroundings, should be seen here as *a frame* or a system of frames imposed on things that the Cartesian paradigm considers external.

The *frame metaphor* is one of the central posits I shall draw on (see Chapter 7). Note that a frame obviously does not produce the framed thing, and yet it does do something with the thing framed – it somehow conditions the thing's accessibility, just like frames imposed on paintings: their goal is to expose the painting hanging on the wall, as if delivering it to the viewer. In due course I shall provide a more technical characterization.

To sum up this part, it turns out that spilling more ink on phenomenology, something that might have been regarded as a detour in this locative ontological study, has elicited one of the key ideas to be developed further on – the idea of cognition as expanding the boundaries of the self, as framing, which is a genuine locative notion. Therefore, *being more serious about experience* means not just the mere acknowledgment that experience should somehow be accounted for, since this is a claim that representationalism also makes and, admittedly, struggles with (see Chalmers 1996 and the whole debate on qualia). Instead, it is a more profound acknowledgment that analyzing experience, just as in the case of seriousness about embodiment and environment, invites us to reconsider the most fundamental building blocks of our conceptual framework for capturing cognition, the mind, the mind-world relation, and *the specific locus* – the main target of this book – where this relationship is set up.

4.6 The experienced Umwelt

Now I shall add something to this rendering of 4E by referring to von Uexküll. Clearly, the locative underpinning of the concept of Umwelt is even more explicit, so that we do not have to interpret it in terms of location – it is already there: a particular Umwelt is clearly a specific locus. According to von Uexküll, the Umwelt is like a bubble surrounding the organism, thus something the organism is *in*. We read:

> All that a subject perceives becomes his perceptual world and all that he does, his effector world. Perceptual and effector worlds together form a closed unit, the Umwelt.
>
> (von Uexküll 1934/2010, p. 6)

The only controversy here is whether the Umwelt should be interpreted as a domain of experience, which would link the locative aspect of 4E to the phenomenological aspect as sort of a summary of all our considerations in this chapter.

Feiten (2020) distinguishes two readings of Umwelt. According to the first, an Umwelt is "that subset of physical properties which are accessible to the perception and action of an organism based on its physiology." Therefore, it is to be understood as a realm defined solely in terms of physiological-behavioral loops. If so, "subjective experience is lost," Feiten writes, "and the specific physiological makeup of a single organism is still fully within the scope of a purely external, quantitative description" (Feiten 2020: 3). Meanwhile, following inter alia Thompson (2007), Feiten strongly aligns with what he dubs the phenomenological reading, according to which "the Umwelt refers to the phenomenal world which an individual organism constructs for itself (...) (Feiten 2020: 2)." As such, it "constitutes the sum total of the subject's experience" (Feiten 2020). However, the process of Umwelt creation is not conscious, and because of that "the meaningful objects and the space in which we encounter them appear to us as objective reality" (Feiten 2020).

Two things stand out here. First, we are told that Umwelten are actually constructed by organisms. This is of paramount significance, since cognition is here portrayed explicitly as a *productive* endeavor. It brings forth something new in the world, and this groundbreaking idea developed by von Uexküll would become central for Varela et al. (1991) under the term "enactment" (see also Rolla & Figueiredo 2023).

Second, Feiten says that the Umwelt consists of experiences which constitute a specific *locus*. This is especially important for us here. We read that "the subject span open the spatial dimensions of its own experiential world, somewhat like opening an umbrella" (Feiten 2020: 3).

The umbrella metaphor is, indeed, very apt, for it covers two crucial aspects: as for the issue of the productivity of cognition, the creation of an Umwelt is portrayed as *expansion*, just like Husserl's specific outward movement; an expansion of the self, as described by Zahavi. But more than that: the closed umbrella is correctly referred to as an umbrella, although it does not perform the proper function assigned to it, which makes it, strictly speaking, a potential umbrella or a thing with the potency to serve as an umbrella. Therefore, if we metaphorize cognition regarded as Umwelt-creation in the same manner, it is like *actualizing a certain potential*, too. Finally, as for the locative aspect, opening the umbrella means occupying more space, which can be understood as setting up a certain new domain.

The only thing I am more skeptical about is Feiten's use of the objective–subjective distinction which traditionally mirrors the internal–external divide, thereby pushing the whole Umwelt terminology back to the Cartesian fixation on inwardness. But this is clearly in opposition to all the key aspects of von Uexküll's theory which Faiten so finely elicits. So, it seems more accurate to abandon the subjective–objective framework: von

Uexküll, just like Husserl, aimed at a conceptual architecture that is free of this dichotomy (whether they were successful, whether or not it is possible to abandon this architecture in the first place, remains a further question).

I propose that the Umwelt is not so much a bubble whose internal sphere is barred from the external realm, which would support the subjective–objective conceptualization, but rather that it is a frame imposed on the organism's physical surroundings; a frame making those surroundings accessible to cognition *in a specific way*, as if through a specific lens. Combining this way of thinking with Feiten's umbrella metaphor we end up with something like this: Imagine a device which opens up like an umbrella, but once opened, it rolls out a web, like a spider web, around you. In effect you see everything through this web which frames your access to the surrounding stuff, perhaps bringing some aspects of it to your attention, but it is still the same stuff that you are surrounded with, not some projection inside a bubble. So opening this web-like framing "umbrella" results in a modification of your location, but it does not actually move you from one physical locus to another. Moreover, it is an *actualization of potentials* – your potential for developing certain cognitive structures and a potential on the side of your surroundings to manifest themselves in specific manners.

Finally, this idea of *cognition as actualization* of a certain potential is quite clear in what I regard as the key thesis of autopoietic enactivism, namely the *enactment thesis* insisting that "cognition is not the representation of a pregiven world by a pregiven mind but is rather the enactment of the world and a mind on the basis of a history of the variety of actions that a being in the world performs" (Varela et al. 1991: 9).

4.7 Abandoning the bifurcation of realities: From Plato to 4E

Positioning 4E with respect to Cartesian cognitive science requires at least a brief analysis of the former's place in the broader philosophical landscape. We saw in Chapters 1 and 2 that computationalism and representationalism are grounded in serious philosophical debates on the nature of cognition going back as far as Plato. Some of the issues discussed there will, therefore, recur below, especially the idea of perfect knowledge and how Plato, Descartes or Kant approached it.

In this context the latest book by Johnson and Tucker (2021) stands out. The authors make an effort to go beyond ritual denouncements of Descartes and his dualism, and to place 4E (they do not use this label explicitly though) against a wider philosophical backdrop. The key thing is what they (following John Dewey) refer to as the "bifurcation" of reality in traditional philosophy, thus "the dualistic logic and corresponding ontology" (Johnson and Tucker 2021: 26), as a result of which reality is split into two separate segments: one populated with perceived, ever-changing material things, and one accommodating genuine beings which are eternal and intelligible, e.g., Plato's ideas. This split is mirrored by two kinds of knowledge: an inferior knowledge referring to the perceived and temporal domain, and a superior knowledge pertaining to eternal beings. Eventually, true knowledge

> must be of what is, of that which is for all time, in all places, eternal and complete. Such knowledge (…) must be based on understanding the essences of things that make them what they are and govern their interactions in the world.
>
> (Johnson and Tucker 2021)

This ontology of bifurcation is most famously spelled out in Plato's allegory of the cave (*Republic* Book VII, 514a–520a). People chained inside the cave are only able to observe shadows on the wall – shadows cast by real objects outside. According to Plato, this illustrates our epistemic position. The manifest image of the world we are faced with turns out to be composed of mere projections of real beings. The metaphor suggests that while the shadows are flickering and flat, the actual beings must be more stable and more multidimensional, thus containing more information. Actually – according to Plato, as I interpret him – they are perfectly stable structures, independent of time, contain all the information existing in the universe and are the referent of perfect knowledge.

Now, gaining perfect knowledge must mean being able to see these real objects, the ideal forms outside the cave. This indicates that knowledge itself is modeled as a kind of *seeing*, a purely intellectual vision, one might say. So, according to Johnson and Tucker, "Plato appropriates and extends the common conceptual metaphor KNOWING IS SEEING. Ideas are understood metaphorically as visible physical objects, (…) and the 'light of reason' shining on idea-objects is what makes knowledge possible" (Johnson and Tucker 2021: 28).

This understanding of knowledge stresses the idea of perfect epistemic reliance, thus the ideal of irrefutable belief that would lay the groundwork of science. This focus, built upon the Platonic ontology of bifurcation, comes to the fore in the origins of modern philosophy, according to Johnson and Tucker, in Descartes. He was bent on finding contents that cannot be doubted, and "psychologically, this amounts to transcending any anxiety that might arise from indeterminacy and ambiguity in experience. This is an impossible task because, as we will see, the anxiety of doubt is built into our deepest systems of motivational control" (Johnson and Tucker 2021: 35).

The key thing for Descartes was the capacity to grasp an idea in mind *clearly and distinctly*. Famously, he found the unshakable, undeniable basis in the *thinking* self, whose existence, due to the very fact of thinking, cannot be doubted: *the self* manifests itself clearly and distinctly once we engage in stepwise methodical analysis in the course of first-person meditation, when we discard anything that may be epistemically unreliable. This may even include mathematical truths which were initially the model of epistemic reliability for Descartes.

Finally, Johnson and Tucker also mention Kant, who – as I already pointed out following Allison (2006) –

> gives up the idea that we can know reality as it is in itself, and recognizes that we can only know things as they appear to us through the mediation of our perceptual organs and the organizing conceptual patterns and processes of our minds.
>
> (Allison 2006: 39)

Kant's main idea was that "our world manifests knowable category relations because such relations are imposed by human understanding as conditions for experience of any object" (Allison 2006: 40). This means, that "we can know our world precisely because we had a hand in constructing it" (Allison 2006). Therefore, Kant made a major step away from the ideal of perfect knowledge and what this knowledge is about. First, we are in no position to know reality as it is independently of our cognitive pursuits; we can only know the "shadows." Second, the conditions of intelligibility are not defined by ideal forms placed in a realm apart from the manifest world; instead, they are our own creations.

And yet "our own" does not refer to empirical subjects, to *living* creatures as they are, with all their cognitive and volitional factors intermingled. The subject here is transcendental in the sense that it is a theoretical fiction capturing *subjectivity as such*, the conditions of possibility of any cognitive pursuit. Hence, in his approach Kant was still, according to Johnson and Tucker, a devout proponent of intellectualism.

Therefore, Kant is a pivotal figure in pulling our pursuit of knowledge away from the fixation on a universe of ideal objects, but at the same time – Johnson and Tucker underscore – his emphasis on the subject lines up with Descartes' theoretical ego-centricity. Therefore, Kant denied the Platonic "bifurcation" of reality and fully acknowledged the *manifest realm* as the only knowable domain, but at the same time he came up with his own transcendental bifurcation. For we end up with his peculiar reference to the noumenal world which is not knowable but somehow referred to. Moreover, Kant also, in his idiosyncratic manner, upholds the Cartesian bifurcation by stressing the difference between what is accessible to the self and what is barred from the self. Here Johnson and Tucker rely on Rorty's (1979) reading and hold that

> Kant denied knowledge of things in themselves, but he secured the possibility of shared knowledge by regarding the outer world perceived by our senses as knowable just insofar as it was structured by concepts arising from the formal character of the inner world of thought.
>
> (Rorty 1979: 41–42)

Note the spatial language used in the latter quotation, which comes directly from Rorty, who articulates the idea in an even stronger manner by claiming that Kant puts "outer space inside inner space" (Rorty 1979: 137). I shall come back to this.

All that being said, if Johnson and Tucker were asked what 4E is fundamentally about, they might provide the following answer: It is essentially about getting rid of all kinds of traditional bifurcations of reality: there is a single dynamic, evolving world with creatures capable of cognition in it; creatures trying to deal with their surroundings not by means of any perfect knowledge, but rather by using necessarily imperfect, situation-dependent know-how.

Now, I am not going to argue against Johnson and Tucker's (2021) diagnosis. However, I propose to re-read their historical overview so as to recognize 4E not only as opposed to certain trends in traditional philosophy, but also as their continuation, especially given the issues discussed in Chapter 1 (see Werner 2023). This is in connection with the question of the world's intelligibility and the recognition that qua cognizers we are not only doers but also understanders who sometimes seek a "safe refuge" from our worldly engagements so that we can "slacken" the intentional bonds with our surroundings in order to reflect on them.

In contrast to Johnson and Tucker I propose that the most important thing about Plato's allegory of the cave is the recognition of the fact that the world we are familiar with, the everyday world which as a whole may not even pose an intellectual challenge, *is* – precisely *as a whole* – a certain manifestation or presentation. This is by no means an obvious thing to problematize. Borrowing two terms from Husserl, we may say that our "natural attitude" to things takes them for granted, meanwhile "bracketing" this natural attitude sees them as somehow *related to us* (for more on this specific recognition see Werner 2022b).

Note that this is exactly what Varela, Thompson and Rosch do when they speak of fundamental circularity. We are, they say, "awaken in a world" that is "not made, but found" but at the same time "it is also our structure that enables us to reflect upon this world" (Varela et al. 1991: 3).

Therefore, aside from what Plato did with this fundamental recognition and what consequences he derived from it, there is, I claim, one fundamental continuity between the Platonic allegory and 4E, mediated especially by phenomenology. Namely, a completely new and all-encompassing look at the surrounding world which functions as the background for *all* the reflection that comes next.

Crucially for us here, note that Plato's model of the manifest world and of our epistemic position in it is articulated in explicitly locative terms, and in this respect it anticipates von Uexküll's notion of Umwelt. In both cases the point is not only that what we are acquainted with *is* a certain cluster of presentations; the claim goes further: this cluster of presentations *constitutes a certain place*, a certain specific *locus* for us. Von Uexküll imagines it as a bubble around an organism in which the organism is in some sense locked up. The cave-dwellers portrayed by Plato also do not merely *happen* to be located in a specific setting; instead, their epistemic position is constituted by the location they are in. In other words, their situation *qua cognizers* is defined not only by what they perceive, but *where they are*, and *because* they are contained in a specific way, they perceive reality thus and so.

The cave-dwellers' position is *constituted* by the fact that they are *in a particular environment* (not one that Plato would praise, advocating for their escape, but that is a different issue). Hence, the cave-dwellers, however strange it may sound, are coupled with this environment even though Plato was not very generous when it comes to granting them opportunities for action (at the end of the day they are still chained).

Plato's model is hardly in the enactivist/embodied spirit – a member of 4E might fret – but, interestingly, it reveals certain 4E-friendly aspects if, with the benefit of hindsight, we compare it with what would happen around the 17th and 18th centuries (see Werner 2023). For there comes Descartes who, via Augustine, still works within the (Neo)Platonic model, making a sharp distinction between what manifests itself in cognition and an assumed genuine reality. And yet the locative setup he brings is radically different. According to his account, our epistemic position is not determined by the fact that *we* are *placed* thus and so, e.g., in a cave, in an Umwelt-like bubble, chained inside or free to move around and explore, but instead by the fact that we have our inner self *in us* and *there* we find flickering "shadows" made of percepts. While in Plato we had a mind located in a cave, beginning with Descartes we have a cave located in the mind, which Dennett (1991) aptly called the "Cartesian theater" – a theater, like a cave, but a theater *in us*, not a theater *we are in*. The difference, therefore, is rather dramatic and, surprisingly, Plato's locative model turns out to be much more in line with 4E.

That being said, Descartes is definitely not a hero for 4E. However, there is a different aspect of the founding father of modern philosophy – hardly a surprising one, although frequently overlooked. I am thinking of Descartes' decision to consider the first-person meditational stance as a source of valuable epistemic insight. His seriousness about experience, by no means obvious nowadays within Cartesian cognitive science, is, all things considered, very much in the spirit of Varela.

Noteworthily, Descartes was not only the first thinker to take the subjective perspective seriously, perhaps with the exception of his direct inspiration, Augustine, but he took this route in a historical context in which an inward move might have seemed the least likely to provide any valuable insight, i.e., in the context of Galileo's third-person ideal of mathematics-based science. And yet Descartes, a mathematician himself, decided to adopt the meditative stance where he found it to be the appropriate method. Isn't this akin to 4E's phenomenological commitment to experience? For Varela and his followers, it is of paramount significance that experience not be treated as an inferior source, a repository of folk psychology, something epiphenomenal and reducible. Therefore, in this particular respect, at least the Varelian tradition within 4E is a continuation of the meditative tradition championed by Descartes (given rise by Augustine). The continuity is even more striking when we consider that Descartes does not prioritize the first-person stance, but that his endorsement of the third-person, scientific standpoint is also unequivocal. This leads to a combination that is by no means frequent, and yet it is just like the one endorsed by Varela: the third-person and the first-person must collaborate in the proper study of mind (see e.g., Varela's 1996 neurophenomenology project).

Clearly, Descartes' conception of cognition has different locative commitments than 4E and Plato. I am referring to Descartes' idea of a cave/theater in the mind and not the mind in a cave. But take into consideration the following thought experiment: what if we take Descartes' meditative method and his endorsement of the first-person perspective but abandon his locative commitments and "transplant" his focus on experience to Plato's cave allegory? It would obviously be something different from Descartes' original proposal, but also something different from what Plato wanted to say. For Plato did not have the notion of subjective experience, grounded in the idea of an inner self owed to Augustine. On the other hand, as already stressed earlier, Descartes did not have the notion of environment, and was therefore, in a sense, destined by the scientific *Zeitgeist* of his time to draw a sharp line between the objective and the subjective.

Combining the Platonic recognition of the peculiar "environmental" plug-in of cognition with Descartes' first-person focus on experience brings us to the idea, perhaps only a hint of an idea, that experiences are not planted *in our heads*, but rather that we are placed *in the realm which experiences* somehow contribute to. This is a completely different locative setup. Instead of being locked up in the head, experience turns out to be constitutive of the specific *locus* in which a creature capable of cognition *is located*. This would be very much in the spirit of 4E.

The question is, what kind of location are we talking about? What kind of locus is constituted by subjects engaged in experiencing their surroundings? If it is not the "Cartesian theater" in the head, nor the "objective" realm of evaporation and volcanic eruptions, to cite Lewontin (2000), the puzzle becomes quite intricate. I shall develop an ontology of the cognitive niche to answer this conundrum.

4.8 Conclusion

After having dug into the locative commitments of the Cartesian tradition, this chapter finally yields a more detailed (yet, of course, hardly exhaustive), articulation of what makes the 4E a considerable alternative.

First and most importantly, 4E takes cognition not only as something that a living creature *does*; instead, cognition belongs to the very fabric of what the creature *is* as an autopoietic/autonomous system capable of maintaining its integrity, defining its own "space" of realization, and creating a shared locus in collaboration with other systems, where they impact in an open-ended process the autopoietic processes of one another.

Moreover, an autopoietic/autonomous system does not just happen to be placed here or there; instead, the system is structurally coupled with its surroundings, thereby bringing forth a certain system-specific environment. Therefore, the system and its environment co-determine each other.

Finally, given structural coupling, experience is not just an epiphenomenal addition to the system's dealings with its environment; instead, experience is a medium through which the surroundings are brought forth and serve *as an environment*. The environment presents itself always *qua experienced* thus and so.

The chapter also discussed the relationship between 4E and a broader philosophical tradition, which would merit a research project in its own right. In short, the usual villains in the eyes of 4E such as Plato or Descartes exhibit some 4E-friendly aspects, e.g., Plato's emphasis on his own specific understanding of the environmental plug-in (the cave allegory) or Descartes' devotion to experience, while their "flaws," for lack of a better term, require a historically sensitive re-reading.

The latter goes back to certain themes from Chapters 1 and 2 and is especially interesting if we realize how consequential a fact it was that neither Plato nor Descartes had the concepts of environment and ecological location at their disposal. Therefore, the author of *Meditations on First Philosophy* was unable to solve the problem of how the realm of extended substances, measurable in "objective" mathematical terms, fits together with the realm of cogitations or cognizable entities, measurable in terms of, for example, intensity (of an impression), clarity and distinctness (of a thought), certainty (of a belief), etc. Introducing a conceptual framework organized around the concepts of environment, structural coupling and embodiment, all tied to one another, opens the door for a major paradigm shift, which is what the 4E preachers hope for, but also for a shift grounded in the philosophical tradition.

Taking all this together, we end up with the loose but crucial idea of cognition as an endeavor that not only adds to the functioning of a system but actually makes the system what it is. And of cognition that not only mirrors external objects, but *actualizes some potential in them*, brings them from one state to another. Both of these productive functions have a key locative dimension: cognition, as part of a broader set of processes of maintaining the system's autonomy, of structural coupling, and of experiencing, brings forth a specific locus – a unique locative footprint of the cognitive system and a unique locative mark of its functioning.

The key question we are faced with now problematizes *the specific kind of locus constituted by cognitive systems* engaged in structural coupling with their environments, experiencing them, and thereby enacting them. I will define this locus further on in terms of the cognitive niche.

Note

1 Strictly speaking Zahavi refers to Husserl's description of the performance of *epoche*, which is not identical to phenomenological reduction but part of it.

5 The Cognitive Niche

A Primer

This chapter addresses the ontological specificity of environments *as loci*. Here and there some of their features have already entered the picture, especially the fact that they gravitate around points of reference occupied by living creatures. They *surround* the living creature thought of as their "center of activity," to use De Jaegher and Di Paolo's (2007) phrase, and thus are not mere spaces where entities simply lie scattered. This "centeredness" now needs to be unpacked in greater detail, especially when it comes to the cognitive functioning of living creatures. I will argue that cognition defines its own "centeredness," i.e., a cognition-specific locative architecture, which means a cognition-specific environment. Its proper elicitation I take as a necessary condition to put the paradigm of ecological cognition on solid conceptual footing.

Environments are ontologically peculiar, since on the one hand they are *out there*, so to speak, thus they are *real* in the sense of not being subjective projections of the Cartesian subject, while at the same time they remain somehow *relative to* their inhabitants, as if "cut out" to fit their specific measure(s). This means that environments have a special mode of being, defined by locative relations occurring inside them, and this shall be my main concern later on. This chapter, therefore, inaugurates a more systematic study of specific loci suitable *for* cognition and determined *by* cognition. Since this sounds quite lofty as a declaration, it must be stressed that – as in previous chapters – the ambition behind these considerations is strictly limited to providing a general theory of cognition-specific or cognition-determined location (locative ontology), leaving the empirical sciences of cognition to do their job.

The key term I shall exploit is "niche," whereas "environment" shall be reserved for bigger clusters of niches. While it makes little sense to speak of the environment of a single organism, it makes perfect sense to speak of the niche (token niche) of a particular mouse, hawk, bear, beaver or human. Therefore, the aim now is to make the first step toward an abstract ontological study of niches and their tenants, with a special focus on so-called

DOI: 10.4324/9781003580997-5

cognitive niches. This specific realm, the cognitive niche, is supposed to serve as both the domain of behavior, thus active structural coupling, as well as a "safe refuge" for reflection and understanding, as I metaphorically put it in Chapter 1.

5.1 Introducing niches and their ontological specificity

A niche can be first characterized as a volume of space occupied by a living creature. The intuitive examples that come to mind are a bear's cave or a worm's cavity. However, the identification of a niche needs to consider not only *places* but also the *conditions* to be satisfied if a creature is to thrive there, or the relations obtaining between the organism and its surroundings (see Grinnell 1917; Elton 1927). Lewontin points out that "*ecological niche* is a technical term universally used to denote the complex of relationships between a particular species and the outside world" (Lewontin 2000: p. 44; see also Lewontin 1983; Laland et al. 1999).

The focus on conditions rather than places has been championed especially by G. Evelyn Hutchinson (1957). He proposed that if we take into account any two "ecological factors" x_1, x_2 relevant to a given organism *o*, e.g., temperature and the amount of water, then measure them along the standard Cartesian coordinates, and finally define some limit values for these factors, we obtain a delineated "space" within a system of coordinates. This "space" is an abstract characterization of the niche – or at least of a part of it – required by *o*. Now, if we take all ecological factors $x_1,\ldots, x_n$ that are relevant to *o*, thereby adding new dimensions to the system of coordinates, completing this job would mean that an "*n*-dimensional hypervolume is defined, every point in which corresponds to a state of the environment" (Hutchinson 1957: 416) which permits *o* to exist. This *hypervolume* Hutchinson calls the fundamental niche of *o*.

Smith and Varzi (1999) come up with a useful distinction: a niche *token* is a fragment of the real world, an actual place. On the other hand, a niche *type* is not individuated by its address but by certain abstract features spelled out in terms of Hutchinsonian conditions. These two characterizations are complementary: if a niche type is to be realized, it must be realized somewhere, thus by some niche token.

Due to the above-mentioned correspondence between niche tokens and niche types, a suitable *ontological* enterprise can be characterized as a study of the most general conditions characterizing niches *qua beings* of a specific type, which means studying very abstract niche types. Therefore, there is no clash between what biologists or scientists from other disciplines are doing and what a philosopher aims at, insofar as the former concentrate on niche tokens and relatively concrete conditions defining these tokens (thus actual habitats), while philosophers concentrate on *the most abstract* conditions, yet remain informed by empirical findings. In this spirit, what I am about to roll out is a certain empirically informed ontology of the cognitive niche; in fact, of the process of constructing a cognitive niche.

Speaking of the latter, the phrase "niches as beings," which specifies the target of an ontological study, might suggest a rather static picture in which we are interested only in the final product and ignore the fact that niches are the result of a constructive effort undertaken by living creatures. These creatures are capable of changing their position in the world and transforming parts of their physical surroundings. Birds building nests and mouses digging cavities are intuitive examples. Now, one might claim that the pursuit of *niche construction* is ontologically irrelevant, and the only thing we should address here is what it means for a ready-made nest to serve as a bird-specific locus, thus niche as a product. This would not be right, I believe. In doing so, we would neglect the dynamic development of niche construction theories that has taken place in recent years.

Niche construction is defined as "the process whereby organisms actively modify their own and each other's evolutionary niches" (Laland et al. 2016: 192; see also Lewontin 1983; Odling-Smee 1988, 2024; Odling-Smee et al. 2003). Based on the latter, here is the initial ontological presupposition underlying this study: Each niche is *a product* of specific *acts* of niche construction.

Here I adopt Twardowski's (1912/1999) classic distinction between *acts* and *products* in its ontological rendering. This means that our most general inventory of *what is* includes acts as irreducible ingredients of the domain, and that what comes into being as a result of an act is not reducible to the latter.

This has consequences which are going to inform how I plan to proceed. Smith and Varzi (1999) introduce the relation "x is a niche for y" as a primitive notion. Then, as is usually the case in formal ontological theories, they unpack this primitive relation by means of an assortment of axioms. Meanwhile, assuming that a niche is a product of niche construction, I take a different route. What I am about to provide is quite unusual in the ontological literature, for it is an ontological "representation" or "simulation" of the *evolution* of niche *construction*, singling out several pivotal points in the process, beginning with niches determined by a relatively simple setup of locative relations, through more and more complex ones, up to cognitive niches which have, as we shall see, an intricate and unique locative architecture.

The distinction between niche *construction* and niches *as products* contributes to the fact, nicely elicited by Smith (2001), that from the ontological point of view, ecological phenomena in general are rather messy.

This is because to get a sense of what they are *qua beings* we need to take into account different kinds of objects, relations, processes, actions, boundaries, etc. This means that constructing an ontological account of ecological phenomena requires a bold step into an extremely rich universe without Occam's razor, thus without any presumed strategy of reduction.

That said, Smith rightly emphasizes that when

> modern-day philosophers turn their attention to ontology they begin not with Aristotle but rather, in almost every case, with a set-theoretic ontology of the sort which is employed in standard model-theoretic semantics. Set-theoretic ontology sees the world in atomistic terms: it postulates a lowest level of atoms or urelements, from which successively higher levels of set-theoretic objects are then constructed.
>
> (Smith 2001: 79)

Meanwhile, taking the Aristotelian approach, as argued for by Smith, means that when setting off on an abstract conceptual analysis we should instead start from the mesoscopic objects we know from our everyday surroundings and *take them for what they are*, instead of reducing them upfront to something simpler. This includes living creatures and their habitats.

I do not want to insist on whether Smith's estimations as to how many philosophers take the atomistic set-theoretical route are correct (there is a project devoted to the ontology of everyday things by Thomasson 2007 or the naïve metaphysics of Fine 2017). The important point is that from the "atomist" perspective, what is of most interest to us here seems to be excluded from the picture, namely complex entities such as environments, organisms, systems capable of cognition, etc.

Part of the reason why some philosophers adopt the atomistic strategy, according to Smith, is their desire to follow science. The problem is, I would add, that these philosophers have a very peculiar sense of "science" in mind, with physics as their model. Meanwhile, disciplines such as, say, population ecology, geography or ethology are sciences too, and yet they *do* study the mesoscopic level known from familiar everyday experience. Therefore, a reference to "science" does not necessarily justify atomism, which is in fact a kind of preestablished reductionism. And while this "atomism" may not have been that surprising before Darwin and the vibrant development of the biological sciences in the 20th century, it may be somewhat more of a surprise and even a disappointment these days. As I already pointed out in the preceding chapters, it is no wonder that Descartes did not develop a more environmentally plugged-in concept of *res cogitans*, given that he could not have come up with the notion of environment. Moreover, the *Zeitgeist* of the 17th-century Galilean scientific revolution clearly favored ontological "atomism" – as Smith points out – and a sharp division into *internal* and *external* (see Husserl 1970 and Putnam 1987). However, insisting on such a "clear and distinct" worldview nowadays seems to be a non-starter.

Why is this relevant to the project undertaken in this book? Provided that Smith is right, some degree of hostility toward the traditional ontological discourse, which can be gleaned from the writings of some major proponents of 4E (e.g., Johnson & Tucker 2021), is partly justified on the part of those who consider 4E a major philosophical breakthrough. They simply do not see much utility in ontological considerations preoccupied with set-theoretical "atomism" and – I would add to that – various other presumptions tacitly made and rarely discussed, like the sharp *objective/external versus subjective/internal* distinction. Therefore, there is a need not only for greater openness on the part of 4E (and representationalism too, for this camp does rely on some traditional ontologies, although it rarely makes it an issue), but also for a certain reorientation of contemporary ontology, which would render it more self-aware of its preoccupations and possible alternatives.

Smith's diagnosis also applies, to some extent, to the locative ontology proposed by Casati and Varzi (1999). This is especially clear when they draw a distinction between integrated wholes and entities lacking the quality of wholeness. In their approach, we either have a thing whose solid integrity is granted by more or less homogenous matter, alternatively by some sort of "glue," or, at the other extreme, scattered parts maintaining no integrity at all, as in the case of a broken cup. The cup is either a unified whole or, once it becomes divided, it ceases to exist. Therefore, it seems that environments whose wholeness must be thought of differently cannot be taken into account. Methodologically this move is understandable – it is reasonable to start an ontological project from relatively simple cases and not complicate the initial picture too much. Here, however, we want to deal with ontologically peculiar ecological interactions, therefore, a different strategy of constructing an ontology is required.

Casati and Varzi (1999) are perfectly aware of the fact that their theory excludes more complex notions of wholeness or unity, such as functional, teleological and causal unities which seem to be exactly what constitutes *systems*, including the cases that interest us here, i.e., cognitive systems and their environments. Yet, Varzi's collaboration with Smith takes a different path around the same time, when they come up with a groundbreaking niche ontology in Smith and Varzi (1999).

Thus, building on Smith (2001), I propose that the first ontological characterization of *acts* of niche construction sees them as a subtype of a broader category of *physical-behavioral units* (a term borrowed by Smith from Robert Barker 1968). We read:

> The mesoscopic environment, the setting of our actions and perceptions, that into which, from moment to moment, we precisely fit, is not homogeneous. It is divided on a plurality of levels into natural units which may repeat themselves (may exist in many copies), from place to place and some of which may be such as to possess definite, salient boundaries of different sorts. Thus the mesoscopic environment is marked by the presence of substances of different sorts (buildings, rooms, walls, bricks, tables) standing in stable relations to each other. But this environment is marked also by the no less overwhelming presence of what Barker calls physical-behavioral units, recurrent types of settings, which serve as the environments for the everyday activities of persons and groups of persons. Examples are: my Friday afternoon class, Jim's meeting with the Dean, your Thursday lunch, the plumber's visit, Gloria's drive to work. Each of these is marked by certain stable arrays of physical objects and physical infrastructure, and by certain stable patterns of behavior on the part of the persons involved. Physical-behavioral units are in this sense two-sided. They are built out of both physical and behavioral parts.
>
> (Smith 2001: 79)

Physical-behavioral units are "transcategorial," thus composed of objects belonging to multiple ontological categories (objects, processes, events; material, mental, social, etc.). Moreover, in a physical-behavioral unit, the relation

> between participant and setting is to different degrees one of reciprocal co-determination. Each participant has two positions within the unit: first, he is a component which thus goes to form the unit; second, he is an individual whose behavior, and whose very nature, is itself partly formed by the unit of which he is at any given moment a part.
>
> (Smith 2001: 81)

Given this co-determination, we end up with a view that clearly goes against the Cartesian categorial dichotomy between that which is internal to the subject and that which is external. Arguably, what Smith writes about co-determination must sound appealing to the ears of any 4E advocate.

With all that in mind, I also follow Smith and Varzi (1999), who provide the following initial outline of the domain *produced* by acts of niche construction:

(i) An environmental niche takes up space, it occupies a physical-temporal locale, and is such as to have spatial parts. Within this physical-temporal locale is a privileged locus – a hole – into which the occupant of the niche fits exactly.
(ii) Environmental niches are unitary. A typical niche enjoys a certain natural completeness or rounded-offness, in contrast to its arbitrary undetached parts and to arbitrary heaps or aggregates of niches.
(iii) An environmental niche has an outer boundary: there are objects which fall clearly within it, and other objects which fall clearly outside it.
(iv) Environmental niches may have actual parts that are also environmental niches, and they may similarly be proper parts of larger, circumcluding environmental niches.
(v) An environmental niche is not simply a location in space; rather, it is a location in space that is constrained or marked by certain functional properties of temperature, foliage density, federal jurisdiction, etc.
(vi) An environmental niche may overlap spatially with other environmental niches with which it does not share common parts.

(Smith & Varzi 1999: 220–221)

This means that while a niche has a specific location, as (i) indicates, it is quite specific in terms of what belongs to it and what does not, and where it ends, which is what (ii) and (iii) state. This specificity is determined by the niche's function, according to (v), and this function may differ for different living creatures. This means that niches cannot be said to just be regions of space, which is what (vi) stresses. In other words, speaking of regions without mentioning functions misses the point. Finally, (iv) teaches us that niches are complex, thus some of them can be decomposed into smaller segments that are also niches. As already mentioned, here I take "niche" to refer to simple units, thus ones that are not composed of niches themselves, while "environment" captures more complex clusters thereof (this, however, is simply a terminological issue).

Going further, Smith and Varzi (1999) introduce another key distinction, that between *niche base* and *niche medium*. The latter refers to what is *actually* part of the niche from the perspective of its tenant, while the former is the physical stuff that the niche is made of, not all of which is part of the medium. This is likely similar to what Lewontin (2000) had in mind when he distinguished environments from the "physical conditions from which environments may be built," and when he stressed that "the actual process of evolution seems best captured by the process of construction" (Lewontin 2000: p. 48). These "physical conditions" refer to the niche base and what is constructed is the niche medium.

The concept of the niche base is assumed here as given. It can only be "defined" in the ostensive manner – the niche base is what you have under your feet, to put it in a somewhat simplistic manner.

Given the latter, I propose that the niche *medium* can be anything – substances as well as states of affairs, processes, etc. – that is *relevant* to the niche tenant. If the niche tenant is an autonomous system, relevance is determined by its conditions of autonomy. Therefore, assuming that the concept of autonomy is given, and that the umbrella term "condition" is also set, I propose that an entity is relevant to a niche tenant if it is necessary for it to maintain its autonomy.

Understood in this manner, "relevance" refers to tenant-specific conditions Hutchinson (1957) talked about. This abstract, "Hutchinsonian," approach makes room for different kinds of niches defined by *different sorts of relevant conditions*. This is not necessarily limited to strictly physicochemical, physiological or geographical factors, which are what a biologist would likely be most interested in. The relevant conditions include not only things such as temperature, food availability, humidity, shape of the terrain, but also factors referring, e.g., to social interactions, problem solving. In other words, by stressing the condition-relatedness and relevance of the niche (niche medium), Hutchinson, but also Smith and Varzi, in a sense create incentives to define conditions that transcend the biological domain, strictly defined, in the direction of social phenomena. In this spirit, niche construction theory also speaks of, e.g., cultural or narrative niches (Laland et al. 2001; Laland & O'Brien 2011; Kendal 2011; Heersmink 2020, de Carvalho & Krueger 2023; Coninx 2023), thereby rendering the concept of niche a tool of social science (for criticism, see e.g., Wallach 2016).

However, one might argue that what is missing *in-between* the biological and the social domains is a properly *cognitive* domain, and that we can conceptualize cognition in niche terms too, thus define conditions for a given living creature or niche tenant that *refer exclusively to its cognitive capacities*.

5.2 Toward cognitive niches

To get an initial sense of what is at stake (see Werner 2020), think of the following setting: suppose we have an organism *o* whose only sense is hearing and whose sense organ is sensitive to sound waves between 15 Hz and 20 kHz. Now, *o* is surrounded by *a*, *b*, *c*. Suppose that *a* is relevant to *o*'s metabolism, e.g., *a* is another organism that can be eaten by *o*, and *a*'s vibrations produce waves with a frequency of around 50 Hz; then suppose that *b* is irrelevant to *o*'s metabolism and the frequency of its vibration is 17 kHz; finally, *c* is also relevant, and it vibrates with a frequency of 70 kHz. If this is the case, *a* certainly belongs to the material base of *o*'s niche – it can be eaten, so it's clearly relevant, and moreover it can be heard, so getting *a* is a real option. However, with *b* and *c* things become more complicated. For it seems that *b* also belongs to the base of *o*'s niche insofar as it can be heard, despite the fact that it is metabolically irrelevant. On the other hand, *c* should also belong to the base of *o*'s niche, given that it is metabolically relevant, and yet we may have doubts due to the fact that *o* is incapable of perceiving *c*. We have here a problem with the proper delineation of which elements of the niche base, the material world around *o*, should be taken as parts of *o*'s niche medium and which should not. Cognition places large numbers of things in view, to put it in simple terms, a great many of which are not, or so it seems, relevant in any manner at least at a given moment. Time and circumstances can make a difference, however, for cognition also makes it possible, one might stress, to get in touch with something that may be of some use in the future, in a different context, etc. Therefore, it may seem reasonable to also include entities that afford potential opportunities, not necessarily only actual ones, in the niche medium. On the other hand, however, there is the risk of a kind of slingshot effect resulting in virtually everything that can be cognized entering the niche medium.

Here is a more real-life and very straightforward depiction (based on the one provided by Smith and Varzi 1999; here following Werner 2020). Suppose we have a bear, its cave, a bat living in the same cave, a snail suddenly getting into the cave, and finally the air filling the cave. The snail belongs to the base of the bear's niche as a "recognized" candidate for food, while the bat is likely "recognized" by the bear, too, but also completely irrelevant (bears don't eat bats, nor the other way around). The air, on the other hand, clearly belongs to the base of the bear's niche, as a necessary condition of the bear's metabolism, but most likely bears (unlike humans living in smoggy cities) do not "problematize" the presence of air; it is not cognized by them. This setting is simplified, as it neglects the fact that at the end of the day we don't know *what it is like* to be a bear, a snail, not to mention a bat, how these creatures perceive one another, and where the line dividing cognition from non-cognitive functioning actually lies. Nonetheless, this can at least give us some initial sense of how different the assortment of niche conditions can be, if the mentioned dividing line exists somewhere.

In this context, we may speak of a *cognitive* niche as a specific realm established *by* and *for* a specific organism's cognitive pursuits. A cognitive niche would be determined solely by conditions referring to the organism's cognitive capacities. In contrast, we could also speak of a niche determined solely by conditions referring to the organism's metabolic needs or, more broadly, to its maintenance of integrity and self-production – its autopoiesis. This distinction could clarify the picture just presented. Namely, while the snail belongs to the base of the bear's metabolism-related niche, for lack of a better term, as potential food, and it also belongs to the base of the bear's cognition-related niche, the bat belongs to the latter but not to the former (more on this distinction in Werner 2020). Finally, the air filling the two animals' shared apartment belongs to the former, but (usually) not the latter. Provisionally speaking, the term "cognitive niche" could therefore refer to all that a given organism is capable of getting "in touch" with by virtue of its cognitive apparatus.

The term "cognitive niche" is not new though. It was originally proposed in the late 1980s by John Tooby and Irven De Vore (1987) to do justice to the specificity of human cognition, and much later picked up by Steven Pinker (2003, 2010) and Andy Clark (2005, 2006, see also Bertolotti & Magnani 2017 for an overview, and Stotz 2010 or Sterelny 2007, 2012 for similar views). The core idea behind this original use is that humans have "the ability to create and maintain cause–effect models of the world as guides for prejudging which courses of action will lead to which results" (Tooby & De Vore 1987: 2010). Given the fact that

> there are an infinitely large number of possible sequences of behavior (…) 'behavioral flexibility' is an insufficient characterization of our innovative adaptive pattern. Our cognitive system is knowledge or information driven, and its models filter potential responses so that newly generated behavioral sequences are appropriate to bring about the desired end.
>
> (Tooby & De Vore 1987)

Andy Clark gives a different definition, according to which cognitive niche construction is defined as:

> … the process by which animals build physical structures that transform problem spaces in ways that aid (or sometimes impede) thinking and reasoning about some target domain or domains. These physical structures combine with appropriate culturally transmitted practices to enhance problem-solving, and (in the most dramatic cases) to make possible whole new forms of thought and reason.
>
> (Clark 2005: 256–257)

Note that Clark does not prioritize humans. But what is more important is that while Tooby and De Vore seem to remain within the representationalist paradigm, putting stress solely on *internal* models, Clark defines the cognitive niche in more enactive and ecological terms. First, he speaks not so much of niches themselves, but rather of niche *construction*, which is the approach I shall follow here, as already announced. Moreover, what makes a niche *cognitive* in Clark's account is not a structure "in the head" but a structure in the world – an external structure that is supposed to contribute to internal information processing.

If Clark can be considered a member of the 4E camp at all, he is surely not an anti-representationalist crusader. This means that he has no problem with the notion of *internal* cognitive processing. And yet, much in the spirit of his (and Chalmers's) famous extended mind hypothesis (Clark & Chalmers 1998), he also seeks external vehicles of cognition in addition to internal ones, and the concept of cognitive niche is supposed to cover these.

However, while following Clark's focus on the construction of cognitive niches, I would like to begin my own inquiry by emphasizing the following issue: when it comes to Clark's view, it remains to be explained in each specific case what makes a particular *niche* cognitive and not another kind of niche, but he assumes that we already have an idea of what *cognition* as such is, and therefore what cognition "expects," as it were, from its environmental placement. Meanwhile, I believe, the original proposal by Tooby and De Vore (1987) is more interesting in the sense that their idea of *modeling causal chains* promises at least a partial answer to the question, somewhat neglected by Clark, of what *makes* a given niche, thus a specific locus, *cognitive*.

As I explained in Werner (2021b), it is one thing to ask how something *becomes* the base of an organism's metabolism-related niche, to use this provisional term again, thus the niche that enables the organism to run the physicochemical processes keeping it alive, and another to ask how the same stuff *becomes* the base of the organism's *cognitive* niche, thus the one that enables the organism to exercise its cognitive capacities:

> As for the first question, it is critical that a certain substance be digestible, for example. As for the second question, by analogy, we need to know how the organism's *cognitive*, not the metabolic, apparatus takes aim at things in the surroundings, thus how some things become *cognizable*. And, clearly, cognizability differs in this respect from digestibility or other metabolic factors, be it e.g. tolerability of microbes by the immune system. The bear's metabolism decides that the bat living in the same cave is irrelevant, yet the bat is likely part of the bear's cognitive niche insofar as the bear can see its winged housemate. Hence, the question is how a given portion of reality *becomes* or starts to serve as the base of a *cognitive* niche.
>
> (Werner 2021b: 6309–6310)

The question of cognizability refers to how the organism cognitively "consumes" things, as Millikan (1984) might say, as opposed to more standard consumption, so to speak. Meanwhile, Clark's reference to "problem spaces" assumes that a particular fragment of the world has *already* been recognized or constructed as a problem space, and thus made into a medium of a *cognition*-specific kind. Recalling Lewontin (2000), it should be clear that "problem spaces" are not like volcanic eruptions. In order to make sense of the vocabulary of "problem spaces," we need cognition as an already active factor, that somehow transforms, for lack of a better term, some pieces of the niche base in step with the cognitive toolbox of specific living beings. Thus, as I argued in Werner (2021b), Clark's conception begins when the cognitive niche medium *already exists*, but it does not answer how such a medium *comes into being* in the first place.

So, Tooby and De Vore's use of the notion of representation is not something I follow here, but their key idea, as I see it, is that it is *constitutive* of *cognitive* interactions that they *uncover, trace and exploit cause–effect patterns*.

To be clear, I am obviously not about to decide from vantage point of my armchair what the actual mechanisms of cognition and cognitive niche construction are, leaving these problems to be studied empirically. Instead, my theoretical attempts are directed solely toward eliciting some fundamental features of the architecture of cognition-related *loci*; to be precise – the *locative architecture* of cognitive niches. For over the course of this investigation I am arguing, as it was already flagged several times, that there *is* a certain *specific locative dynamic behind cognition* thought of as an embodied and environmentally plugged-in phenomenon.

5.3 The cognitive niche as an embodied model: Selection by reconstruction

Here is a viable heuristic that can clarify how modeling without representation might work. We can safely assume that the physical reality surrounding us consists of an enormous abundance of causal chains. Consider the room or a different space in which you are reading this book:

> Asked about the causal chains that exist in this space, you will likely list a great many of them, including the power of gravity working on you, your computer and the books around you, and how the table you are sitting at intervenes in this causal chain by preventing the books from falling. You will also list the cause-effect bonds between your hands and the table or book, etc. But what about the water evaporating from flowers on the windowsill? What about the emission of CO_2 caused by your

> fireplace? And what about the causal chains between the evaporation and the CO_2 emission, and tomorrow's smog in your town? How about the airwaves made by the butterfly you see outside and tomorrow's hurricane in the Philippines?
>
> (Werner 2021b: 6310–6311)

One thing you can learn from this imaginary exercise is that the majority of causal chains around you may not even be under your consideration –

> not just because you haven't paid attention to them, but also because there may be no single ready-made setup of these chains waiting to be mapped. The point is, therefore, that you are actually facing a *selection* of causal chains, distilled, as it were, from the tangled causal vortex of the niche base.
>
> (Werner 2021b: 6311)

So the idea I'm putting forward here is that this selection or *specification* of causal chains might have something to do with the pursuit of cognitive niche construction. In the paper I mentioned above, I likened it to preparing a sample in the laboratory with a certain reagent, where you can see certain causal relationships because you bring them out by adding an extra chemical substance. Note that cognition in this sense would be like an actual intervention in the structure of the world; something called "structural coupling" in the 4E literature.

However, this process of selection is not like food preferences, which are determined by the functioning of the digestive mechanisms of a given animal; instead, it must be specific to cognition. Metaphorically speaking, what is the cognition-specific reagent in the process of niche construction, understood as the specification of causal chains?

Tooby and De Vore's key idea is that cognition, unlike food preference and the like, is about "modeling." And despite the fact that they originally spoke of internal models, i.e., internal representations, I see no reason in principle not to try to exploit this idea at a deeper level and at the same time at a more "primitive" level of cognitive sophistication, so to speak. The ability to represent is clearly an advanced cognitive tool from the perspective of the evolutionary history of cognition (see Feinberg & Mallatt 2016). However, we might also think of these more "primitive" connections between the living being and its environment as a kind of "modeling."

Consider an everyday case (see Werner 2021b): for example, if you have a bookshelf without side walls or other supports, the books at either end are likely to fall to the floor. You can "model" this frustrating causal chain in many different ways, e.g., by measuring how far from the edge the last book has to be in order not to fall off. However, if you add side walls to the bookshelf, this is also supposed to "model" *the causal chain you want to avoid.*

So the idea is that if there is no internal representation, as is especially the case in relatively primitive cognitive systems, the only way to "model" the world is by interacting with it, especially by changing the world itself. We can, therefore, speak of embodied models as distinct from representational models. This is in line with Rodney Brooks's (1991) famous dictum that the world is its own best model.

Someone might argue, however, that specifying or "distilling" causal relations in the way just described requires internal representations because it relies on perception, and therefore all external or embodied models depend on internal ones. If so, cognitive niche construction adds a new layer to the quest for representation, but cannot provide a non-representational or pre-representational explanation of what cognition is as such – the argument concludes.

The point to be made in reply, from the 4E perspective, is this: at the most fundamental level, modeling causal bonds cannot mean simply representing them because prior to this there is *nothing to be represented.* The realm to be represented must first be specified, and cognitive niche construction is exactly how that comes about. There may be, and in relatively advanced cognitive systems there surely is, some internal processing, but it is impossible to say, for example, that the internal state x stands for a structure y in the external world without y's being singled out from the messy causal maze. And the idea put forward here, in step with 4E's "seriousness" about embodiment, is that this "specification" happens by means of some actual "work" performed by the cognitive system as an entity coupled with its surroundings. This being said, the story, of course, is not about the individual effort of a single system creating the world from scratch, as the "worldmaking" doctrine would preach (Goodman 1978). Admittedly, we are dealing here with a sheer idealization of what in reality was a long evolution of niche construction, which means a co-evolution of living creatures and niche structures which are in large part inherited and only at times, here or there, transformed (see, e.g., Sterelny 2012). Nevertheless, the terminology of niche construction, which is very much in line with the 4E spirit, at least makes it possible to problematize the said co-evolution. Meanwhile – and this is the core difference – representationalism *takes the represented realm as already being there*, just waiting to be represented.

When Varela, Thompson and Rosch (1991) tell us that a living creature "brings forth and specifies its own domain of problems to be solved" and that "this domain does not exist 'out there' in an environment that acts as a landing pad for organisms that somehow drop or parachute into the world" (Varela et al. 1991: 198), this can be read as the process of cognitive niche construction thought of more or less the way Tooby and De Vore (1987) described it, yet without their representationalist baggage. In effect, in this interpretation the cognitive niche is about the "distillation" of causal bonds from the causal vortex by a living creature by means of direct engagement and interventions within this vortex ("enactivist interventions," as Gallagher 2017 might call them). Here, for example, Di Paolo et al. (2017) provide a formal model of simple perception, thought of, at the most "primitive" level, as the specification of sensorimotor invariants, i.e., simple perturbations that remain relatively stable over the course of bodily movement (which somehow harks back to Hainz von Foerster's 1976/2003 notion of *Eigenforms*). This is precisely about *how* certain specific causal connections between the cognitive system and its surroundings build up a relatively stable environment whose familiar layout is filled with mesoscopic things, processes, etc.

On the other hand, my decision not to reject the "model" terminology upfront may be controversial to advocates of 4E. This is because of the suggestion implicit in the notion of *a model*, even an "embodied" one, that we are in fact dealing with something abstract. Perhaps not yet with a full-fledged symbolic representation, but also no longer with a pure physical intervention into the stuff surrounding the system. Simply put, models require some (initially small) degree of decoupling from the world (which is what Ramsey 2007 called universality; see Chapter 3). This might be seen as a betrayal of the key tenets of 4E, all predicated on the concept of structural coupling. The worry is that once we start talking about cognition in terms of "models," the system capable of cognition is no longer structurally coupled with its surroundings. This is because – it might be argued – if we agree that part of the system's cognitive processing may be run off-line, so to speak, there is no limit to be imposed *a priori* on the scope of such processing. At the end of the day, we may end up with the idea of an advanced cognitive system thought of, *in principle*, as an entirely off-line computer, thus with the traditional Cartesian subject or at best with PSS, and with no need for the niche terminology whatsoever.

This is a subtle, yet crucial issue. On the one hand, the "abstractness" attributable to our provisionally posited "embodied models" which are supposed to make a niche specifically cognitive must not abandon 4E's "seriousness" about embodiment and environment. This means that we have to stick to the notion of structural coupling. On the other hand, however, without this "abstractness" speaking of "modeling" would be empty, and we would still have no idea how to provisionally capture the specificity of *cognitive* niches. For not all physical transformations performed by a living creature in its surroundings count as "models," thus as acts of *cognitive* niche construction. Without this controversial "abstractness," the concept at stake would be redundant.

Therefore, the question we want to equip ourselves to address is this: what are the specifically *locative* marks of *cognitive* niche construction thought of as embodied modeling, i.e., what are the locative relations between the living creature and its surroundings that the pursuit of cognitive niche construction, spelled out in terms of embodied models, brings forth?

It is beyond the scope of this study to say exactly how this most primitive "abstraction" attributable to embodied models is realized, i.e., whether the mechanism underpinning it is computation in the classical sense, or predictive processing as Friston (2009) imagines it (see also Allen & Friston 2018), or something else; or perhaps we are dealing with some other kind of information processing altogether. The only thing I can do and plan to do here – although this is something that I believe to be crucial for a proper grasp of cognitive niche construction – is to elicit the *locative* "architecture" underlying the expected "abstractness" of embodied modeling, and thus the "abstractness" of *cognitive* niche construction.

First note that embodied models, as understood here, do not in fact reflect causal bonds but *patterns* thereof. Recall the simplistic example of the bookshelf: in fact, the transformation introduced into the world by the bookshelf is not about specific books falling on a specific floor; it is about *any* book that can be put on a shelf, or perhaps even *any other thing of comparable size and weight* and *any* floor or ground that the cabinet can be placed on. Therefore, the embodied model intervening in the causal bonds surrounding a cognitive system singles out or – if someone prefers to put it in a more constructivist manner – establishes *a pattern of causal bonds* that may be of some use to the system. Otherwise, thus if a model was only about one particular bundle of causal chains, it would hardly be of any use. Organisms benefit from relatively stable structures and the relative predictability of their surroundings (recall Friston 2009), which requires at least a primitive awareness of what we humans would refer to as *kinds* or *types* of things, processes, events and *patterns* thereof. When these are "modeled," although not necessarily "in the head," an organism can impose a "web of significance" on the world (De Jaegher & Di Paolo 2007) as part of a process that 4E refers to as sense-making. Note that the very idea of *imposing a web of significance* suggests the kind of modeling we are talking about here.

That said, note one thing about our simplistic example: the bookshelf model does single out or establish a pattern of causal chains by *creating a specific locus* for the things whose causal bonds are to be "modeled." Just as with the wine glass, an example exploited several times before, here the bookshelf has the *capacity* to accommodate entities, and this capacity, this "offer," as Gibson (1979) would put it (see 5.4 below), must be limited to specific types of things; it has what I have called and provisionally characterized as *locative capacity*.

Here is, therefore, what I propose regarding the peculiar "abstractness" of cognitive niches thought of as embodied models: what *makes* certain interventions of an organism in its surroundings "abstract" and yet still structurally coupled, thus not detached as off-line representations "in the head," is the fact that by means of these interventions the organism *creates new locative relations* between selected entities. Therefore, they are not just interventions into causal bonds; what matters is that these interventions *create new loci for things in the world.* In short, the "abstractness" boils down to the fact that as a result of embodied modeling, thus actual interventions, a new and relatively stable *locative architecture* emerges. The model singles out or establishes *patterns* of causal bonds in the sense that the latter now "fill" certain locative connections between things like water flowing within the limits of a river basin (all of this will be explained more technically in the following chapters). I, therefore, propose that if we are to describe cognitive niches as embodied models, we must pay attention to the kind of locative relations that are characteristic of the cognitive niche.

However, there is one thing that is unfortunately missing from the picture proposed by Tooby and De Vore, and thus also absent from my 4E-friendly re-articulation of their cognitive niche theory. Namely, if it is a cognitive system that casts its "web of significance" upon its surroundings, then the cognitive niche thereby created must be, as it were, *centered around* the said system so that the latter acts as a "center of activity" in it (De Jaegher & Di Paolo 2007). Therefore, we have to be able to articulate not only the locative relations between *things* within the medium of the cognitive niche, but also the already flagged "centeredness" of the cognitive niche whose locative architecture is somehow "anchored" in the location of the niche constructor/tenant itself, thereby making the latter a point of reference for everything around it.

5.4 The cognitive niche as a realm of information: Gibson's ecological approach

In the previous section, I tried out the concept of modeling as a potential introductory characterization of the cognitive niche, emphasizing the fact that even when embodied, such models must in some sense abstract from the concrete stuff that a living creature is dealing with at a specific moment, and therefore specify not so much causal bonds themselves, but rather patterns thereof. For only insofar as it fits a pattern, a particular causal bond can *mean* anything to the living creature, thought of as the "center of activity" in a given realm.

However, speaking of patterns is not sufficient if we are to identify a particular niche as *the* cognitive niche of *a specific* organism or autonomous system. As said, we need to account for the peculiar "centeredness" of the cognitive niche. This is not an easy task, for it is one thing to say how a particular bundle of causal relations affects a particular organism, and another to describe how *a pattern* of causal bonds can have anything to do with this organism. There is no affection or perturbation in the literal sense of the term that a living creature undergoes as a result of bumping into a causal *pattern*.

The idea I propose states that if we are to account for how patterns of causal relations render an organism the "center of activity" within a given environment, we must be able to single out a specific setup of relations between the *location of* the organism and *the locations* of things it is affected by. There must be some – as I like to put it metaphorically – locative architecture underpinning the causal network that the organism is engaged in. But what sort of architecture?

In addition to the original posit of Tooby and De Vore (1987), I will now try out another interpretation of the concept of cognitive niche, which, as I see it, spells out both of the features of cognitive niches uncovered so far: their "meaningfulness" as well as their "centeredness." I am thinking of the ecological psychology of perception proposed by James Gibson (1979). Since Gibson is frequently cited by 4E authors as one of the movement's antecedents, his insight may provide a link between the "model" conceptualization tested above, which isn't perhaps that appealing to advocates of 4E, and one that is likely more bearable. For Gibson's proposal is spelled out in terms of direct and loopy links with things as they manifest themselves through the organism's actions. These manifestations Gibson calls *affordances*. He does not use the term "cognitive niche," but he does speak of niches filled with affordances, so there is a strong tie between his conceptualization of perception and the niche talk I am pursuing here.

Gibson's proposal does not appeal to *internal* information processing. However, this does not mean that the concept of information as such is abandoned. On the contrary, it may prove quite useful. For what really matters for him is the question of *how much information is delivered by the environment*, and how much depends on the cognitive system. As Miłkowski (2017) emphasizes, there is no a priori assumption in computationalism regarding this issue, and therefore it can be taken in either direction, thereby even opening the door to a computationalist reading of Gibson (see Rowlands 1999; and Chemero 2003, 2009 for a different view). For example, Marr (1982) and a large number of cognitive psychologists underline the informational scarcity of the environment and thus the need to postulate internal representational processes to fill the gap. Gibson takes the opposite approach, arguing in favor of the environment's informational abundance, which makes the need for representations minimal.

The central notion in Gibson's ecological theory of perception is *optic array*. The key thought behind this conception, as Chemero (2009) nicely articulates it, is that because "perception does not involve mental addition of information to stimuli, yet is able to guide behavior adaptively, all the information necessary for guiding adaptive behavior must be available in the environment to be perceived" (Chemero 2009: 23). Hence, speaking of the optic array points to a certain organization of the environment, thought of as a realm of information.

Here is how this is supposed to work. While in Marr's (1982) view visual perception starts from and builds upon the retinal image, Gibson's claim is that it begins a step earlier, we might say, thus when the perceiver finds itself in a realm filled with objects *and* with rays of light. These rays move between the surfaces of things, creating a certain dynamic nexus of reverberations so that each point in it is characterized by a specific nest of light rays coming from all directions, and each of these nested rays has a certain characteristic such as angle, frequency, etc. which in turn makes each such nested point a complex and unique mixture. Therefore, as Rowlands puts is,

> we can imagine an observer (…) as a point surrounded by a sphere, which is divided into tiny solid angles. The intensity of light and the mixture of wavelengths vary from one solid angle to another. This spatial pattern of light is the optic array. Light carries information because the structure of the optic array is determined by the nature and position of the surfaces from which it has been reflected.
>
> (Rowlands 1999: 33–34)

But what does it mean that the optic array "carries information"? How is information generated in the optic array? This is not a question we can target properly here, although even a provisional answer would elicit a certain important fact about the locative architecture of environments. According to Rowlands's reading, information is *nomic dependence*. This means that the structure of the optic array attributable to a particular perceiver depends "in a lawlike (i.e., nomic) way on the structure of the physical environment" surrounding the said perceiver. And due to this dependence, "the optic array carries information about this wider environment" insofar as the optic array is "*specific* to the environment" (Rowlands 1999: 34–35). Now, since speaking of the "structure of the environment" refers to how things are placed with respect to one another, I would say that the informational character of the optic array rests on a specific locative architecture of the environment.

Since perceivers are not passive recipients of stimuli but active samplers, by picking various fragments or segments of the optic array that are of use to them in performing specific actions, the perceivers' movements elicit certain patterns within the optic array. These patterns are co-determined by the arrangement of the environment itself, and by the perceiver's movements. If so, the perceiver is also able to elicit certain invariants inside this domain. I already referred to such invariants above (recall Di Paolo et al. 2017, who provided a model of how these invariants are singled out).

Interestingly, Rowlands calls the optic array "a *locus* of information for suitably equipped creatures" (Rowlands 1999: 36; my highlight). However, the nature of this locus, thus the issue of location as such, does not stand out for him as something to be reflected on in its own right. Meanwhile, the optic array cannot be thought of, in my understanding, simply as a realm filled with physical entities and light waves. More is needed to make sense of it. This is because the realm in question would *not be an array* of any sort, just like water circulation or glacial periods do not by themselves constitute environments, had it not been "centered" around something(s). An optic *array* must have some direction(s), and this requires, formally speaking, that a *point of reference* or "point of view" be singled out. And as I pointed out with regard to Tooby and De Vore, this "centeredness" requires careful study.

Someone might say that this is exactly what Gibson postulated: there are *points* in the array characterized uniquely by the qualities of the light rays they nest, relative to each point, e.g., the angle of a given light ray, its reverberation path, thus the line of objects it "met" along the way.

I agree that the idea of *nesting points* is close to what I am arguing for here, yet my claim is that Gibson's characterization is not sufficient. Such a point must *actually* be a point of reference or *serve as* one. And, crucially, not every point picked by theoretical fiat from the vantage point of an external observer is an *actual point of reference*. The reason why that is so, as well as why I have just highlighted the words "actual" and "actually," has to do with the distinction between the standpoint of an observer and a standpoint that is internal to the domain under investigation. Of course, if we look at a given domain of objects and light rays as external observers, we can specify the properties of the domain from the perspective of any randomly chosen point, but there is nothing that makes this randomly selected point a "possessor of a perspective on the world," so to speak. This is the key issue: as external observers we can define and attribute a "perspective" to any point we like within a space of our choosing; however, points themselves are *just points*. There is nothing about them that makes them points *of reference* inside a given realm when they are *not* mapped from the vantage point of an external observer. The question now is what makes some points *in* a realm points that the realm is "centered around."

To get a sense of what I am aiming at, imagine a sky with clouds being moved by the wind in just one direction. Certainly, there is a point, actually many points, in the sky relative to which *we* can measure the speed of the moving clouds or their size, or classify them as cirrus clouds, cumulus clouds, etc. But here comes a question: what is it that determines the *resolution* of that point's perspective – formally speaking, once a point is fixed it is possible to measure clouds from its angle, but it is also in principle possible to get a more fine-grained image and measure the movements of clusters of molecules composing the clouds. And this can still be done with varying degrees of resolution, so that once a cloud is "recalibrated" as a swarm of molecules there could still be an observable "contour" of the swarm resembling the fuzzy boundaries of what previously appeared as a bulky cloud, or no longer any such contour shows up, so that any reference to a "cloud" would now be baseless. Needless to say, there are certain nomic correlations at each level, but the correlations that Gibson talks about, those carrying information for a potential perceiver, are not present at every level. Perceivers, at least known ones, operate at a specific level of complexity. In other words, it is only with respect to a specific range of resolutions or calibrations that *it makes sense* to speak of potential *perceivers*. Now, who or what decides on the resolution of a given nesting point?

Faced with this puzzle, we either assume that the perceiver makes the "calibration" for some specific purpose, or we may need to single out some *relations inside the domain itself* that set up the resolution appropriate for perception. If we attribute this competence to perceivers, there is no rationale for speaking of nesting points or points of reference because there is no explanatory gain from introducing these notions. All there is to be said should be said about the cognitive machinery of the perceiver.

This is not a conclusion that Gibson would accept, and we should not accept it either. For talking about the optic array around a nesting point was supposed to explain how it is possible that the cognitive system finds itself in an informationally rich environment that is *not* merely a product of *its own internal* processing (as Marr 1982 and representationalists following him would have it). Meanwhile, we ended up with the internal processing as the only relevant factor.

What applies to resolution applies *to any other characteristic*, such as a point's "reach" or "scope," meaning the range of qualities of surrounding things that are available to that point. A priori, the point where I am sitting right now could be used to measure not only the speed of the cars passing by the building, but also the speed of wind on Mars. And yet, admittedly, the latter measurement would make little sense.

The general question is what determines all the factors that make up the unique perspective of a given point, so that the surrounding part of the world is indeed an *array*. Let me repeat – a point is just a point; therefore, a point must somehow *become* a point *of reference*. And it is by no means a trivial question how that happens and what it means.

So, if we are to say anything about how a given point actually *becomes* a point of reference within a given domain without referring to an external observer or to the internal information processing performed the actual perceiver, the story must not be only about the point itself. It must be about this point *and* a cluster of relations in the domain. To be specific: I advance the idea that it must be about certain specific *locative* relations that make the physical realm in question a domain of *ecological* ties, not just causal bonds.

Adding locative relations to the picture makes it possible to provide the Gibsonian nesting points with more substantial characteristics, yet abstracting from the peculiarities of the physics of optic arrays, light waves and the way the latter travel. The idea that I will set forth later on states that it is the specific locative capacity of a point that makes the latter *a point of reference*. This point of reference in turn renders a surrounding configuration of objects, electromagnetic waves or what have you (depending on the "calibration") a genuine *array* (be it *optic* or of any other kind). This abstract architecture shall be unveiled in the subsequent chapters.

On the other hand, while maintaining this abstract stance, we must not ignore the role played by the perceiver or, more generally, the cognitive system. While Gibson's idea of the informationally rich environment goes against the notion that information is produced by the internal machinery of the system, the system has a critical function in this story. For the foundational notion of ecological psychology is that this informationally rich environment delivers system-specific pieces of information, as if "messages" for appropriately equipped perceivers. And here comes another crucial posit by Gibson, the one that he is likely most famous for.

Once certain points of reference materialize, the agents *occupying* these points do not just stumble across a particular thing or another. What they actually perceive are what Gibson calls *affordances*. These are opportunities for action. Metaphorically speaking, they are "offers" made by perceived entities to agents. For example, I do not perceive a wooden stick as a mere bulk of wood matter; I perceive it *as* a potential tool to support my body or to hit somebody who is attacking me, etc.

There is no ready-made list of affordances, given changing circumstances and the fact that the affordances one receives depend on one's capacities and needs. This makes affordances rather peculiar ontologically – something that Gibson himself also stressed – since they are neither objective nor subjective in the Cartesian sense of the term. On the one hand, they cannot be deemed entirely external if being external means being fully mind-independent or free of any intervention on the part of the perceiver. On the other hand, however, they are not in the perceiver's head – they are external in the most straightforward sense, i.e., they await the cognitive system in the surrounding world (see Heft 2001; Chemero 2003; Stoffregen 2003; Bruineberg et al. 2019).

This ontological peculiarity is a really powerful point, since it blows up, figuratively speaking, the Cartesian worldview from within, which is something that 4E welcomes eagerly. However, the strategy followed by Gibson, in my reading, is quite intricate and artful. It starts from the Cartesian internal versus external divide, positing an informationally rich *external* realm. This is in opposition to Marr (1982) and the cognitive psychology mainstream, who claim that informational abundance is born on the internal side. Nonetheless, the general Cartesian architecture seems to be intact. Yet at the end of the day Gibson reaches a point when the Cartesian framework can no longer stand. Affordances are beyond *internal versus external*, thus also beyond the *subjective versus objective* distinction; they just don't fit the framework, as if calling for a different one.

From this perspective, it becomes crucially important to conceptualize properly what the category of *occupying a point of reference* in a given domain means; what the cognitive system is doing there. It seems that there is some informational potential nested at a given point, and the task of a cognitive system is to *actualize* that potential, as if opening a computer file stored on a disk.

Let us consider this last comparison in more detail. Assuming, for the sake of this illustration, that the computer file itself is a series of bits that are ultimately grounded in physical entities in the hardware of the computer, what is required to actually make it a *graphic* file, for example, is a program, software. What the latter does is *actualize* the potential of *presenting something*, such as the image of a beloved face, to someone. By analogy, cognitive systems can be thought of as factors that "open" nested pieces of information at a given reference point in their environment.

From this perspective, cognitive niche construction may be thought of as the process of nesting potential information and then opening/actualizing it. Now, as with the actual processes responsible for embodied modeling, the mechanisms responsible for how cognitive systems "unpack" the information potentially available in their environment(s) need to be studied empirically by biologists, (ecological) cognitive psychologists, etc., and thus cannot be decided from a philosophical armchair. Yet, as before, a proper job for the philosopher is to unveil the locative architecture underpinning the notion of *occupying* a point of reference; in other words what kind of change in the structure of locative relations is brought forth by the presence of a cognitive system. This completes the previous task which was focused on the notion of a point of reference.

The task is therefore twofold: first, to identify the locative architecture that is involved in the most abstract idea of an environment, a portion of space organized *around* a point of reference; second, to elicit the structure of locative relations between a cognitive system standing at that point of reference and the entities that the system deals with.

5.5 Conclusion

Following the extensive discussion in Chapters 2–4 of how representationalism and 4E see the cognitive system's placement in an environment and the system's own locative footprint, this chapter had one major goal. It was to introduce the concept of a cognitive niche in a way that would be intuitive but also grounded in the relevant literature. Some comments were also made on why referring to niches, environments or physical-behavioral units proves problematic from the point of view of contemporary ontology. The latter is important given that a suitable ontology of the cognitive niche is the final target of this book.

I outlined and re-interpreted the original posit by Tooby and De Vore (1987) whose key idea was that cognitively advanced systems (they basically mean humans, but I propose to generalize this following Clark 2003, 2005) create and exploit *cause–effect* models of their surroundings, which makes their environment genuinely informational in nature. The behavior of such a system or agent is, therefore, not only flexible but first of all information-driven. Cognitive niches are thus best understood as realms of information. While Tooby and De Vore adopted the representationalist model of cognition, I have proposed a different (provisional) account in which the models they talked about are not representations, but actual interventions of the system in its surroundings. Cognitive systems, structurally coupled with their environments, transform their surroundings (and therefore also their own functioning as part of an open-ended loop of structural coupling) in such a way as to "distill" or "specify" *patterns* of cause–effect relations, and such transformations give rise to cognitive niches. I have called these embodied models. However, Tooby and De Vore do not say much about the locative architecture of cognitive niches, especially how we are to conceptualize the "centeredness" of these specific loci, i.e., the fact that they are attributable to cognitive systems functioning in them as "centers of activity."

In this context, Gibson's conception of informationally abundant environments has been proposed as a plausible alternative (perhaps supplementary) explanation of what the cognitive niche thought of as a realm of information is. It has one advantage over Tooby and de Vore's original posit. Namely, it explicitly problematizes and aims to account for the quality of "centeredness" attributed to niches. Since embodied models, unpacked in terms of perceptual or sensorimotor invariants, can also be accommodated within the Gibsonian framework, we obtain quite a compelling conceptualization of the cognitive niche. We have thereby come closer to our target, that is to say a better conceptual grasp of what an environment *suitable for* and *determined by* cognition is.

That said, we need to go further in order to fully exploit the potential of the cognitive niche terminology understood in the Gibsonian-ecological and 4E-friendly sense. Strictly speaking, we are still in need of a more detailed and general theory of locative relations underpinning the "centeredness" of the niche, which shall empower us to unveil the *locative specificity* of cognition.

6 The Basic Ontology of the Bounded Locus

The time is ripe to finally set out on the announced ontological analysis. This chapter introduces a number of basic concepts such as exact location and boundary, which are then used to define open and closed objects, various kinds of connection, containment and framing, among other, posits. Special attention is devoted to the notion of boundary, which results in a novel classification of boundaries, crucial for further analysis of niches.

The final goal of this part of the investigation is to come up with a suitable definition of the concept of bounded locus, intuitively introduced in Chapter 1. This means characterizing the relation "*x* is a bounded locus for *y*." Note that I do not speak of bounded loci *of y*, since that would suggest that *y* is as if *in possession* of its own bounded locus. Meanwhile, there may be other entities in *x* too, just like there are many toys in a box and many people in a building. On the other hand, "for" alludes to a certain service that the bounded locus provides to its occupants, which is a good indicator of its functional character. The latter is significant as I proceed, in the final part of this chapter, to discuss two kinds of bounded loci – containers and frames.

It should be stressed, however, that developing a full-fledged formal ontology of location is not my goal here – unlike in the seminal works of Achille Varzi, Roberto Casati, Jerzy Perzanowski and Barry Smith (see Perzanowski 1993; Smith 1996; Casati & Varzi 1999; Smith & Varzi 1999; Varzi 2007; also Kleinschmidt 2014, 2016) which I am going to rely on. This is a study in applied ontology in the sense that it is dedicated to a better understanding of specific phenomena; in our case – systems capable of cognition, operating within a certain cognition-specific niche (environment).

Therefore, what this chapter brings forth can be dubbed a Basic Ontology of the Bounded Locus, which is going to be developed in Chapter 7, eventually producing a Basic Ontology of Niche Construction. What is worth emphasizing, however, is the fact that the latter is *not* the only possible development of the former. This means that the Basic Ontology of the

DOI: 10.4324/9781003580997-6

Bounded Locus can also be developed further by someone who wants to come up with an ontological treatment of the mind conceptualized in more Cartesian terms. *A priori*, the conceptual framework to be rolled out here is open to multiple specifications, and does not rely on any presumptions in this respect.

As for the conceptual framework to be presented, it can be referred to as *minimal*, which means involving only those notions that are necessary to succeed in the flagged task – unlike the *general* locative ontology of Varzi, Perzanowski and others – while on the other hand the list of concepts available in the literature shall be significantly extended to appropriately capture the phenomena we are interested in.

6.1 Exact location and parthood

The imaginative exercises conducted in Chapter 1 targeted an intuitive, but logically complex notion of location referring to various kinds of bounded loci as exemplified by cases such as "the toy is in the box" or "the wine is in the glass." Now, armed with this introductory recognition of the rich variety of *being-in* relations, the focus must be shrunk in the first step of a proper ontological investigation and move from the whole scene, composed of an entity placed in a certain broader setting, to the entity itself. We must think of the location of this entity on its own, *its own* address, not relative to any other entity, container or whatever. This is the most logically primitive notion of location called *exact location*, or, more precisely, the primitive relation of *being exactly located*, which carves up the address in space occupied solely by the entity in question and by nothing else (Casati & Varzi 1999).

Think of any physical item in your everyday surroundings. The key thing now is to realize that it occupies not only a segment of a certain broader locus, like a box or a room, but that it first and foremost occupies a unique portion of that locus *filled exactly* with the entity in question. Think of a pebble thrown into the water. There is a portion of perceivable physical space occupied by the pebble and *not* by the water, and there is a portion of space that you occupy on a bench in a subway no matter how slender you are, no matter how humble you are and how mindful of your neighbor's comfort. You cannot help producing a certain hole in the air, figuratively speaking, and *filling* it *perfectly* with your body. Every material entity occupies such a hole in which, technically speaking, it is *exactly* located (this understanding of place comes from Aristotle, see e.g., Smith 2001 for a more detailed overview). This means that a thing is related to the carved-up portion of space in which it is exactly located, "like a liquid in an urn relates to the urn, or the hand relates to the glove" (Smith & Varzi 1999: 218).

Following the seminal work of Roberto Casati and Achille Varzi (1999), I take *being exactly located* as a primitive notion. Therefore, there is a primitive relation "x is (exactly) located at y" that is assumed as given. This enables us to define regions in a straightforward manner (see also Smith & Varzi 1999):

(1) y is a *region* if there is an object located there, i.e., if there is such x that x is exactly located at y.

However, the word "region" can be ambiguous in everyday speech, so when I sometimes refer below to the *exact locations of* things, I am strictly speaking referring to the regions at which they *are exactly located*, as defined in (1). The relationship between things and their regions (exact locations) is quite special, since on the one hand regions/locations in general do not depend on any specific thing – the very same region/location can be occupied by numerically different, but spatially identical entities. On the other hand, regions or exact locations generically depend on things, as Smith puts it, in the sense that it would make little sense to speak of regions if there were no objects at least potentially located there.

Now, another crucial thing is that regions may have parts, just like the things located in them. Mereology, i.e., the formal theory of parthood, is therefore the second theoretical ingredient we need. Following Casati and Varzi (1999) I take *being part of* as the second primitive concept. Hence, I assume that we all understand what it means that x is part of y, e.g., that my cat's leg is part of the cat's body; that a spout is part of a teapot; that Texas is part of the United States; that my kitchen is part of my flat.

The parthood relation was studied by Aristotle, yet it had to wait until the 20th century to become the target of a more disciplined investigation. The pivotal moves were made first informally by Husserl (1901/2000) and then formally by Stanisław Leśniewski (1916/1992), Leonard and Goodman (1940) and many others who would follow (see Simons 1987; Varzi 2007; Fine 1999; or e.g., McDaniel 2010 for a nice philosophical introduction).

There is controversy as to whether the concept of *part* or that of *proper part* should function as a primitive. I follow Casati and Varzi (1999) here, and pick the former. Now, we can easily define the latter (assuming the notion of identity as given):

(2) x is a proper part of y if x is part of y and x is not identical to y.

Things may share parts. We then say that they overlap:

(3) x overlaps with y if there is z such that z is part of x and part of y.

If things do not overlap, they are disjoint.

Then, there is an axiom that opens room for defining the crucial concept of mereological fusion. First:

(4) For any condition φ, referring to a property, there is an entity composed of precisely all the things satisfying φ (all the φ-ers).

Now we can define the entity called *fusion*:

(5) x fuses all the objects satisfying the condition φ iff each of the objects satisfying φ is part of x, and x has no part disjoint from each of the objects satisfying φ (this formulation paraphrases the one in Kleinschmidt 2014a).

Since it is possible to define an entity based on any condition, the range and the very ontological sense of the notion of fusion is a matter of controversy, but that will not concern us here (for more see e.g., Varzi 2007). What is important is that having mereological fusion set, we are able to define four standard Boolean operators:

(6) A sum of x and y is the fusion of such z that z is part of x or z is part of y.
(7) An intersection (a product) of x and y is the fusion of such z that z is part of x and x is part of y. Intuitively, this is what x and y share.
(8) A difference x minus y is the fusion of such z that z is part of x and z is not part of y. Intuitively, this is everything in x that has nothing to do (mereologically) with y (it can be all of x if they don't share any parts, or just a fraction of x).
(9) A complement of x is the fusion of such z that z and x do not overlap. To put it simply, it is the domain comprising everything except x.

Exact location and parthood enable us to speak of mereological relations between regions, and thereby also between things *defined fully in terms of their regions or exact locations*. For example, if I am to account for my being in the room, it is not only about my exact location, since being in the room is more than just occupying my unique "hole" in the universe. Certainly it is not about parthood, for I am not part of the room. However, *my location* is *part* of the *location of* the room. Therefore, the first intuition that comes to mind is that when a thing is located inside a different thing, we are dealing with a parthood relation between two regions, *not* between two things.

Yet this is still not enough to do justice to some of the peculiarities of the relation of *being-in* identified by linguists and brought up in Chapter 1. In each of these cases we had a certain complex setup of entities, like the wine plus the glass or the fly plus the glass, or the top pearl plus the bowl, and what determined their peculiarity was the way the boundary or boundaries of the whole complex were drawn. The top pearl is in the bowl only if the boundaries of what is referred to as "the bowl" somehow surrounds the entire pile of pearls. The wine in the glass is actually *in* the glass if the boundary of the glass functions also as the boundary of the portion of wine, which seems to have no stable boundary of its own. Finally, the fly is in the glass only if the boundaries of the glass restrict the movements of the fly in some way.

The driving intuition behind these cases is that being-in is a specific situation where it is not the things themselves but rather their locations (their regions) that compose a certain temporary whole or unit. The notion of wholeness turns out to be quite challenging, and requires the addition of a third primitive to our minimal ontology: that of *boundary*.

6.2 Introducing boundaries and enclosement

Parthood is not enough if we want to articulate what makes some collections of parts a single *whole*. What is the difference, we may ask, following Smith and Varzi (1999), for example between a broken cup whose parts are scattered on the floor, and the whole cup. They write:

> We should like to talk of things that are connected, or of a piece, on the one hand, and distinguish them from scattered groups or aggregates and other gerrymandered beings, on the other. It is impossible to account for this difference on the basis of mereology alone. More generally, mereology cannot account for some very basic spatial relations, such as the relationship of continuity between two adjacent parts of an object, or the relation of one thing's being entirely inside or surrounded by another. To provide a systematic account of such relations will require a topological machinery. We shall assume here an apparatus closely corresponding to ordinary topology, though constructed on a mereological basis. The central concept is the concept of boundary as illustrated by the outer surface of a sphere, the edge of a table, or the borders of Japan.
>
> (Smith & Varzi 1999: 222)

This means that speaking of parts and fusions is not identical to speaking of parts and wholes, for in principle we can compose a fusion out of any entities, e.g., we can postulate a fusion of my leg and planet Mars. Yet, at least as long as the familiar world around us is concerned, we see wholes as fundamentally different not only from scattered sets of elements but also from *ad hoc* collections. Therefore, mereology alone is too weak to account for wholes and additional theoretical tools are needed to perform that job.

This means that there needs to be a certain *foundation* that grounds the unity of all the parts of a given entity insofar as the entity in question is to be considered a whole. And the concept of a boundary is intended to capture the idea of such a foundation. We might say that wholes are not only collections of parts; they are collections that "care" about their distinctness from other entities and thus "maintain" a certain barrier or at least a demarcating line delineating the collection from its surroundings.

One crucial caveat is needed though, before we move on. Smith and Varzi refer to "topological machinery" and I follow their steps here; however, I consider the said "machinery" insufficient, too, if we are to account for a genuinely ecological phenomenon of niche, especially when it comes to ecological cognition thought of in term of cognitive niche construction. This is because what really matters in the latter story must seriously engage *active interactions* between a niche tenant/constructor and its surroundings, and their evolution, which is not a phenomenon that can be captured by "mereotopology," to use Smith's (1996) term, alone. To put it differently, one might argue that some of the notions to be defined below, e.g., reference points, enclosement, push the open door since their proper characterization has already been provided by topology and its philosophical reworkings. Yet, I disagree – although "mereotopology" provides us with the most fundamental concepts and insights, what we need is not only an ontological (mereological) reworking of various topological concepts, but an ontological effort that deals with genuinely *ecological* senses of surroundings, enclosements, boundaries, etc. And, in my reading, this ecological perspective is missing or incomplete in the existing theories and conceptual frameworks. A preliminary conceptual framework of the expected kind is to be provided below.

Following Smith and Varzi (1999), I take the relationship "x is a boundary for y" as primitive. Note that we have "boundary for" here, and not "boundary of." Why so? This is to indicate that speaking of a boundary does *not* necessarily mean speaking of a maximal boundary, thus a full setup of delineations attributable to a given thing. One can refer to just one boundary, e.g., the one delineating Germany from France, but not the one delineating Germany from Poland.

An entity's maximal boundary is not a primitive concept, yet it can be easily defined as the fusion of that entity's boundaries:

(10) The maximal boundary of x is the fusion of all such y that y is a boundary of x.

This opens room for a variety of further derivative concepts. First we shall need:

(11) The closure of x is the sum of x and its maximal boundary.
(12) The interior of x is x minus its maximal boundary (it is, so to speak, x stripped of its boundaries).
(13) The exterior of x is the interior of the x's complement.

While all the previous chapters gave us a provisional idea of how the concepts of *interior* and *exterior* prove crucial when it comes to the mind-world relationship, how cognitive systems relate to their surroundings, etc., here we begin to arm ourselves to tackle these puzzles with greater precision.

Going further, we can now speak of internal parts:

(14) x is an internal part of y iff x is a proper part of the interior of x.

Then, there come two crucial notions unpacking the intuition regarding the openness and closedness of certain things in the world:

(15) x is closed when x is identical to its closure. Intuitively, when referring to x's closure adds nothing to referring to x itself.
(16) x is open when it is identical to its interior. Intuitively, when it has no boundary.

Crucially, *not being closed* does *not* mean being open and *not being open* does *not* equal being closed. There are objects, actually plenty of objects – some crucial for this analysis – that are *partially open* and *partially closed*. Therefore, closedness and openness are two extremes on a continuum.

We can now define several notions that unpack how things may be connected with one another. This step is crucial, since within the ontology to be proposed cognition will be defined as a kind of connection. The structural coupling which 4E talks about shall be seen as a connection, but recall that in his representationalist account Newell (1980) also explicitly spoke of connection between the physical symbol system and its surroundings.

Let us begin with the standard generic notion which may be found in the literature. The baseline is this:

(17) x and y are *directly* connected if they share a part (overlap) or share a boundary (thus their closures overlap).

However, we shall need a more specific connection, i.e., one defined solely in terms of boundaries:

(18) x and y are *directly* but *externally* connected when they do not overlap and share a boundary.

We can read the latter as portraying situations when two entities are "sewn together" by a shared boundary.

Finally – and this will also prove quite crucial when it comes to some of our goals – entities may also maintain a remote connection:

(19) x and y are *remotely* connected when they are not directly connected but there is z such that x is directly connected to z and z is directly connected to y.

The above characterization is a bit of a simplification, however, for it is possible for two entities to be remotely connected with more intermediary objects, not just one. This is because I take it as an axiomatic property of remote connection that when x and z are remotely connected and z is remotely connected to y, then x is remotely connected to y too. Therefore, whenever remote connection shall be brought up from this point on, it may also refer to longer chains of connections.

It may also be useful in some contexts to speak of connection without specifying its kind. This shall be connection *simpliciter* taken as a generic umbrella term:

(20) x and y are connected (generic) if they are either directly (externally or by overlap) or remotely connected.

A further crucial concept that marks the difference between scattered swarms and wholes is self-connectedness:

(21) If x is the sum of fixed entities $z_1, \ldots z_n$, then x is self-connected when any z_i and z_j belonging to $\{z_1, \ldots z_n\}$ are connected (generic; i.e., they are connected in either of the defined manners) with each other.

The above gives us the most basic conceptual scaffolding, in most cases following the literature. From this point on, however, I would like to come up with several additional concepts. In the first place, and quite crucially given the subject matter of this investigation, I propose to speak of exclusively *locative* connection, already flagged in the previous chapters, in particular when I tried to demonstrate how non-trivial and challenging a posit the concept of a reference point in a fixed domain is. Locative connection is likely the weakest form of tie, for while being predicated *of objects*, it is defined fully *in terms of their regions (exact location)*.

(22) x and y are in locative connection when the exact location of x (the region where x is exactly located) is connected (generic) to the location of y (the region respectively).

As the weakest kind of connection, locative connection is built into any other kind of connection, which means that for any of the previously distinguished kinds of connection, if x and y are connected, they are also in locative connection. For example, if they share a boundary, they are also in locative connection. But not necessarily vice versa.

As weak as it is, the concept of locative connection is quite useful. Just think of everyday examples of relative locations expressed in everyday speech by phrases such as "at," "on" and "near". If John is sitting in a room on the right side of James, there is no actual connection between the two gentlemen, and yet they are tied in some weak sense – they can abut each other, especially if one of them falls asleep, bored by a lecture, and leans on the other. But even if nothing of the sort happens, we may want to be able to spell out that weak bond between them somehow. It would be quite plausible to say that while John and James are not themselves connected, quite obviously, *the exact location of* John is externally connected (perhaps only remotely) to *the exact location of* James. Therefore, it is possible to posit the following generalization of the case:

(23) A relative location of x with respect to $y_1,\ldots, y_n$ can be individuated by the unique setup of locative connections x maintains with $y_1,\ldots, y_n$.

The "setup of locative connections" means that unlike in the case of John abutting James, where one locative connection was enough to report how the two gentlemen have to do with each other in terms of their placement, sometimes we may need a more complex structure of locative connections that occur in a particular setting. For example, if I want to report that, say, my friend Boleslaw was in the same theater as King Charles III, which is supposed to express how close he was to His Majesty, I may need a swirl of locative connections that would represent a more distant locative connection between the two men.

Finally, the last crucial notion at this stage is *enclosement*. Let this be the first step specifically geared toward grasping the notion of container which, as we learned in Chapter 1, proves crucial in the philosophy of mind. However, perhaps contrary to what Ryle or Popper might expect, containment is a complex concept, requiring some preliminaries. Containment is a special kind of enclosement which obscures access to the contained entity (recall the analyses of Tyler & Evans 2003). Meanwhile,

I argue, "obscuring," which also needs to be characterized in more technical terms, is just one exemplification of a more general condition in which one entity, the enclosing one, somehow *conditions* access to another entity, the enclosed one.

This is meant to define the structure of the proto-scene for "in" as described by Tyler and Evans (2003), yet without any further presuppositions as to the nature of the "conditioning" in question. Moreover, enclosement does not even have to exemplify the intuitive "geometrical" structure that we tend to associate with the ordinary idea of enclosing something. Recall the example of the pearl at the top of the pile – it is not geometrically enclosed by the bowl, and yet it is enclosed in some more general sense.

Casati and Varzi (1999) propose the following definition:

(24) *x* is enclosed by *y* when for any *z*, if *z* is connected to *x*, *z* is also connected to *y*.

I propose to call Casati and Varzi's posit *strong enclosement* which naturally captures situations of a more "geometrical" character, to use Talmy's (1983) phrasing again. For example, containment in a box clearly satisfies (24). However, the pearl case does not do that exactly. Therefore, I also propose *weak enclosement* which makes non-trivial use of the concept of locative connection:

(25) *x* is enclosed (weakly) by *y* when for any *z*, if *z* is connected (generic) to *x*, *z* is in *locative* connection to *y*.

This imposes a weaker condition on *y*'s enclosing capacities in the sense that *y*'s "intervention" in *x*'s connection capacity, so to speak, is weaker. This concept, I believe, describes the pearl example. The bowl does not mediate the top pearl's connection, in the sense that anything connected to the pearl must also be connected to the bowl; nonetheless, in order to gain access to the top pearl one cannot avoid setting up *some kind* of remote connection with the region occupied by the bowl. Intuitively speaking, if the bowl is, for example, moving, this clearly impacts one's ability to grab the top pearl. To put it differently, the bowl sets up conditions for anything "willing" to get access to the pearl, but *not* in the sense that one needs to get access to the bowl first; the bowl is just a precondition of the pearl's very being there, ready to be seen or grabbed. (25) aims to capture this relatively weak constraint imposed by *y*.

From this point on, I shall employ (25), which means that any time I refer to *enclosement*, I shall mean weak enclosement, if not explicitly stated otherwise.

Now, enclosement can be further weakened when we allow for its being partial:

(26) x is partially enclosed by y when (25) applies to some objects in the given universe.

As a complement of the latter, we also naturally obtain:

(27) x is *fully* enclosed by y when (25) applies to all objects in the given universe.

One thing is clearly missing in this short discussion on enclosement, and the reader might even have a feeling that the picture drawn so far is incomplete without it. What I mean is the concept of boundary. For isn't it the case that in the relation of enclosing, one entity finds itself within the boundaries of another, and that these very boundaries are responsible for how the connections maintained by the enclosed entity are conditioned by the enclosing one? My answer is negative: enclosement is a more general concept, and yet – indeed – if we are to make further progress in this analysis, we need to pay more attention to boundaries. This is because the primitive notion of boundary introduced and exploited above is not sufficient. Think of the pearl in the bowl example again – if we are to articulate the peculiar sense in which the *pearl + bowl* compound is bounded, we need to know more about boundaries. That is because, quite clearly, the boundary of this compound is different in kind from the boundaries of the pearl and the bowl by themselves, and is not even a simple sum thereof.

Note, however, that the challenge here is obviously not about how we store pearls. The stakes are much higher and concern the status of what Smith called physical-behavioral units. This is because the *pearl + bowl* unit is a very simple exemplification of a much more general idea whose most complex exemplifications (at the other extreme) are the environments or niches (as well as cognitive systems, according to 4E); i.e., entities whose status depends on locative relations. The question is therefore: what are the boundaries suitable for such units?

6.3 Questioning boundaries

There seem to be three fundamental intuitions underpinning the notion of boundary, all of which have already been flagged. The first is that boundaries have to do with discontinuities. If it is possible to indicate a point or set of points (a line) where one object ends and another begins, this is a good indication of the two entities' being delineated by a boundary.

That said, we must not forget that two entities may also be "sewn" by a boundary, like neighboring countries, two parts of a shirt, or a fly able to sit on a water surface thanks to surface tension. Therefore, connection is the second intuitive association with the concept of boundary.

The third fundamental intuition associated with the notion of boundary has to do with the idea of *wholeness*. It seems quite intuitive to distinguish between entities maintaining some sort of integrity and collections of entities that do not together compose anything. Therefore, we need the concept of boundary in order to articulate what it means for some complex beings to form a unity; for *many* elements to be is some sense *one*.

Now, having assumed the three intuitions behind the primitive concept of boundary, there are plenty of things whose boundaries, if any, are problematic and therefore require deeper philosophical scrutiny before we move on to discuss the kinds of boundaries that are applicable to mind, cognition and niches. This is even more pressing when we realize that a boundary may not necessarily be a clearly discernible line, but something more contextual. It may not be a visible barrier with bulk, so to speak, like a wall or a cell membrane, but a more abstract entity determined by a set of conditions (think of the boundary of a tiger's hunting territory). Here, in addition to the primitive notion assumed as given, we need to refer to a derivative or complex concept of boundary. A more detailed investigation of some puzzling examples is necessary precisely because the boundaries relevant to cognitive systems and their niches, as we shall see, are among these more derivative cases.

To begin, the first question of concern to a philosopher working in the field of the ontology of boundaries is whether or not boundaries are *real* (large parts of this section come from Werner 2021b). For it seems at least *a priori* possible to approach all boundaries as a mere *façon de parler*, i.e., as entities brought forth by thinking, speaking or perceiving. This is, roughly, *anti-realism* with respect to boundaries. Characterized negatively, *realism* denies anti-realism and holds that at least some boundaries are produced by nature itself.

This debate draws on the distinction between genuine or *bona fide* boundaries and *fiat* boundaries proposed by Smith (1996; see also Varzi 2011, 2016). The distinction appeals to the observation that there seems to be a clear difference between "natural demarcations," which "would exist even in the absence of all delineating or conceptualizing activity" (Varzi 2016: 51), and those that seem artificial and thus depend on the action of perceivers or thinkers. The latter are dubbed *fiat* boundaries. Indeed, there must be something more essential, it is assumed, in the division between the stony surface of a mountain and the conventional, rather blurred boundary between the mountain and the piedmont. Generally, surfaces of things are usually seen as *bona fide* boundaries, while configurations of things are frequently delineated by *fiat*.

Think of living creatures as autopoietic/autonomous systems for which maintaining boundaries is not a contingent feature, but rather one of the factors that constitutes them as "bounded self-producing units engaged in traffic with their environments, where this traffic includes sensing and adaptive response" (Godfrey-Smith 2016: 780). The maintenance of a boundary is a definitional feature of autopoiesis and autonomy. Thus, organisms "need to have boundaries, to prevent movement towards thermodynamic equilibrium, but also need to ensure traffic across them" (Godfrey-Smith 2016: 778). This applies both to simpler as well as more complex organisms, thus those having bodies, where a body can be understood as "a collection of matter that, thanks to internal forces (cohesive, adhesive, gravitational, etc.) constitutes a unitary whole endowed with an identifiable boundary that separates it from its surroundings" (Villalobos & Razeto-Barry 2020: 8). It may seem, therefore, that "the boundary of the body is defined by the properties of the material that constitutes the physical unity itself, and not merely by some distinction (…) made by the observer" (Villalobos & Razeto-Barry 2020). This suggests that the boundary of a living creature is a good example of a *bona-fide* boundary.

However, there are cases that – although they certainly should not convince us that bodily boundaries are *fiat* – should nonetheless prompt us to reflect on the distinction between *fiat* and *bona fide*. A simple illustration of the somewhat indefinite nature of bodily boundaries is supplied when we consider cavities. As Keijzer and Arnellos put it, "animals have an internal gut in some form or other, where food items are digested inside the body but outside of the cells" (Keijzer & Arnellos 2017: 432). Therefore, the boundaries of the body *as a whole* cannot be identified with, say, the total sum of all the boundaries of the cells composing the tissues, thus with the actual matter of the body, contrary to what Villalobos and Razeto-Barry suggest. The cavities, although actually also filled with matter (air, for instance), are not, *qua cavities*, "collections of matter." From the ontological perspective, they are unusual entities, namely *holes* (see Casati & Varzi 1994 for a formalized theory). As such, they make the distribution of different sorts of matter *inside* the body possible. Therefore, these cavities, *qua holes*, somehow partake in the body, together with their somewhat less specified boundaries, thereby rendering the issue of the body's boundaries quite intricate and puzzling.

Moreover, if one considers the body as "a collection of matter" first and foremost, and takes skin as the paradigmatic bodily boundary, one needs to take into account internal tissues, i.e. mucosa, covering the internal cavity walls as well. For they delineate the actual material that the body is composed of from the material that happens to enter the body. Yet, they can hardly be compared to walls that merely separate two regions insofar as one of the very purposes of mucous membranes is to secrete specific chemical complexes, such as mucins. Hence, separating the tissue from its *products* seems rather artificial given that the latter play crucial roles, e.g., as parts of the immune system. Therefore, when speaking of the mucous *boundary*, arguably, one should speak of the tissue itself *and* the secreted chemicals. If so, however, then not only *physical* factors, strictly speaking, determine the boundary of a *living* body. The boundary at stake turns out to be a *functional role* played by several concentrated (*concatenating*, as Villalobos & Razeto-Barry 2020 put it, borrowing the term from linguistics and mathematical logic) as well as more dispersed entities rather than a clear-cut physical barrier. One might, therefore, argue that there are many factors determining the boundaries of the body and that they can be "drawn" in different "places" depending on the circumstances.

Finally, it is also a well-recognized fact that "multicellular organisms have vague boundaries with respect to which *cells* are parts of the organism and which are not" (Godfrey-Smith 2016: 781; emphasis added). A good illustration is provided by cases of symbiosis when, for example, environmentally acquired bacteria become part of a larger organism's digestive tract (see Pradeu 2011, 2012, 2016; O'Malley 2014). Symbiosis can be characterized as a long-lasting relationship between two organisms belonging to different species (McFall-Ngai 2002), or, additionally, as a long-lasting interaction that is beneficial to one of them and at least neutral for the other. The most familiar examples include the 10^{14} bacteria living in the human gut (Lee & Mazmanian 2010). Now, it is by no means clear whether or not they count as part of the hosting organism, and thus unclear where the boundary between the organism and its environment lies. Yet the organism is unable to actually maintain its metabolism without the bacteria, so treating them as external can also be considered an artificial *fiat*.

Therefore, the alternative proposal set forth by Pradeu (2011), following Burnet (1969), is roughly that the boundaries of complex organisms are not identical to the physical barriers established by the skin and are not the mere sum of the boundaries of all their constituents. Pradeu (2011) proposes to define an immunological criterion, namely that if there is a complex organism x, any cell or multicellular complex that is tolerated by x's immune system, thus satisfying the specific *conditions* imposed by the immune system in question, should be considered part of x, thereby justifying speaking of an *immunologically drawn boundary* between the organism and its immediate surroundings. The emphasis is placed upon the *conditions* establishing the boundary. The latter is not a single thing but a *role* played by many different entities engaged in the functioning the immune system.

Now, the cases invoked might compel somebody to endorse anti-realism; i.e., to hold that all boundaries within the biological realm are in fact determined by conventional fiats attributable to observers and scientists. But such a radical move would be too hasty, as the boundaries in question, however fuzzy, really *mean* something to the entities they delineate: it is *fundamental* for an organism to be bounded. The definitions of autopoiesis and autonomy already make it clear. The fact that this boundedness can be realized in a plurality of ways makes it no less critical. But can a realism based on the *bona fide* versus *fiat* distinction accommodate this plurality? It seems that a *bona fide* boundary, as originally defined by Smith (1996), cannot exist under one condition and disappear under another.

What is suggested here, therefore, is that speaking of multiple conditions establishing boundaries in diverse contexts or at different levels of complexity (call it *pluralism* with respect to boundaries) does not necessarily commit one to anti-realism (see Varzi 2011). Rather, it would seem that the distinction between realism and anti-realism based on the *bona fide* versus *fiat* dichotomy is too coarse to provide an adequate ontological account of the biological realm. And therefore, I presume, also of the realm of cognition.

The next question is whether the cases invoked above convey a more general message about familiar entities and their boundaries, including not only entities populating the biological realm but also the broader domain of complex material objects. After all, even some biological entities seem to be "wrapped" in clearly defined *surfaces*. For example, there appears to be a clear line delimiting the apple from the air around it.

Based on what has been said so far, it won't come as a surprise that some members of the 4E camp, such as Varela, Thompson and Rosch (1991), would strongly argue against the notion of bona-fide boundaries of things. This is because – they claim – there may be *different conditions* determining the surfaces of things, relative to the cognitive apparatus used. We read for example:

> But how are we to specify what counts as a surface? How are we to specify its edges, boundaries, texture, and orientation, if not in relation to some perceiver for whom these distinctions are relevant?
>
> (Varela et al. 1991: 167)

In a completely different context, namely in discussion with Smith's view of realism, Varzi formulated a somewhat constructivist account of surfaces in the following way:

> (...) the boundaries that strike us as "natural" are likely to reflect for the most part our cognitive limitations. Thus, earlier I mentioned the

> surface of an apple as an instance of a bona fide boundary (...). Physically speaking, however, we all know that an apple is not the solid, continuous substance that it seems to be. It is a smudgy crowd of tiny particles frantically dancing in empty space, and speaking of its surface is really like speaking of the surface of a swarm of bees (...). There are no such boundaries in the bona fide world. All involve a fiat demarcation whereby a plurality of smaller things are circumcluded and assembled by our cognitive system, bridging the gaps and connecting the dots. And what goes for apples goes for human bodies, water droplets, rocks, trees, chairs, and so on (...).
>
> (Varzi 2016: 56–57)

To substantiate this point, note first that when it comes to objects and their surfaces, humans are decidedly vision-centric creatures. Therefore, *visual* objects and *visible* boundaries serve as templates for the general conception of what *an object* is, what its boundaries are, and what perceptual acquaintance with these boundaries (surfaces) means. This fact stands out clearly, especially to those researchers who pay attention to other channels of perception, such as the auditory or olfactory systems.

Michael Kubovy and David Van Valkenburg, known for their studies on auditory perception, observe that "[l]anguage itself may lead us to believe that objects are visible by definition" (Kubovy & Van Valkenburg 2001: 98), and they refer to the *Oxford English Dictionary* to prove their point. Indeed, the term "object" is defined there as "something placed before the eyes, or presented to the sight or other sense" (Kubovy & Van Valkenburg 2001);[1] hence "other senses" are invoked, although somewhat marginally compared to the emphasis upon "eyes" and "sight." Meanwhile, Kubovy and Van Valkenburg hold that when it comes to perceptual channels other than vision, *the very criteria of objecthood* may change.

Consider how hearing is usually described. For example, when it is said "John hears a bird," one likely imagines a man and a bird sitting somewhere in a tree. If asked to draw this situation, one would quite likely add a line between the bird and John, showing the sound wave created by the bird's vocal organs reaching John's ears. But this image presents the scene *as it is seen* by an external observer, a primarily vision-centric creature. As a result, there is a *visual* bird, thus an object delineated by boundaries drawn in visible space, which *happens* to also produce sounds. However, if this external perspective is abandoned and an attempt is made to determine the actual relationship between the two entities, then there is no reason to prioritize visual over any other kind of perception. In order to be true to hearing thought of as a cognitive process in its own right and *as it actually occurs between two parties* (not in front of an external observer equipped with vision), a vision-independent idea of objecthood is required to capture the entity that is heard. And, going back to the example, it is by no means obvious that the boundaries of *this* entity will be identical to the boundaries of the "visual" bird.

In this context, Kubovy and Van Valkenburg (2001) came up with the concept of an *auditory object* whose objecthood is not defined in terms of space (visible space, to be precise) and time, but primarily in terms of time and frequency. This means that the cognitive system may decide whether or not a given sequence of percepts constitutes an object by first taking into account what is perceived to be the pitch of the sound. Of course, in reality many other things are taken into account, such as the sound's intensity and timbre. Yet, frequency is the key factor and sufficient to provide the illustration required here.

Therefore, the conditions determining the boundaries of auditory objects differ. Kubovy and Van Valkenburg make a very clear point on this matter:

> Another phenomenon characterizes visual objects: the formation and assignment of edges (...). Let us suppose that any object, be it visual or auditory, must have an edge or a boundary.
>
> (Kubovy & Van Valkenburg 2001: 103–104)

> Likewise, in audition, we find edges in pitch, and edges in time, but not in space. The claim that there are edges in pitch may seem strange, but a moment's thought will show that the idea is quite natural. A biologically important source is periodic, at least over short periods of time. Therefore, it is characterized by a fundamental frequency that can be thought of as its lower edge in pitch (...). It is further characterized by the shape of its leading edge in pitch-time, its attack, and its trailing edge in pitch-time, its decay.
>
> (Kubovy & Van Valkenburg 2001: 110–111)

But the same applies to all the other senses. In other words, this suggests that the seemingly natural and bona-fide boundaries of familiar things are not as un-negotiable as it may seem at first.

Now, this could be read, again, as inevitably leading to some sort of anti-realism. One can conclude that, in many cases, speaking of boundaries and surfaces is, to use an apt comparison by Simons (1991), like speaking of the "flat top" of a fakir's bed of nails. But does it mean these boundaries are *not real*? Suppose that Simons's words are taken literally for a moment: if one is actually sitting on a fakir's bed, there are surely *conditions*, determined by the construction of the bed on the one hand and by the sensitivity of the sitting person's nervous system on the other, establishing, *for this person*, the point at which sitting on the bed starts to really hurt. So there certainly is a "line" between the sitting subject and the bed that the subject does not want to cross, and the fact that it depends on the conditions referring to the machinery of the subject's nervous system *does not make it less real*, at least insofar as being *not real* means being some sort of merely imaginary entity. The boundary just described is certainly not merely imaginary.

I do not hereby wish to advocate for a new meaning of the term "real," reducing it to the functioning of a cognitive apparatus. However, the point is that insofar as the *criteria* used to distinguish real things and their boundaries from fiats do appeal to a cognitive apparatus, the *bona fide* versus *fiat* distinction no longer seems so clear-cut. Therefore, there emerges a difficulty pertaining to such qualifications as "bona fide," "natural" or even "real." If they are to be the opposite of fictions or epiphenomena, it is clear, as indicated above, that there are boundaries resulting from "bridging the gaps and connecting the dots," as Varzi puts it, that nonetheless can hardly be thought of as *not* real, at least insofar as "real" implies "having real consequences," thus having the capacity to influence a course of action. If, however, "real" cannot refer to anything that comes into being as the outcome of an interaction, but instead must be pregiven, as Varela et al. (1991) would have it, then a large group of consequential boundaries (listed above) must count as fiats. This, however, of itself seems a purely theoretical fiat.

A provisional diagnosis proposed at this point is that the *bona fide* versus *fiat* distinction is founded on the idea of a "detached" subject, as illustrated by Varela and collaborators in the already cited passage in which they speak of the "traditional wisdom" which states that the "environment in which organisms evolve and that they come to know is given, fixed, and unique" and that "organisms are basically parachuted into a pregiven environment" (Varela et al 1991: 198). Thus, one is faced with the following alternative: either one accepts that there are pregiven (or ready-made, as Putnam 1987 would say) boundaries in reality, and that the subject "parachutes" into the said realm and proceeds to create additional boundaries by drawing *fiat* lines, or one agrees with those who claim that since there are no pregiven boundaries in the pregiven world, the "parachuting" subject draws them *all* as fiats.

Meanwhile, the real source of friction here is the idea of the "parachuting" subject. If, in line with what 4E commands, we reject this idea, the whole puzzle of boundaries will have to be reconsidered. The latter is what I plan to do.

6.4 Re-introducing boundaries

I shall now re-introduce the notion of boundary (following Werner 2020a). To begin, arguably, for each *complex, structured* entity there are some *locative requirements* to be realized in a specific medium. As Chapter 1 figuratively put it, things have their locative footprints. However, boundaries are not necessary for all such locative footprints. Homogeneous mixtures, which by the way were also studied ontologically by Llored and Harré (2014; see also Fine 1996), provide examples of structures that clearly have spatial requirements but are not so concerned with any particular "architecture" of the region they occupy. If ones mixes a bit of glucose and water, the glucose molecules will push and shove to win some space amid the water molecules, and the mixture will thereby occupy more space than water alone. But the glucose molecules will not be particularly "interested" in maintaining stable bonds with each other; they disperse easily, which is the reason why we call such a mixture homogeneous.

In contrast, think now of a micelle with a portion of surfactant introduced into a water solution. Due to their surface tension the two substances set up a relatively stable structure of a micelle, clearly delineated from the water around them. Here is a viable heuristic: if two structured entities are supposed to couple, they sometimes "negotiate" where one of them *ends* and the other *begins*, as during peace negotiations between two neighboring countries. And the "negotiated" line sets the *conditions* of their further interactions. They "negotiate" a certain "architecture" of the realm of their interactions. This means that *once the boundary is set*, all relations occurring between the two entities are somehow mediated or conditioned by the established boundaries.

Hence every complex entity needs an address, yet *some* entities need more than that. Namely, some *interactions* between such entities bring forth further, *relatively stable structures* which in turn can influence subsequent events and interactions. What this means is that for *some* interactions between structured entities, the IN versus OUT distinction is critical. Think of the cell and its interactions with the medium and with other cells. Hence the line dividing the two coupling structures must be a critical issue they "negotiate" if they are to coincide in space.

All that being said, here is the core idea I shall be unpacking more technically in due course: it is possible to think of boundaries as *factors specifying the domain of possible interactions*; thus, making the surroundings of a given entity suitable to that entity's capacities and needs. First of all, if a given realm is supposed to serve as a domain of possible interactions between a cognitive system and specific segments of the latter's surroundings, it must be (at least) *relatively* stable; one might say – organized and predictable to some degree. The key word here is "possible." For speaking of *possible* interactions brings up different scenarios of action, some of which become actualized. Meanwhile, in a completely unstable and disorganized realm it would not be possible to come up with any *scenarios* of action at all. Going back to our introductory reflections on Tooby and De Vore's (1987) notion of the cognitive niche, the domain of possible interactions is one in which certain *patterns* of cause–effect bonds are specified, singled out or modeled, with boundaries playing a crucial role.

Therefore, a cognitive niche is, among other things, determined by a specific setup of boundaries; an architecture thereof. According to the proposal to be set forth, boundaries are crucial not only for the system's self-production and self-maintenance (for its autonomy), thus for the relative stability of the system itself, but *also for the relative stability of the system's dealings with its surroundings.*

To play this role, however, boundaries must be understood in a new way. The *bona fide* versus *fiat* distinction is of no use in this new context.

Here is the first distinction I propose instead:

(28) The *interactional* boundaries (*i*-boundaries) of *x* are boundaries that exist in virtue of *x*'s interactions (structural coupling when *x* is an autonomous system) with another such entity *y* and thus can exist only insofar as *x* interacts with *y*.[2]

Metaphorically speaking, interactive boundaries are like stop signs indicating where the territory occupied by one structured entity ends and the territory of another entity begins.

If so, then we can also think of the complementary concept:

(29) The pregiven boundaries (*g*-boundaries) of *x* are boundaries that are determined solely by *x*'s own structural features.

This distinction is, of course, a theoretical fiction. For example, the boundaries of organisms, especially of complex organisms such as animals, can be seen as exemplifications of both kinds of boundaries, therefore, each attribution of a given boundary to a single type is a certain idealization performed in comparison to the relevant attribution of a different boundary. For example, while immunological boundaries (a provisional concept drawing on Pradeu (2011, 2012)) are natural candidates for *i*-boundaries, skin is a *g*-boundary in comparison to the immunological barrier. This, however, does not change the obvious fact that skin also requires specific conditions in the animal's surroundings, e.g., air pressure, in order to play its boundary function. Yet, it does not seem plausible to simply classify all organismic boundaries as *i*-boundaries, for if we were to make this theoretical move, we might lose the capacity to articulate certain crucial functional differences between the various barriers delineating a living creature.

Furthermore, arguably, there is something special about the boundaries of *organisms*, whether they are *i*-boundaries or *g*-boundaries. Godfrey-Smith emphasizes that "the special features of subjects are organizational"

(Godfrey-Smith 2016: 776). This means that "part of what we have to understand is a certain kind of *unit*" (Godfrey-Smith 2016; emphasis added). Therefore, all the various processes that *organisms* comprise at *different levels* of complexity are parts of a *unified system* constituted by a unified set of conditions or a unifying organizational *principle* or power. To get a sense of what this means, consider the following two of Daniel E. Koshland's Jr. (2002) seven Pillars of Life, as he calls them:

> The first pillar of life is a Program. By program I mean an organized plan that describes both the ingredients themselves and the kinetics of the interactions among ingredients as the living system persists through time. For the living systems we observe on Earth, this program is implemented by the DNA that encodes the genes of Earth's organisms and that is replicated from generation to generation, with small changes but always with the overall plan intact. The genes in turn encode for chemicals – the proteins, nucleic acids, etc. – that carry out the reactions in living systems.
>
> (...)
>
> The third of the pillars of life is Compartmentalization. All the organisms that we consider living are confined to a limited volume, surrounded by a surface that we call a membrane or skin that keeps the ingredients in a defined volume and keeps deleterious chemicals – toxic or diluting – on the outside.
>
> (Koshland Jr 2002: 2215)

Compartmentalization is realized by different systems of boundaries, which explicitly relates to the issues we have been discussing here. However, a particular compartmentalization must be determined, as everything else in the living creature, by the "program" Koshland Jr. emphasizes in the first quote. Therefore, taking the two Pillars together, it makes sense to speak of systems of boundaries as realizations of the "program," which – when generalized as part of our applied ontology – leads to a new kind of boundary.

To get a better grasp of this proposal, compare the organism with a structured entity of a different kind. For example, if we take a plastic Lego brick, it turns out that the conditions establishing complex Lego structures, houses or vehicles, do not maintain any non-contingent relationship with the conditions active at the chemical level of molecules which make the *plastic* itself possible. We can rephrase it this way: it is irrelevant from the perspective of the structure realized at the chemical level whether the chemical structure in question constitutes a Lego brick or something else, and whether that brick is a component of a house or another assemblage because the factors active at the "higher" level and determining different structures there have no influence on the factors operating at the "lower" level. Whether one uses Legos to make a house or a train has no effect on the chemical structure of the Lego bricks used. On the other hand, it doesn't really matter for the structures composed of Lego bricks whether they are made of plastic or another kind of material. Of course, one may have certain preferences, e.g., preferring plastic to metal, but a variety of other materials would do just as well.

Meanwhile, in the case of living creatures, there *are* of course different conditions active at different levels of complexity, but what seems to make organisms unique is that all levels of complexity *work in concert* toward a single goal (maintaining the system's autonomy), and even the most basic level of chemical reactions between cells contributes to the execution of the more sophisticated metabolic or sensorimotor functions. In effect, the organism is a *unitary* machinery or system committed to remaining out of equilibrium with its surroundings, transforming energy, developing, reproducing, behaving, etc.

Getting back to our main topic, all this means that while there *can* be many different setups of *g*-boundaries and *i*-boundaries, determined by different conditions, between the organism and its environment, all of these diverse boundaries – in line with Koshland Jr.'s first Pillar – *form a unified system* governed, as it were, by *a unifying principle or program.*

Therefore, there is a need to define another type of boundaries:

(30) The *principle/program-based boundaries* (*p*-boundaries) of *x* are boundaries determined by *x*'s unifying principle/program *p*.

The concept of *program* goes beyond the limits of applied ontology and thus is taken here as given, together with all the other notions introduced earlier, e.g., autonomy or structural coupling. Actually, the autonomy conditions that 4E talks about may be considered as one of such "programs."

A natural complement of the *p*-boundary is the concept of *free* boundary, for lack of a better term:

(31) The *free* boundaries (*f*-boundaries) of *x* are boundaries that are not determined by any unifying principle governing the functioning of *x* as a whole.

Now, one might ask how the two proposed typologies relate to each other. I shall not dwell too much on these pure possibilities (or impossibilities) since, as I mentioned, my purpose is to formulate an applied ontology of cognitive systems and their environments, not a general theory of boundaries and locations. I shall, therefore, limit the scope of this analysis to combinations that may prove useful given the actual goals of this investigation. We, therefore, have:

g-boundaries	*i-boundaries*	
(I)	(II)	*p*-boundaries
(III)	(IV)	*f*-boundaries

Consider the following provisional examples:

Category (IV) includes, in my understanding, what Smith (1996) called *fiat* boundaries, thus those that are grounded in an entity's interactions while at the same time maintaining no close ties with the entity's internal principles (if any). For example, delineating a parcel of land and calling it "Texas" has little to do with the objective, physicochemical and geographical features of the said parcel and is only relevant to the fact that the parcel in question stands in relation to a certain group of people.

Category (I) most likely falls into Smith's *bona fide* category. These are the boundaries that things have only in virtue of their own structure and independently of their interactions. However, insofar as these boundaries are independent of interactions, and insofar as cognition *is* a kind of interaction (not mere "copying" nature), they remain unknown to us. In other words, we have good empirical reasons to claim that the cognized boundaries of things are at least to some extent dependent on how we cognize them (recall the distinction between visual objects and auditory objects brought up earlier in this chapter), and that we do not have access to any other boundaries. Nonetheless, things *in themselves*, to use the Kantian phrase, i.e., the stuff that reality is composed of independently of how it presents itself to cognizers, may have boundaries that are clean and clear of any influence from perception, interaction, categorization, etc. There is no reason to deny the latter belief, although we cannot actually validate it either.

On the other hand, we may also consider (II), and actually this is *the key scenario* if we are to provide a proper interpretation of the shift to the mind-*in*-a-place paradigm advocated by 4E. Here a thing is wrapped in boundaries that on the one hand are grounded in the nature, thus the "principle" of the thing in question, while, on the other hand depend on its interactions, *including cognition* (if a cognitive system is involved). This is the key innovation introduced by 4E, although never spelled out explicitly in this manner – namely, positing cognition as a kind of "worldmaking" activity, to use Goodman's (1978) famous term, which however is not about projecting something from scratch, imposing a structure on some formless gunk, but grounded in the dynamics of system–surroundings interactions which give rise to a variety of bounded structures: cognizers on the one hand, and their cognitive niches on the other. Providing this dynamic with a suitable ontological rendering is the goal of the present endeavor.

Organisms should perhaps belong to both (I) and (II), since all of their boundaries, most likely, must be program-governed, and yet some of them, as I have already shown, are also determined by the organism's interactions with its environment. What makes organisms special, at least provisionally, is the fact that both their *g*-boundaries and their *i*-boundaries *are* necessarily also *p*-boundaries, meaning that the unifying principle(s) determine the conditions, for example, the prerequisites, of any boundary "negotiations" with surrounding entities. In other words – and this is the more general message that we must take to heart here – a boundary's being interactional does *not* mean that it is free of any internal-to-the-system determinations. The governing principle(s) of the system can "design" certain *i*-boundaries thought of as the above-mentioned prerequisites for locative "negotiations."

All of the above claims are provisional, however, since each of them merits an ontological study in its own right, not to mention the need to refer to empirical studies if a proper ontology of organismic boundaries is to be provided. There is no place here to conduct such a sweeping investigation, but part of it shall be done in reference to cognitive systems and their cognition-specific environments.

That said, the key question to be addressed by this ontological study does not concern organisms as such, but cognitive systems – be it representational systems engaged in the pursuit of information exchange and computation, or autonomous systems involved in structural coupling. What kind of bounded loci are they? What kind of boundaries do they maintain: *g*- or *i*-boundaries, *p*- or *f*-boundaries? What kind of bounded locus is their environment and what type of boundaries do we find there?

Note that these are reformulations of the concerns elicited already in Chapters 1–4. We are getting closer now to addressing them. This shall be done in Chapter 7.

6.5 Further conceptual amendments: *i*-openness, *i*-closedness, *g*-openness, etc.

Given that we have four new kinds of boundaries, our ontological landscape becomes somewhat more complicated (which is a birthmark of physical-behavioral units elicited by Smith 2001). This is because for each of the notions in sections 6.1 and 6.2, we now have four variants, so that for any entity *x* we obtain:

(32) The *i*-closure of *x*, is identical to the sum of *x* and all the interactional boundaries (*i*-boundaries) of *x*.

Analogously, we can define *g*-closure, *p*-closure and *f*-closure. This allows us to amend the relevant definitions of open and closed entities, as a result of which we obtain the following alternatives:

(33) Any *x* is either *i*-open or *i*-closed or partly *i*-open.

Analogously, for *g*-openness, *g*-closedness, *p*-openness, etc.

Note that this produces a significant bulk of possible combinations of boundaries that a single entity can maintain, and a considerable variety of openness- or closedness-related qualities that it can possess. For in principle, I assume, any combination of the above-mentioned kinds of boundaries and qualities is possible, although this merits a more in-depth formal-ontological inquiry. For example, *x* may be *i*-open and at the same time *g*-closed, which means that *x* has its own, structurally determined pregiven boundary whether or not it interacts with anything, yet there is no *specific* boundary "designed" for the sake of *x*'s interactions, thus one that *x* would "negotiate" with other entities. One might argue that in this case the *g*-boundary plays the role of an *i*-boundary, but still an entity's function or role needs to be conceptually distinguished from its nature. Therefore, *x* is in this case *i*-open despite being *g*-closed.

Further on, *x* may be *i*-closed and *p*-open, which means that either the principle governing *x*'s structure does not determine *x*'s boundary, or *x* simply lacks a principle, and yet it has some boundary added to it independently of that principle (which makes it also an *f*-boundary) – think, for example, of a swarm of bees which, it seems, has no *p*-boundary whatsoever, meaning that it is a *p*-open entity, but usually it is delineated by perceptual *fiat* (we see the swarm as a kind of "cloud" that is blurred but nonetheless begins and ends somewhere), which suggests *i*-closedness insofar as cognition is thought of as a kind of interaction.

In addition to all of the above, given the plurality of kinds of boundaries, we also end up with quite a number of subtypes of external (direct or remote) connection: if we have *i*-boundaries, we could speak of *i*-connection; and respectively for *g*-connection; *p*-connection and *f*-connection.

If so, we eventually also have *i*-enclosement, *g*-enclosement, *p*-enclosement and *f*-enclosement.

Some of these scenarios or qualities may be redundant and empirically unlikely, but since each case would require separate discussion and careful analysis of actual, empirically recorded instances, I leave all these *a priori* possibilities open. Only some of them shall be exemplified in the ontological "reconstruction" of the evolution of (cognitive) niche construction, which I am about to unfold in Chapter 7.

6.6 Fulfilment and locative capacity

Equipped with the basic concepts of locative ontology, and having discussed the puzzle of boundaries in greater detail, we are now in a position to tackle more complex structures. This means not only an entity's exact location, thus the "hole" filled exactly with the thing in question, but also how the entity in question can fill a locus established by other entities, composing a kind of physical-behavioral unit or (as I prefer to call it) *ecological unit* with them – a new object constituted not by direct ties between the entities *themselves* but rather by specific relations between *their locations (regions)* which we usually characterize in terms of *being-in*. Therefore, the final goal now is to introduce the concept of *bounded locus*, already illustrated in Chapter 1 in reference to the work of the linguists Vandeloise (1991, 1994), Herskovits (1986) and Tyler and Evans (2003).

Recall the examples of wine in a glass and a fly that happens to have gotten into the glass. One might say that the former is a simple case in which being in the glass can be unpacked in terms of touching or abutting. Yet, first, these two notions are by no means trivial and also require some elaboration (see Casati & Varzi 1999), and, second – they do not seem to be constitutive of being-in exclusively. The sad scenario of the glass breaking and the wine spilling on the floor also involves touching, and yet is not an exemplification, at least not a standard one, of a bounded locus. On the other hand, the poor fly does not touch the glass at all while clearly being *in* it. Therefore, the *glass + wine* and *glass + fly* compounds require some more work, not to mention units such as *cave + bear* or *morning traffic + me driving*.

A good move is to appeal to relations between regions, not things themselves. For example, it may seem that the exact location of the wine is a proper part of the exact location of the glass (almost identical to the latter), and the same applies to the fly. But is this condition actually satisfied? I have already pointed out that between the *actual matter* that the glass is made of and the fly (its matter) there is something that *looks* like empty space that is in fact filled with air. Therefore, the location of the fly can be considered a proper part of the location of the *fly + glass* compound only insofar as we consider the (supposedly empty) *region* filled with air to be *part of the glass* too. It may seem obvious that this region *is* part of the glass since it is the very nature of a glass to "provide" *space within it* to other entities, such as wine, water or flies, more or less in the sense in which Gibson spoke of affordances. The glass affords to other things the possibility of *filling it*. So the supposedly "empty" region must be part of the glass, for otherwise the very idea of *filling the glass* would make no sense whatsoever.

Fair enough, but what happens if we abandon the glass reference? The actual material parts of *this thing* (let us stop calling it a "glass" for the moment) occupy a certain region. For the sake of the argument, let us call it the "substantial" region (the exact location of the physical substance that the entity in question is made of). It turns out that what we *intuitively* take to be the *interior of the glass* does not belong to this substantial region. Therefore, the location of what we previously called the *glass* cannot be only the sum of the locations of its actual material parts. The location of *the glass* must somehow also encompass the space to be filled. But what region *exactly* is encompassed in this case? Another interesting illustration from Chapter 1 – the pearl in the bowl – shows that there is no obvious answer. The top pearl is intuitively said to be *in* the bowl, yet "geometrically" it is not. Therefore, the region to be filled when we speak of something being *in the bowl* may extend beyond what we would otherwise regard as the empty *space inside* the bowl.

Smith and Varzi (1999) were aware of these problems. To resolve them, they invoked the notion of cavity. It is a feature of a great variety of real things, not only glasses, that they have cavities, thus specific "holes," as constituents of their structure. "Holes" are peculiar constituents, for they do not by themselves have objecthood, but piggyback on solid things, so to speak. The best example is the animal body which contains an internal cavity responsible for letting certain substances in (through, e.g., breathing and eating) and letting others out.

A solution proposed by Smith and Varzi, among other conceptual posits, refers to the notion of compact closure. First, the authors distinguish between objects that have connected boundaries and those that have disconnected ones. Members of the first group are clearly cut off from their surroundings, while the boundaries of members of the other group are more or less scattered, or at least divided into segments. For example, the boundary of a rock is connected, while the boundary of a pile of rocks is disconnected. Provided that this distinction is made, the compact closure of an object is characterized as "the smallest entity whose boundary is connected and which includes the object as part" (Smith & Varzi 1999: 231). Hence, when it comes to the glass in our example, we can say that what we refer to as *a glass* is a certain quantity of physical substance taken as part of its compact closure. Speaking of *a glass* refers to such compact closure, not to the material substance alone.

Practically, speaking of the smallest object with connected boundaries implies drawing the shortest "line" in a place that lacks a proper boundary.

Therefore, the glass becomes topologically closed by the imaginary straight line at the top, between the two rising material edges.

This solution, although formally correct and arguably applicable to a variety of cases, is not satisfactory. To understand why, just consider the pearl in the bowl example again. Or think of the same glass, but this time filled with sand or blueberries. If we put in as much of it as possible, like we did with the wine, we will end up with a different line, thus a different closing boundary. This time, the line is likely to be curved and to extend beyond what Smith and Varzi (1999) would consider to be the boundary of the relevant compact closure. But is there any *a priori* reason to prefer a straight closing boundary to a curved one? Moreover, is there any *a priori* reason to seek *any* closing boundary?

We are naturally inclined to think that *some* boundary must finally be drawn, for otherwise the glass would not be *a glass* at all. However, if we were to imagine some intelligent creature living on another planet, with a different cognitive and sensorimotor apparatus, seeing a glass for the first time at a welcome party on Earth, it would by no means be obvious to that creature that the thing we refer to as a "glass" also contains a portion of supposedly empty space, and therefore that the object in question *needs* an additional boundary (closure). It is likely that the quantity of matter composing the object would stand out as a perceivable substance to our extraterrestrial guest, which is what I already alluded to above when speaking of the "substantial" location of the glass, but there is no reason to assume that the extraterrestrial would have *any* preconceived idea not only as to where the "missing" boundary should be drawn, but also of the fact that there *is* in fact a "missing" boundary.

To further illustrate this point with a more mundane example, think of a cavity drilled in the rocky side of a mountain. If we consider this particular part of the mountain as *a cave* in which a bear could live, therefore as a potential habitat, a niche, it will be a partially bounded entity requiring closure. But if we are interested in what the mountain is made of, and not in potential shelters, e.g., we are drilling for limestone to build something, we will perceive that very same part of the mountain as an entity with somewhat irregular but connected boundaries. There will be no hole and, therefore, no need for any closure. Hence, holes are what they are if we want to put something in them, it would seem.

Therefore, as already flagged, we need to account for the fact that some entities not only have *their own* exact locations, but also a certain *locative capacity*: that they can somehow *intervene*, for lack of a better term, in the surrounding realm and impact the locations of other entities. Crucially, "offering" a locative capacity to other things is not about having a particular shape or structure. Arguably, some structures or shapes may seem more likely to possess this quality, but this is a highly contextual issue so we cannot say anything about it as part of this ontological investigation. The goal is to account for what locative capacity is, while the question of which entities actually possess it is an empirical one.

Here is my proposal:

(34) The locative capacity of x is the sum of regions *such that* all things (exactly) located in them are in locative connection with x.

For example, if we consider the actual matter that a glass or a bowl is composed of, we can also point to specific regions in the world such that if something is located in those regions it will be externally connected to the location of the matter the bowl is composed of. In other words, however unnatural it may sound, the matter composing a bowl has a locative capacity that "expects" pearls, fruits and a variety of other entities, as Figure 6.1A shows (and therefore affords something to them), yet not all entities. This means that there are regions in the world (those we would intuitively regard as the interior of a bowl plus some portion of regions surrounding it; see Figure 6.1B) such that whenever something is located in them, it is in locative connection – and in *locative* connection only! – with the matter that the bowl is made of.

Of course, it is not a priori decided which regions belong to the locative capacity of a given entity and which ones do not (e.g., in Figure 6.1B, the said portion of regions could be extended or cut down; their "shape" depends on the entities actually located in a given realm; generally we should not stick too much to this or any other depiction of locative capacity which is thought of a very abstract concept). This specification is context-dependent (relative to a fixed set of objects surrounding x).

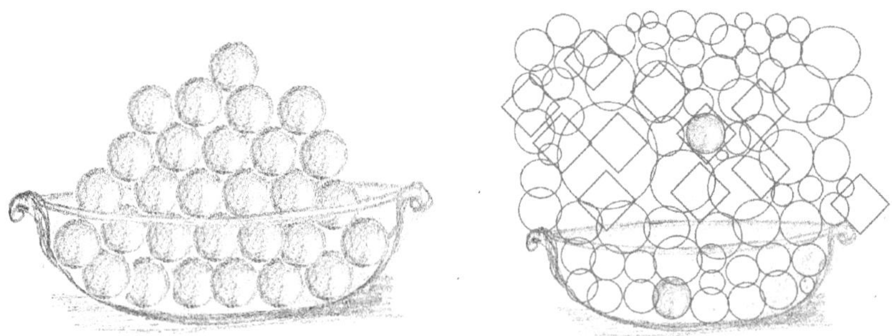

A B

Figure 6.1

With the latter caveat in mind, I propose:

(35) The fulfilment of x equals the sum of x and its locative capacity.

Note that the boundaries of fulfilment have not been specified yet. This shall be our next step: to simplify somewhat, we can say that *bounded loci* are *bounded fulfilments* (see below). Meanwhile, let us appreciate the abstractness of the concept we have just defined, for this is the most general schema of an *ecological unit*. Examples of the latter include not only boxes in which toys are hidden from the eyes of children or the glasses and bowls we have examined several times now, but also various kinds of natural habitats: a cave, a hole burrowed by a worm in the soil, a nest or a loosely defined jumble of branches in a tree, surrounded by other branches so that a squirrel can be safe there from birds of prey. Our apartments with us and our stuff inside them are also ecological units in that sense, and by the same token, so are whole towns, the infrastructure we build, etc. Having a conceptual grasp of ecological units is, therefore, important because speaking only of the substances they are composed of would be insufficient, and having a purely abstract grasp of their locations would not be sufficient either. We need to capture their locative relations, with some selected entities possessing this specific capacity, as I put it provisionally, to *intervene in the locative realm*, thus with entities having locative capacity.

6.7 Bounded locus

The key idea I propose is this: a bounded locus is an ecological unit in the sense outlined above, equipped with boundaries. Let us begin by characterizing closed and partly open, *or* partly closed fulfilments:

(36) A closed fulfilment of x is identical to the sum of x and its locative capacity, such that the sum is a closed object.
(37) A partly open fulfilment of x is identical to the sum of x and its locative capacity, such that the sum is not a closed object.

The two definitions above can be read as stipulations that a fulfilment cannot be a fully open object – it must have a boundary, even if it is not entirely closed. However, (36) and (37) do not specify the kind of boundaries a fulfilment must possess, therefore we may have *g*-fulfilments or *i*-fulfilments; *p*-fulfilments or *f*-fulfilments.

That said, we can now move on to our main target: defining a bounded locus. However, the variety of contextual cases, some of which were elicited by means of the examples above and in Chapter 1, suggests that we require several concepts of a bounded locus, not just a single one. As with the concept of connection, the bounded locus *simpliciter* shall be introduced as an umbrella term.

If we take "*x* is a bounded locus for *y*" as a generic relation, we must first characterize the concept of a *closed* bounded locus, so the context "*x* is a closed bounded locus for *y*." I propose:

(38) *x* is a closed bounded locus for *y* when *x* is a closed fulfilment (strictly speaking when *x* = the closed fulfilment of *x*) and *x* encloses *y* (fully or partly).

This means that *x* and *y* make up a closed ecological unit in the sense given above, and crucially that *x* mediates the connections that its filler *y* can maintain with other entities — those not bounded by *x*. Remember that enclosement stands for a situation in which *all* or *some* connections set by *y* must be mediated by *locative* connection with *x*. Therefore, when *x* is a bounded locus for *y* and the former fully encloses the latter, *y* can maintain connection only with entities that are also within the locative capacity of *x*. Intuitively, if you have a toy in the box and you want to grab it, you need to put your hand into the box. In the case of partial enclosement this applies to some but not all entities that *y* would like to connect with.

Next, we have:

(39) *x* is a partly *open* bounded locus for *y* when *x* is a partly open fulfilment and *x* *partly* encloses *y*.

Given all these kinds of boundaries and enclosement, we have a wide range of bounded loci: *i*-bounded locus or *g*-bounded locus; *p*-bounded locus or *f*-bounded locus.

Recall the pearl in the bowl example again. Herskovits (1986) proposed that a certain causal factor is responsible for why we regard the top pearl as located in the bowl. Compare this case to a situation in which a pearl is suspended on a string from the ceiling and hanging over the bowl in the exact same location as the topmost pearl in the pile. Clearly, nobody would say that this suspended pearl is in the bowl. The pile, therefore, according to Herskovits, indicates a certain causal relation between the top pearl and the bowl, which serves as a pivotal additional factor making the top pearl be *in* the bowl in some derivative sense.

This is still not sufficient, however. Let us imagine that there is no pile but a different arrangement between the bowl and the pearl still located at the same address in the universe, such that the direction of causal connection is still the same as in the pile of pearls scenario. For example, the pearl is attached by a thin rigid wire to the sides of the bowl, and as a result is suspended over the bowl. This hardly counts as being *in* the bowl nevertheless.

What this last case tells us is that, however, significant the causal bond (its direction), it is crucial that the said causal bond fit into a specific *locative pattern*. Otherwise, it bears no relation to *being-in*. I propose that there must be a *sequence of connected regions* in order for *being-in* to obtain. As for the original example, the specific causal bond between the pearl at the top of the pile and the bowl renders the latter a bounded locus because of the specific locative arrangement, i.e., the bond obtaining between entities whose locations (regions) are connected. Causation here fills in the pattern created by a *particular arrangement* of connected regions. This arrangement is precisely what I regard as the locative capacity of the bowl. The bowl is an open bounded locus for the top pearl because the pearl is within the locative capacity of the bowl and the bowl "mediates" some (though not all) connections maintained by the pearl with the other entities. Thus, there are connections maintained by the pearl that require the connected entities to also be within the locative capacity of the bowl.

But let us leave the pearl, which was supposed to propel our imagination forward, and think of ecological phenomena such as niches and territories. A niche built/inhabited by an organism, which can serve as the prototypical example of an ecological unit while at the same time being very confusing ontologically (as pointed out by Smith 2001; see Chapter 5), also counts as a bounded locus. It clearly intervenes in the organism's connections, encompassing its tenants, and therefore is not just *a* place where the organism *happens* to be located. The bond between the niche and its tenant clearly involves a certain vortex of causal bonds between the organism and the surrounding entities, which arguably includes entities placed outside of the niche, with there being a certain *pattern* of causal ties determined by the niche. Therefore, niches are defined by their locative capacity at the most fundamental level, and by a more complex capacity to serve as bounded loci. This intuition shall be unpacked more technically in the next chapter.

Before we move on, however, the conceptual framework just rolled out must be supplemented with a couple of notions alluding to a more dynamic aspect of ecological units. Once this is done, we shall be able to define two kinds of bounded loci in terms of *how* they intervene in the capacity of their occupants to maintain connections with non-occupants.

6.8 Containers and frames

Within the proposed framework, as it stands now, either something *is* or *is not* closed, open, connected or disconnected, etc. This is especially confusing with respect to connection and relative location (the variety of subtypes thereof), since it seems rather intuitive, if not utterly trivial, that complex entities in the familiar world, especially living creatures, change their position, establish or break off connections, etc. As a matter of fact, a similar dynamic was suggested implicitly when I introduced the notions of enclosement and of bounded locus. For the intuitive message underpinning these ideas goes more or less like this: if x is a bounded locus for y and you want to get access to y, you need to somehow take x into account, i.e., you need to be (at least) in locative connection to x. Yet, to *be* in locative connection to x is not a precondition for your getting access to y in the sense that you can only connect with y in one way or another if you *are* tied to x. Instead, *becoming* tied to x, at least in the form of locative connection, is something you cannot avoid *at the moment* you are getting in touch with y. All this is about *becoming connected*, not so much *being* connected.

Let us return to some of the examples from Chapter 1. In at least some of them we clearly saw that the relation of being-in played an additional role for the entities in question, which was not merely about providing an address. For example, being *in prison* refers to a more or less permanent state of confinement, thereby endowing the said facility with the function of providing this peculiar service to prisoners. To take a different case, being in a state of war refers to a situation or state which also proves to be a specific kind of confinement, but this time the relevant role is conferred on an arrangement of people, things, processes, events, etc. Quite contrary to being "in touch" or "in light of," where the role involves exposition, the very opposite of confinement.

The conceptual toolbox of contemporary philosophy offers several ways of unpacking the main idea that I am about to put forward, including Molnar's (2003) metaphysics of powers or various theories of causality (e.g., Woodward 2003). There is no space and actually no need to dwell here on the details of either of these posits. Instead, based on the study conducted by Sloman et al. (2009), I take two locutions to be understandable: "x enables/allows y" and "x prevents y."

This is not about causal relations proper, but rather about an entity's capacity to *create conditions* in which something is *more or less likely to happen.* For example, I can give my child some amount of money, thereby enabling her to make a variety of purchases, but I do not make any of the actual purchases (it is up to my daughter whether she buys a book or a cosmetic, or buys nothing and keeps the money). In this case, *enabling something* means *setting the stage for something to come into being* but not causing this thing to actually arise. This capacity is crucial, yet rather weak (it's close to Woodward's 2003 interventionist causation, applied by representational mechanicism; recall Chapter 3, but also directly informed by Perzanowski's 2004 formal ontology of "makings" such as the modal relation of "making possible").

Meanwhile, the opposite capacity is quite strong. It means creating or contributing to the creation of conditions such that something is very unlikely to occur (in extreme cases its occurrence becomes impossible). Hence, it is not only about blocking a particular occurrence (of a given entity, event or action at a given moment), e.g., when a policeman is preventing the actions of a criminal. Instead, it is about creating conditions in which certain actions are practically impossible, or highly unlikely. To take a politically charged example, consider gun laws in relation to the individual bravery of a police officer: the intention, or ideal outcome of these laws is to create conditions in which certain forms of violence are highly unlikely. To consider a different scenario, I can confiscate all of my child's money as a form of punishment, thereby ideally making all purchases impossible.

Finally, we arrive at the point where two core notions can be re-introduced, starting with that of containment. Recall how crucial the notion of a container was for certain interpretations of the traditional views on cognition – those of Ryle, Popper and Lakoff and Johnson. It was also central for the cited linguists, since they all regarded the relation of being-in, not quite rightly in my view, as referring to some sort of containment.

I propose that the basic idea behind containment is this: Containers *are preventers of access*, which means that they are bounded loci that create conditions for their occupants in which it is less likely or, in the strongest case, impossible for the latter to *get access to* or to *be accessed* by some or all entities that are not co-occupants. For example, the crucial aspect of hiding a toy in a box is to make it impossible for the child, or any other person, to access that toy. At the opposite end, the goal of putting a burglar in prison is to make it impossible for that person to have access to fellow citizens and their property.

Admittedly, this may not seem a groundbreaking posit when exemplified by toys in boxes. But note that it also applies to more situation-dependent conditions. Let us go back to the idea of situational being-in, discussed earlier, and imagine something more local than being in a state of full-fledged war. For example, if a group of criminals attacks you as you are going home at night, the newly emergent relations between you and these attackers, definitely unpleasant, create an invisible boundary around the situation in which you are now unwillingly embroiled. The point is that these boundaries block your ability to get access to possibly useful entities outside the situation, thereby putting you in a dangerous *new environment*. Despite the fact that from a purely topographical perspective, you are still on the same street as before. This situation is clearly a case of containment, but a fully situational one: the boundary established there is not visible or touchable; however, it is certainly *real* in the sense that it really constrains your actions and can have ramifications in your life.

Now, here is the other core concept that shall prove crucial. It goes in the opposite direction and has been mysteriously neglected by philosophers like Ryle or Popper, who were preoccupied with the association of "in" with containing. I mean the concept of *frame*. Frames are structurally identical to containers but *they are enablers of access*. Thus, they are bounded loci that create conditions for their occupants such that it becomes *possible* or *more likely* for the latter to get access to or to be accessed by some or all entities which are not co-occupants.

In contrast to the earlier example of hiding a toy in a box, consider a box with the very same structural properties, but made of glass, and instead of a toy, consider a priceless sculpture: there is a sense in which the sculpture is not hidden but, on the contrary, put on display in the glass box. *Framing* thus works in the opposite direction to containing, while still sharing the same locative "architecture": both are bounded loci.

Framing is also abstract enough to accommodate more than straightforward cases, such as the one just referenced. Note that the glass box, or to be more precise, the museum display case, is located in a broader environment. First of all, within a certain arrangement of entities dedicated precisely to making some things, such as works of art, available to cognition: through vision, thinking, aesthetic experience, etc. Museums are types of institutions specifically designed to *enable a particular kind of access*. Therefore, metaphorically speaking, the notion of frame draws on the basic linguistic intuition referred to as "the cognitive availability sense" of "in," devised by Tyler and Evans (2003) – the intuition that comes into play when we say that something is "in the light" or "in view."

Going further in this direction, we could certainly imagine situations, somewhat in contrast to the unpleasant example of the street fight above, which make reaching for something possible. For example, you may arrange the workspace around you so as to be able to grab a tool just when you need it; a leader may organize the collaborative effort of a group of people in such a manner as to make this collaboration possible and successful thanks to all members having access to one another and to the required resources. Finally, let us reconsider the fifth intuition pump from Chapter 1 in this context. It can now be reformulated as the following question: *can we think of the mind as a frame, and not – as the Cartesian tradition suggests – a container*?

Note that a scenario suggested by the latter question was discussed in Chapter 5. For Clark (2005, 2006), following Tooby and De Vore (1987), speaks of *cognitive niche construction* to describe cognitively enabling environments such as the well-organized workspace invoked above. I shall explore this intuition further in the next chapter (interestingly, pathological forms of niche can do the opposite; see Werner 2021b; Coninx 2023).

Now, to introduce containment and framing into the conceptual framework rolled out earlier in this chapter, we must first clarify what the terms "getting access to" and "being accessed," used above in our intuitive illustrations, actually mean. Recall that Newell (1980) also spoke of "some kind of access" when he referred to the tie between the physical symbol system and its surroundings.

The "access" relation could be taken as a generic, primitive concept, as evidenced by a variety of empirical cases – from E-coli's *access to glucose* to 5G *internet access*. An ontology of access would have to be provided, namely a theory that unpacks the properties of the relation "*x* has access to *y*," beginning with outlining its basic properties qua relation and then proper axiomatization (similarly to the relation of parthood in mereologies). This is not a bad scenario in and of itself, but here it would not be very informative, rendering the entire vocabulary introduced so far rather useless.

I, therefore, propose to understand "access" in terms of *at least* locative connection. The "at least" provision highlights the fact that it may be a more substantial connection, e.g., as when two entities have a shared boundary, which *also* puts them in locative connection. For, as already indicated, all other kinds of connection imply locative connection. However, the latter obviously does not imply the former.

Containment *simpliciter*, as in the case of bounded loci, will be an umbrella term for a family of more specific posits. First, I propose that there is a distinction between absolute and relative containment:

(40) *x* is an *absolute* container for *y* when *x* is a closed bounded locus for *y* and for *all* entities *z* that are external to *x*, *x* prevents a locative connection between *y* and *z*.

It is not entirely clear whether there are any such containers in the world, but it certainly defines a certain ideal for all actual attempts to construct facilities that block access to some specific entities (e.g., radioactive waste containers).

(41) *x* is a *relative* container for *y* when *x* is a closed bounded locus for *y* and for *some* entities *z* that are external to *x*, *x* prevents a locative connection between *y* and *z* (in such a case, we say that *x* is a relative container for *y with respect to* z_1, z_2, etc.).

Think again of the example with the toy in the box. A variety of relations occur between the toy and the box, e.g., there certainly is physical contact between them, thus some force is exerted by the one on the other. But extracting the purely locative aspect of this nexus of real-world relations between the toy and the box also allows us to indicate *what is truly specific about the fact that one thing contains the other*. This abstract structure of containment is in principle independent of (even if necessarily entangled with) these other bonds. For any toy and any box, if a powerful god had miraculously replaced both of these relata with their doppelgängers, containment itself would have stayed structurally and functionally the same, since it plays out between these objects *solely with regard to their respective locations*.

To take a more interesting example, consider a cell enclosed by its membrane: it is closed but the membrane is of course selectively permeable. There is a huge number of specific relations between the cell and its chemical medium, and it is not at all within the limits of a philosopher's competence to theorize about them. And yet, I argue, underneath this variety is a certain locative dynamic, relative containment to be precise, which also needs to be made explicit. And for that purpose, we need a proper abstract ontological vocabulary.

As we approach the proper target of this study, mind and cognition, let me note that Cartesian cognitive science, as Rowlands (1999) dubbed it, indeed seems to bring the notion of absolute containment to the table, insofar as it considers the mind not just as a specific section of reality, but a genuinely different realm, substance or "space." It is either the "space" filled with ideas, impressions or sense data, but not physical entities proper, which was a belief shared by Descartes, Hume, Locke and Moore, among many others; or the space of the "black box" which the behaviorists postulated as a domain we cannot and do not actually need to obtain access to. Recall the fierce debate on qualia within the Cartesian tradition, which was about whether there are any "entities" in the mind that cannot be unpacked in representational or computational terms and which are entirely subjective or private. Note that in locative terms this would mean entities that are absolutely contained inside the mind, which indicates that the idea of absolute containment is somehow still in the air in Cartesian cognitive science even today.

In this context, we can see the fundamental breakthrough promised by the 4E movement, since what it aims at is not just a manipulation of the boundary of the mind or cognitive system, thus not only rendering the mind, still thought of as a container, permeable in some sense, but a major change in the very architecture of the mind–world relation so that it is *in principle no longer about containment*. At the same time, the lack of a proper ontological effort on the part of 4E proponents makes them less aware of a variety of locative options: even containment offers more than might seem, given the variety of different kinds of boundaries, connections, bounded loci, etc. For example, the containment provided by *i*-boundaries must differ from the containment constituted by *g*-boundaries, as the street fight example shows. Interactional or situational factors may suffice for relative containment to emerge even in the total absence of any physical barriers.

Let me stress that given the conceptual distinction made, especially between bounded loci and containers, which are specific subtypes of the former, we can see a difference, as emphasized in Chapter 1, between what Popper called the bucket theory and a more general mind-*as*-place paradigm. As already stressed, the latter does not necessarily boil down to the former. In short, while the bucket theory states that the mind is a container, perhaps even an absolute container, the more general mind-*as*-a-place approach makes the much broader claim that *the mind is a bounded locus of some kind*. In the final chapter I shall argue in favor of a posit that is a variant of the mind-*as*-place approach and goes against the bucket theory – what I call *ecological internalism*.

Going further, think of *framing* again. Being "in a frame" is just like being "in the light," in the sense that frames render entities accessible from the outside. Yet, unlike the light case, which is looser in terms of its boundaries (i.e., it may be hard to decide where a lit area ends), a frame has the clear "architecture" of a bounded locus, and this latter fact makes it a useful comparison for our purposes.

To get an even clearer sense of how framing works, instead of thinking of an antique canvas surrounded by a heavy, gold-encrusted wooden frame, consider the following setting. Imagine a wall covered with small graffiti – letters and tags. There are lots of them so that it is difficult to discern a single tag and differentiate it from the others. But suppose that there is a rationale for distinguishing one, for instance, because it was made by a famous artist. The best way to do it would be to take a simple rectangle of suitable size, made of wood, plastic or whatever material one wishes, and place it on the wall so that it encloses the desired tag. The tag is still on the wall, it has not been removed, yet now the attention of viewers is *directed towards* the tag *by* the frame. Note that attention is not supposed to be drawn *by* the frame itself, but directed *by* it, while the frame itself (or its role) remains in the background. As a result, it is perfectly fine to say that the tag draws attention *via* the frame. Therefore, a frame is all about exposing the framed entity and making it visible, accessible.

Hence, I propose:

(42) x is a universal frame for y when x is a bounded locus for y and for *all* entities z that are external to x, x enables a locative connection between y and z.

Again, as with absolute containment (note that to speak of "absolute framing" would hardly be understandable; the word "universal" is a better fit), it is not clear whether universal frames can really exist. They, nonetheless, define a certain ideal. Perhaps Berkeley had such universal framing in mind when he referred to God as the one who perceives everything in a single glimpse. Perhaps Plato also had a similar idea in mind when he postulated his idea of the Good, central to the *Republic*, as that which makes all of perceivable reality intelligible. Finally, Kant's transcendental subject could also be interpreted as a universal frame or universal *framer*, insofar as it imposes a certain categorial structure on the domain of all phenomena. We could try to interpret a number of classic proposals from this angle, which is a tempting task, although one that would require a separate book.

As for more realistic cases, we have:

(43) x is a *relative* frame for y when x is a bounded locus for y and for *some* entities z that are external to x, x enables a locative connection between y and z (in such a case, we say that x is a relative frame for y *with respect to* z_1, z_2, etc.).

One could argue that the intuitive appeal of the notion of frame is somehow conservative, in the sense that it draws on the rather old-fashioned concept of the work of art. Meanwhile, no frame is needed for Marcel Duchamp's *Fountain*, not to mention *The Gates* in New York's Central Park by Christo and Jeanne-Claude. This argument gives me a chance to emphasize that this category is in fact far more abstract than the initial example suggests.[3] Just as with containment, we should distinguish between prototypical cases of framing, such as that of a rectangular structure attached to a wall covered with tags, and its derivative senses. As a result, framing a given entity can also mean establishing a situation, not only a thing proper, in which the entity is delineated, exposed or highlighted in some manner. To illustrate this, let us stay within the domain of the arts a moment longer. Drawing on Arthur Danto's (1964) idea of the artworld, George Dickie defined a work of art as an artifact on which a social institution (the artworld) has conferred the status of "candidate for appreciation" (see Dickie 1974). In my reading, conferring the status of a work of art on a given x can be conveniently translated as *imposing a particular frame* on x. This means that x, e.g., one of Duchamp's ready-mades, is selected from among a variety of entities and exposed or presented in a particular context, situation or circumstance, so that a new "story" can be told about x (a function performed by artists, curators, critics or viewers). Duchamp's urinal or Christo and Jeanne-Claude's installations in Central Park had to be selected or "captured," and thus *framed* by specific institutions in order to *emerge as works of art*. Otherwise, the urinal would have continued to be just *a* urinal. A certain bounded space, or rather a situation or an arrangement, first had to be delineated (even though the boundaries are fuzzy in this case) to direct viewers' attention, and the selected entities had to be exposed within that space or *brought into view* there as "candidates for appreciation." Given that we have the notions of *i*-boundary and thus *i*-bounded locus at hand, this case can easily be accounted for. And, as it will turn out in Chapter 7, the "innovation" brought to the world of things by cognition, if we can put it thus metaphorically, is a perfect example of interactional or situation framing.

6.9 Anticipating the next step: Container–frame complexes

The exposition provided above is overly idealized. There are two reasons for this: first, we were talking about a single bounded locus and its single occupant; second, a particular bounded locus was conceptualized as *either* a container *or* a frame, but never both at the same time.

That being said, if the notions introduced above are to give us any insight into how the shift from the mind-*as*-a-place to the mind-*in*-a-place paradigm is to be conceptualized, we need to step down somewhat from this level of idealization, and while maintaining an appropriately abstract approach also do justice to real exemplifications of the notions defined.

I, therefore, propose to speak of *container–frame complexes*. Put simply, they perform two functions: they contain *and* they frame. But they do these two things as part of one complex cluster.

I propose to discuss here two of the most fundamental "architectural" functions attributable to a container–frame complex.

The primary function of its external boundaries is to block connections between the occupants and entities external to the system. The complex, therefore, works primarily as a container *when approached from an external point of view*.

The primary function of its internal boundaries, the boundaries that create a specific internal structure within the complex, is to enable connections between the occupants themselves. The container–frame complex, therefore, works primarily as a frame *when approached from an internal point of view*.

I propose that for the container–frame complex to maintain its integrity, a stable, even if not strictly definable, division of labor between its external and internal boundaries needs to be in place. As an illustrative example, consider a state and its immigration policy. The concept of containment reflects the notion that there is always *some* kind of immigration policy defined by the state. The policy may be liberal and welcoming, but this is a contingent (thus manipulable or alterable) condition which – and this is the critical take – does not change the fact that there is *a* border and thus *a* policy. Yet, once a person crosses the border, they find themselves in a sense exposed to new laws, rules, opportunities, and dangers. Simply put, exposed to interactions with other people inside their new country. Therefore, whether liberal or not, the very existence of an immigration policy illustrates the concept of containment (and the concept of a frame, too). Or think of a different example: an art gallery. We could imagine a very conservative institution, housed in an old building and which rarely adds new artists to its collections. But we could also imagine an institution which ventures out into the streets and parks, organizes outdoor exhibitions and performances, and constantly invites new artists from around the world. The latter case does not change the fact that in principle, *there is still a fundamental distinction* between being part of an exhibition and not being part of one, being invited and not being invited, etc. The *internal* activity of exhibiting is possible precisely because the *external* boundaries perform their function.

The intuition behind these examples, when generalized appropriately, should be clear: cognitive systems, the physical-behavioral units that Smith (2001) talked about, and niches, including the cognitive niches I discussed in the previous chapter, should all be targeted as container–frame complexes.

6.10 Conclusion

This chapter was quite replete with concepts. The goal was to define the locative concepts underpinning the preposition "in" which is quite heavily used by philosophers of mind without much reflection. Taking stock of the rich variety of senses of "in" exposed by the linguists brought up in Chapter 1, and inspired by these thought exercises, I moved on to a more technical discussion.

Basic notions of locative ontology were introduced following first of all Casati and Varzi (1999) and Smith and Varzi (1999), and a number of new concepts were defined based on these fundamentals. The pivotal ones included: various kinds of boundaries, including interactional boundaries and pregiven boundaries.

I then defined bounded loci, after a detailed look at what it means for an object to be filled or fulfilled with something else, and what it means for two or more objects to be connected. What stands out especially is the new concept of locative connection. I then moved on to its most frequently discussed specification, namely the notion of containment, and afterward to the crucial notion of framing. The latter is a setting which shares the same structure as containment, but crucially differs from it functionally. While it is the goal of containers to prevent access to the contained entity, it is the sole goal of frames to expose the thing framed, to make it accessible or available. The notion of access was cashed out in terms of locative connection.

Finally, given the fact that real-life cases are hardly exemplifications of one single kind of bounded locus, the provisional idea of a *container–frame complex* was introduced.

What comes next? We shall now ask what kind of container–frame complex cognitive systems and their environments are.

Notes

1 See: http://www.oed.com/view/Entry/129613?rskey=gxnfpb&result=1&isAdvanced=false#eid.

2 This idea is in some sense similar to the one set forth by Avrum Stroll (1979) who distinguishes between what he calls the Leonardo Conception whose outline we can find in Leonardo da Vinci's notebooks, and the Somorjai Conception, named after Gabor A. Somorjai, a modern-day chemist working in the field of surface chemistry. The distinction pertains to surfaces in particular, but it can be generalized. According to the Leonardo Conception, a boundary is shared by two coinciding entities, although it cannot be regarded as their common part. This, as Leonardo stresses, is because the boundary has no substance, no "bulk." Meanwhile, the Somorjai Conception depicts boundaries as real things; as top layers of entities which are aggregates of atoms (see Somorjai 1978). The crucial issue here, though, is the fact that the *i*-boundary comes about as a product of interactions. The latter is therefore a more dynamical model.

3 Many years ago a remark made by Colin Allen prompted me to make this point explicit.

7 The Basic Ontology of Niche Construction

This key chapter lays out an ontological account of niche construction, utilizing the proposed conceptual framework of the Basic Ontology of the Bounded Locus. The goal is to capture the essential traits of cognition thought of as an ecological phenomenon – as a factor determining a specific locus – and thereby to elicit how cognition, at least following the Varelian current within the 4E movement, takes part in the creation of the world *as we know it*, a certain *enacted*, species-specific environment.

I hope to show that among plenty of things to be said about cognition, which are for the most part topics to be addressed by the empirical sciences, there is a certain interesting, and actually quite fundamental dynamic which can be described in abstract locative terms. As already emphasized, cognition has a very specific way of dealing with location, and this chapter finally takes this issue apart.

However, the price to be paid for such an ontological endeavor is its abstractness and thus, one might say, its somewhat artificial character. This is because all empirically available cases, the actual niches of real animals, are in fact *re*-constructions, meaning that there exist innumerable "layers" of niches, one built upon another over hundreds of millions of years, reshaping one another and composing wider environments (which is nicely unpacked in terms of "evolved apprentice" by Sterelny 2012). Meanwhile, insofar as the goal of a traditional philosophical study is to dig into the very *nature* of phenomena, we need to adopt a different angle on the phenomenon under investigation here in order to obtain at least partial grasp of its *nature*.

With this in mind, I shall propose a kind of highly idealized ontological "simulation" of the evolution of (cognitive) niche construction, beginning with the fictional "point zero" where the process sets off, thus where there is no niche at all, and proceed stepwise up to the emergence of cognitive niches. Of course, no such "point zero" can be established empirically. To my knowledge, such an approach to the ontology of ecological or biological phenomena has not been tried, and yet it was inspired by

DOI: 10.4324/9781003580997-7

Godfrey-Smith's (2016) illuminating attempt to single out several pivotal stages in the evolution of cognitive capacities and consciousness. On the other hand, the kind of abstraction and idealization I use, while informal, is similar to, and also inspired by, formal models of simple agents within dynamical systems theory (for some recent work, see e.g. Beer 2023 or Beer & Di Paolo 2023). The goal, therefore, is to provide a genuinely ecological categorization of the relation between the living and cognizing system on the one hand, and its surroundings on the other.

7.1 (Cognitive) Niche construction in a broader philosophical landscape

Before I plunge into this ontological story, I will recapitulate my goals, put forward in Chapter 1 and afterward selectively restated throughout the book, in order to place the planned ontological "simulation" within a broader philosophical context and justify the proposed effort once more.

Already in Chapter 1 I laid out the most general controversy over whether the cognitive system should be conceptualized *as a locus* of some kind or as something that *needs a locus* (an environment). This was the controversy between the mind-*as*-a-place view and the mind-*in*-a-place approach, as it was provisionally articulated. Representationalism – whether tacitly or openly – sides with the former view while 4E adopts and advocates for the latter.

Now, as I tried to show, the rationale for the traditional mind-*as*-a-place view was not a preoccupation with any specific concept of location or with any predefined ontology of mind or soul, but rather a need to account for the fact that we are understanders who not only act in the world, but also reflect on the world as it manifests itself to us. The Augustinian invention of the "inner self," as we learn from Taylor (1989) and Cary (2000), among others, had a moral and epistemic purpose. This means that the question of the kind of location that the mind or soul (cognitive system, to put it in contemporary terms) exemplifies was to a large degree left open. Therefore, its locative-ontological specification in terms of the internal versus external dichotomy which we owe to Galileo and Descartes (see Husserl 1970 and Putnam 1987) is *just one possible* specification – one that, due to the lack of any concept of ecological location must have seemed the only viable option in these thinkers' times. But today, I argued, we can be more fine-grained about the matter, while the adoption of the niche construction terminology opens up a number of new possibilities. The aim is not to throw the baby out with the bathwater – since we still need to do justice to our self-recognition as understanders – but to refine the mind-*as*-a-place model. And once the task has been so defined, we can see that by introducing *i*-boundaries, *g*-boundaries and *p*-boundaries we can obtain a much more complex and nuanced picture of the internal versus external divide which, when nuanced, is no longer a dichotomy. If so, the "safe refuge" for reflection that we are seeking, as I put it somewhat poetically in Chapter 1, can be conceptualized in more ecological terms (see Chapter 8).

7.2 The Basic Ontology of Niches

Drawing on the proposed Basic Ontology of Bounded Loci, this section, similarly, unpacks the fundamental locative features of niches, based on the following assumption:

(44) A niche is a bounded locus.

That is all we need to know for now regarding niches. As for the niche tenant, intuitively, we may assume that it is a living creature or an autonomous system in the sense defined previously, but what we really need for now is solely to concede that:

(45) A niche tenant is a *g*-closed entity such that all its boundaries are *p*-boundaries.

This condition is quite specific, for although it looks very simple, it suffices to uniquely identify potential creators and possessors of niches within the abstract story to be told. First, (45) requires that the niche tenant be closed by at least one setup of pregiven boundaries, thus boundaries that are in principle not dependent of interactions, not "negotiated" with the outside world but determined fully by the internal structure of the complex entity in question. This is a certain idealization, of course, for in real-world cases even physical barriers such as cell membranes depend on external conditions, air or water pressure, etc. in one way or another (as already pointed out in Chapter 6). Nonetheless this theoretical fiction does play a significant role, eliciting a significant feature of living creatures. In more realistic terms it can be put as follows: living creatures have boundaries that are predominantly "set up" by internal factors, independently of the vast majority of interactions the creatures are engaged in within their surroundings (which is in step with the autopoietic tradition).

To be clear, being *g*-closed does not mean that *all* of the entity's *g*-boundaries at *all levels* of complexity close up the entity in question, nor that the entity cannot have *i*-boundaries. Quite obviously, living creatures maintain a variety of *i*-boundaries.

That being said, (45) also requires that all boundaries of the niche tenant, including its *i*-boundaries, be "designed" by *its* governing "program," as Koshland Jr. (2002) puts it. There is no other thing in the assumed universe of our locative ontology that proves as demanding, in a sense. Stressing the fact that the "program" must be the tenant's unique design principle becomes important once we come to the ontological characteristics of the niche: these are also fully determined by a "program," and yet, as we shall see, it is *the tenant*'s "program," *not* the niche's own design principle.

Being integrated by the "program" across all its levels, the tenant can be seen as a specific *system*: it is neither defined as an autonomous system nor as a representational one. It can be both, and yet these concepts do not belong to the proper ontological vocabulary being rolled out here. Nonetheless, the *autonomous* system (which may also happen to become representational at some level of niche construction; there's no reason to join the anti-representational crusade and exclude this possibility) can serve as our best approximation of what the niche tenant is.

As already cited in Chapter 5, Smith and Varzi (1999) introduce the distinction between *niche base* and *niche medium*. The latter refers to what is actually relevant to the niche tenant out of all the stuff surrounding the tenant. Now we can slightly reformulate the notions of niche medium and relevance using the conceptual framework rolled out in the previous chapter:

(46) The niche medium is a mereological sum of all the objects – substances, parts or accidents thereof – that are relevant to the tenant.

In Chapter 5 we decided that insofar as the system in question is an autonomous system, relevance is determined by its conditions of autonomy. And yet, as just stated, autonomy is not a proper part of locative ontology. Therefore, I propose a different definition which is not supposed to replace the one spelled out in terms of autonomy, but rather, first, to climb up even higher in the hierarchy of abstraction; and, second – to articulate a locative counterpart of autonomy-determined relevance:

(47) x is relevant to the niche tenant when x is a necessary condition for the tenant to have a p-boundary as its part; thus, more intuitively speaking – to maintain the tenant's p-boundedness.

This characterization, arguably acceptable to a 4E advocate, makes room for a wide variety of types and levels of relevance, depending on the kind of boundaries in question: either g-boundaries or a variety of i-boundaries.

Within this framework, what is the pursuit of niche construction all about? Here is a guiding idea or a general heuristic to be unpacked over the course of this chapter:

(48) The process of niche construction is a series of acts by which the niche tenant *becomes* connected with a variety of relevant entities in its surroundings.

Therefore, as already flagged in Chapter 5:

(49) A niche is the final product of a process of niche construction.

The emphasis on "finality" is meant to reflect the fact that many new things can come into being as part of the process of niche construction that are not themselves niches. For example, a new dam built by a beaver is not a niche in and of itself, although it is clearly part of the niche that the animal has built. But taking all of these constructive efforts and their products together, a niche can be seen as the final step in the process. This does not mean, of course, that nothing happens once the work is done. Speaking of the "final step" is, of course, a theoretical fiction. In reality, niche construction is an ongoing process.

Here are some further ontological marks of niches:

(50) Niches are self-connected objects.

This means that niches are not simply scattered clusters of things. Instead, they are units (keeping in mind the different kinds of connections defined in Chapter 6).

(51) Niches have external boundaries, i.e., boundaries between the niche medium and its exterior, i.e., what is not part of the niche medium, as well as internal boundaries, i.e., boundaries between the niche medium and the tenant.

Niches are defined by their external as well as internal boundaries. It must be noted, however, that the external boundary of a niche is not necessarily a line delineating two segments of physical space, like the one between the interior and the exterior of a bear's cave. Instead, (51) states that it is the division between the sum of the entities composing the niche medium and the remainder of the niche base. The boundary may, therefore, not be a clear-cut line that we can easily locate in physical space or imagine, but something more contextual and, so to speak, entwined with the complexities of the niche base. Recall the bear's cave as analyzed earlier – the bat is inside the cave but outside of the bear's niche.

Now, an absolutely key issue is *where these boundaries come from*. This is the moment to unpack in locative-ontological terms the fact, stressed many times so far (especially in step with Varela et al. 1991) that niches are *relative to* living creatures; they are not pregiven realms merely inhabited by organisms, but rather organism-*specific Umwelten*. Here is a way it may be put:

(52) All the boundaries of niches are *p*-boundaries (internal and external) determined by the unifying "program" of the niche tenant.

This point renders the unity of a niche dependent on what makes the unity of its tenant possible, on the design "principle" that defines the bounded unity of the living creature.

Further on:

(53) All internal and external boundaries of the niche are *i*-boundaries: with its tenant(s) (intuitively these are the boundaries resulting from "negotiations" between the niche tenant and its immediate surroundings), and with other entities (external to the niche).

Compare this to the analogous condition referring to the niche tenant, namely (45). There the stipulation was that a niche tenant/constructor must have at least one setup of non-interactional, pregiven boundaries, thus that it must be *internally* determined *as a unit*. This condition does not apply to niches. On the contrary – although we might be tempted to think of the non-interactional boundaries of niches, such as the walls of a bear's cave – what is constitutive of a certain thing's *serving as* the niche of a particular system is that the thing's capacity to play that role fully depends on its interactions with the system; it is not a quality that can be sensibly attributed to a thing as such (e.g. the cave wall) without regard for the organism that makes use of it. The stony wall of the cave is what it is – a piece of stone – not a niche boundary, but once the cave becomes a niche base, the wall may also, in some intuitive sense, *become* a niche boundary (in fact, the emergent niche boundary is a *new* entity, not simply the wall itself with a new role – but let us put this subtlety aside for the sake of a more intuitive grasp of the organism-relative character of niches that I am trying to spell out here).

Let me stress that this does not smuggle in a radical constructivist view according to which there are no tenant-independent boundaries of *things* partaking in the niche medium. These are two different things which I shall spill some more ink on in due course. The niche medium is, according to (46), a mereological sum, and (53) makes it clear that *this sum*, not its ingredients, has no boundary independent of its interactions with the tenant. All niche boundaries are therefore *i*-boundaries, but stony caves and *their* boundaries remain what they are, perfectly "objective" things in the Cartesian sense of the term, if you like.

However, all this does not mean that the niche must be internally closed. The relationship between a niche and its tenant may be more complex. I propose:

(54) If x is a niche for y, x is internally p-open to y when it has no internal boundary as its part, which means that the unifying principle p of y does *not* determine any stable setup of internal boundaries for x that are parts of x itself.

(55) If x is a niche for y, x is internally p-closed to y when it has its internal boundaries as its parts, which means that the unifying principle p of y determines the full setup of internal boundaries for x that count as parts of x.

The parthood condition is important in (54) and (55). This is because I propose to distinguish two cases: one, when an external boundary of the tenant *serves as* the internal boundary of the niche. Obviously, there is always a distinction between the living creature and its surroundings, but the key question is whether the boundaries which the tenant possesses anyway *also* establish the distinction the tenant and its niche, or if there is an *additional* boundary or boundaries determined by the unifying principle of the tenant, yet emerging *on the niche side*. This shall prove quite crucial when we discuss niche construction and especially the way a cognitive niche comes into being. For we might think of the internal boundaries of a niche as the niche's *surface* facing the tenant; in other words, the layer that the tenant actually faces when interacting with its niche. In this case the internal boundaries belong to the niche itself and are not merely "borrowed" from the tenant; they are relatively distinct from the tenant and can be *cognized* by the tenant as *given*. Phenomenologically speaking, and returning to what Varela, Thompson and Rosch (1991) dubbed "fundamental circularity," these internal niche boundaries can be experienced as parts of the world we awake in, not something that we produce. This interpretation anticipates claims to be made later; for now, however, we have not yet begun our ontological reconstruction of niche construction.

Further on, I propose:

(56) If x is a niche for y, y is i-closed to x when it has its i-boundaries "negotiated" with x as its parts, which means that the unifying principle p of y determines a stable setup of demarcation lines dividing what belongs to y and what belongs to its niche *for the sake of their interaction*. Otherwise it is (fully or partially) i-open.

This requires some commentary. As (45) stipulates, a system must be non-interactionally closed, i.e. g-closed, for this is a definitional ontological mark of any entity that may be a niche constructor. Put in a more appealing way – it is an ontological mark of living/autonomous systems, full stop. However, g-boundaries are independent of wherever and however the system is located, and having g-boundaries does not mean that each system establishes a *distinct* setup of boundaries "designed" for the sake of interaction with *specific* surroundings. Of course, if the system does not determine such specific i-boundaries appropriate for its interactions with a particular cluster of surrounding entities, its g-boundaries have a say in how the interactions play out, so to speak. However, it may be beneficial to the system to determine more contextual barriers too, and these shall be seen as the system's *i*-boundaries. We should keep in mind that real-life examples always fit these theoretical fictions only to a limited extent, yet think, for instance, of animal bodies such as our own. Each human being is *g*-bounded by the skin (actually by a whole system including skin, but let us keep the picture simple) which is, *ceteris paribus*, independent of any surroundings in which the particular human happens to be placed. We can imagine a scenario, hardly viable but at least thinkable, in which this is the only system of boundaries humans have. If so, some infectious microbes will be stopped for sure, but a great number of them will breach the skin barrier. In contrast, the immune system in principle works as a system of *i*-boundaries protecting us from specific external threats. So in addition to skin, it is beneficial to us to have immunological boundaries too. And the latter cannot be reduced to the former.

Now, let us recall the distinction between containers and frames, which also proves to be a crucial part of the story:

(57) If x is a niche for y and x is an internally closed bounded locus, x is a relative frame for its medium with respect to y.

This means that although serving as a container for its medium with respect to the tenant is not precluded (it may be a function of a particular niche to block the tenant's access to some parts of the niche), it is not a constitutive feature of the niche. On the contrary, it *is* the very function of a niche to expose its medium to the tenant, thus to make it available or accessible. As we shall see further on in relation to the cognitive niche, while its primary function is to make the niche medium cognitively accessible, it is in principle a selective access with limited resolution which can be cashed out in terms of a mix of internal frames and internal containers.

But how about the niche's external boundaries? I propose:

(58) If x is a niche for y, x is a relative container for y and the niche medium with respect to entities that do not belong to the niche medium.

This condition states that a niche would not be what it is if it was composed of external frames only, for one of its primary functions is to secure resources for its tenant and to secure the tenant itself.

Given (57) and (58) a certain general characterization of the niche emerges; one that I shall be working with now in greater detail. Namely, it can be said that *a niche is a container–frame complex* constructed by a living creature in its physical surroundings.

Yet it cannot be just *any* cluster of containers and frames around a living creature. The niche tenant must maintain some kind of unique position as well as some kind of intimate relationship with the said cluster of containers and frames. Using De Jaegher and Di Paolo's (2007) nice phrase, already cited several times, the tenant must be the "center of activity" within the surrounding container–frame complex. However obvious this remark is, it is by no means obvious how we can cash it out within the conceptual framework rolled out here.

Smith and Varzi (1999) propose that a niche tenant is connected to its niche in at least one of the senses of connection that they list. I shall follow them, yet not by adopting the claim directly, since I have made several important distinctions among many types of connection which Smith and Varzi did not discuss. Instead, I shall take their insight as a guiding principle.

Perhaps contrary to its benign appearance, Smith and Varzi's (1999) posit is a far-reaching statement, for what follows from it is that either the niche must be open to its tenant, or the tenant must be open to its niche, or they share a boundary. Otherwise they would not be connected, at least given the conceptual framework within which Smith and Varzi work. I shall follow this idea as well, and build on it, since it proves crucial when it comes to the announced reconstruction of the niche construction process. Namely, niche construction turns out to be about *setting up connections*. The key thing to determine now is what kind of connections these are, for unlike in Smith and Varzi's (1999) proposal, here we have a rich variety of connections.

7.3 The niche–tenant connection

Given that the medium is a mereological sum of objects that are relevant to the tenant (as stipulated in (46)), a system is connected to that sum *as a whole*, and therefore by definition also to parts of it. However, what if we consider these objects not as parts of the medium, but as objects in their own right? What is the relation between them and the system? This question needs to be answered if we are to understand the process of niche construction.

Let me recall the concept of locative connection: two objects are in locative connection (direct or remote) when their exact locations, thus the regions occupied by them, are connected (directly or remotely).

I therefore propose:

(59) If x is a niche and y is its tenant, y is in *locative* connection (direct or remote) with all objects z such that x's medium is a sum of z.

This means that in addition to the connection between the tenant and its niche (strictly speaking the niche medium as a mereological sum), we can speak of locative connections between the living creature which happens to be the niche's tenant and *each* of the surrounding objects that happen to be mereologically summed up as the niche's medium. Let us take a very simplistic and straightforward illustration. If the medium of my current niche is defined as the mereological sum of my laptop, desk, and the air molecules surrounding me, I *am* connected (thus I share a part of a boundary) with *the sum* of these entities, which is taken here as an entity in its own right, but I *am not* connected either with my laptop or my desk (quite obviously I share neither parts nor boundaries with them, yet when it comes to air molecules the issue is more complex, for we would have to employ a mereology of chemical reactions; see Llored & Harré 2014). However, according to my proposal, I *am* in *locative* connection with these two things, the laptop and the desk, meaning that there is a certain pattern of connections between the *region* occupied by me and the *regions* occupied by my laptop and my desk. And these patterns of locative connection cast me in the role of *the point of reference* in my niche. This is due to the fact that the laptop, the desk as well as the air molecules are not beings occupying a random portion of space; they are *around me*, at *my disposal*, within *my reach*, so to speak.

This being said, I propose to augment our Basic Ontology of the Niche by adding the following posit:

(60) If x is a niche for y, and z is a set of objects mereologically summed up as x's medium, y is a point of reference for all members of z.

Therefore, there are *patterns of locative connections* between the niche tenant and any object that happens to be part of the mereological sum serving as that niche's medium. This stipulation proves quite consequential.

We can now think of niche construction as, first, a given system's effort to *set up locative connections* with *relevant* objects in its surroundings, so that the system *becomes* the point of reference in a certain newly carved-up domain. Then, second, we can think of niche construction as that newly created domain's becoming mereologically summed up in the form of the niche medium. What needs to be added is a boundary or many boundaries between the system and this newly constituted complex. So, niche construction is about setting up locative connections and about "drawing" boundaries so that certain things are incorporated into the system's locative capacity and thereby into the realm in which the system maintains its own *p*-boundaries, thus its integrity as a unit.

This preliminary characterization is not easy to unpack in greater detail, however. What I propose is not so much a proper *definition* of niche construction. Rather, I prefer to be as true as possible to the dynamic character of the phenomenon under investigation. So, the goal of the ontological "representation" of niche construction undertaken here is to roughly distinguish several stages in the process, each one individuated by a particular locative "innovation" or "turn." As already emphasized, this is in contrast to the way ontology is usually pursued. For a typical ontological account of a given phenomenon usually takes the phenomenon as already being there (or *not* being there, if one is concerned with non-existents), in the domain of physical entities, mental entities, intentional, ideal, cultural entities or what have you, or at least as a thinkable possibility in one of these domains; in other words as something already determined. Meanwhile, tracing the emergence of something, its *coming into* being, is an ontology of the phenomenon still *in the making*.

7.4 Making the system ready for interaction

To begin with, I propose that the assumed *universum* of the projected ontology (ontological domain) consists of a fixed system S whose integrity and self-maintenance is determined by the fixed principle *p*. We also have an unspecified number of objects $\{o_1, o_2, \ldots\}$. For the sake of simplicity, let us assume that we have a single system dealing with the same set of objects over the entire course of the evolution of niche construction. This is a highly idealized theoretical fiction, of course.

The nature of these assumed objects is not specified. We might say that they are things *in themselves*, or that they are the ultimate physicochemical base of all niches. The system on the other hand is best thought of as an autonomous system, but this does not rule out its being a computational system in the sense of Newell and Simon. The story to be told removes itself from the representationalism – anti-representationalism debate, putting emphasis on the idea that whether or not the system at some point becomes capable of creating internal, off-line representations, the key thing is that *in principle* it is an embodied creature, co-determined by its environment and in turn co-determining its environment.

First we need to single out a portion of the universum that will actually serve as the base for all S's future niches, since, quite obviously, S does not have the entire universe at its disposal, but only a tiny segment of it, placed in some proximity. Therefore, I propose:

(61) F is the mereological sum of fixed entities $o_m,\ldots o_n$, belonging to $\{o_1, o_2,\ldots\}$, selected by S's governing program p, and F is in direct locative connection to S (intuitively speaking, F is the system's direct neighborhood).

Now – crucially – I propose to speak of a starting point, *moment zero* of S's niche construction endeavor, which is artificially postulated here for the sake of the argument and not intended to single out an *actual* moment in natural history. It satisfies the following condition:

(NC0) At *moment zero* both S and F are *i*-open, and F is moreover *p*-open.

This is the moment when co-determination of the system and its environment begins. At the starting point, the two are open to one another in the sense that neither of them has any *interactional* boundary. Of course, the system is, by definition, already established by some non-interactional, thus pregiven (*g*-) *p*-boundaries (following (45)), and there are likely non-interactional *g*-boundaries on the other side too – among the unknown things that are summed up to form F. The point is that the two sides, S and F, have not negotiated *between them* a boundary yet. If so, the principle *p* governing S's integrity, has not yet had a chance to intervene in the system's neighborhood, so to speak. That is why F is also said to be *p*-open, meaning that it has no boundary determined by the system's needs yet.

Noteworthily, we must be careful not to specify the system's neighborhood more than the proposed reconstruction requires, and not even try to imagine it, since at this point it has no cognizable layout, *no presentation* whatsoever. If one prefers to be a physicalist about the niche base, one might provisionally say that the system's neighborhood is a swarm of particles or a soup of chemical complexes, but this is also too much of a statement given the fact that *speaking* of particles only makes *real* sense as part of a certain intelligible discourse, thus when a certain cognizable presentation of reality – the one established by modern science – is already the case. That is why above, as I said above, $o_m,\ldots o_n$ should be treated as things *in themselves*, in a more or less Kantian sense of the term, for otherwise we would not be able to even tell the story.

This assumption also realizes more or less what Varela, Thompson and Rosch (1991) emphasized, namely that while in principle the world and the cognitive system are *not* pregiven but instead *mutually enacted*, this *does not* mean that they miraculously come into existence *ex nihilo*. Varela and collaborators clearly endorse a position beyond the Cartesian realism versus idealism debate. Here we can see that distinguishing *i*-boundaries actually proves quite useful. As I see it, Varela's point on *not being pregiven* actually refers to *i*-openness, not to complete lack of any determination at the level of $o_m,\dots o_n$.

To cast more light on NC0, let me refer to Godfrey-Smith (2016), since he provides a nice analogy. He speaks of two functions of the nervous system. One is widely appreciated and stressed, that is to say the function of coordinating sensory input and behavioral output, which gives rise to the more sophisticated functions then tackled by representationalism. A still more primitive function, he says, is agent-building. This refers to the internal coordination of the parts and functions of a complex living creature so that it can behave *as a whole*. This is in step with what is known as the skin-brain thesis (see e.g. Keijzer et al. 2013) according to which early nervous systems evolved to organize muscle tissue, thus enabling animal motility, and thereby also internally integrating the animal body as a *future* active factor in the world.

Godfrey-Smith writes (referring to the so-called Ediacaran biota living around 600 million years ago):

> Our animal cousins are highly alert to their environment; they track friends, foes, and countless other features of the landscape. They do that because what's going on around them matters; often it's a matter of life and death. Ediacarans' lives show no evident sign of this moment-to-moment engagement with the environment. If so, this makes it likely that our Ediacaran ancestors put their nervous systems – when they had them – to different uses from those seen in more recent animals. Specifically, this might have been a time when the role played by those nervous systems fits (...) the view based on internal coordination rather than sensory-motor control.
>
> (Godfrey-Smith 2016: 31–32)

By analogy, to understand N0 we must also bracket our intuitive understanding of all the complex interactions between the living beings we know best and their surroundings. At this postulated primitive stage, there is no interaction, because the *conditions* that would make interaction possible have not yet been "negotiated" (of course, there are transfers of energy, chemical complexes, etc. across the system's *g*-boundary, but this is *not yet interaction*). In addition, and again analogous to what Godfrey-Smith is talking about, niche construction is in principle a system-building process, but it leads not only to the growth of new structures in the system itself, but also – as a kind of by-product, which later becomes a constructive process in its own right – to the emergence of relatively stable structures in the system's neighborhood. Finally, the idea here is that this reciprocal process of co-creation can be neatly articulated in terms of *i*-boundaries. Namely, new configurations of the system's *interactional* boundaries emerge in the course of niche construction in partnership with the new *interactional* boundaries of its neighborhood (of course, new *g*-boundaries also emerge, but that is not our concern here).

Let me repeat: at NC0, both "actors" in the process of niche construction, the system and its neighborhood, are *i*-open: they maintain no structure that stabilizes their dynamic relations at this point. This is not to say that nothing is happening between them (that would be empirically false). The point is that there are not yet any "negotiated" patterns of these happenings.

Now, I propose that niche construction is a process of mutual co-determination, yet one initially resulting in an *i*-closed *system*; a stipulation which in a sense follows Godfrey-Smith's (2016) elicitation of the pivotal steps in the evolution of organismic complexity (see also Feinberg and Mallatt 2016). The purpose of niche construction at this stage is to provide the resources required for the system's maintenance of its integrity as a unit. Therefore, it is all about building a closed, stable tenant, but *not yet* about building a stable environment (which comes later). Therefore:

(NC1) At the first stage of system-niche co-determination:

(a) there emerges an *i*-closure of S determined by its interactions with F (which is, by definition, a *p*-closure too, for all boundaries that S has must be somehow conditioned by its governing principle *p*) – it shall be called *the first interactive closure* of S;
(b) F is still *p*-open and *i*-open to S (it's open *to* the first interactive closure of S, strictly speaking), meaning that it maintains no *i*--boundaries of its own.
(c) the first interactive closure of S is a relative frame for S with respect to F.

Speaking of the "first interactive closure" stands for the fact that S (and F, too, as we shall see shortly) may have many such structures at various levels of complexity and at various moments in time.

Noteworthily, NC1(c) makes it clear that the *purpose* of the system's newly emerged interactional boundaries is in principle not to contain the system, thus to obscure access to it, but rather to expose it *as a whole* to its neighborhood *also taken as a whole* (unlike in NC5 below). We may figuratively say that S's *g*-boundaries do the job of obscuring access to S's ingredients sufficiently and that there is no need at this point for S's newly established interactional boundaries to join in this effort. Instead, they are assigned a different task, that of *exposing* the system for the sake of new possible interactions, therefore also new "opportunities," so to speak. For having *i*-boundaries is a precondition of the very capacity to spot affordances, as Gibson (1979) might say.

The expression "as a whole" used above is significant. For once the *first* closure of the system is completed, and once there arises for S *as a whole* a new opportunity for engaging in interactions with its neighborhood (recall Keijzer et al. 2013 and Godfrey-Smith 2016 again), the process of co-determination, thus of niche construction, can continue. Note that prior to that point S was considered static and "interested" solely in maintaining its own integrity, chiefly by means of its *g*-boundaries. Hence, S's first setup of *i*-boundaries can be thought of as S's first "attempt" to set up certain *conditions for interactions* with F. These new conditions are precisely what we mean by S's *i*-boundaries: they are still fully devoted to maintaining S's integrity, nonetheless, there is a crucial new aspect – this new setup of boundaries is about keeping the system intact against a range of new perturbations caused by interactions – *by doing something*.

7.5 Preparing the system's neighborhood for interaction

Here is the main thought put in a different form still. Suppose the system living its peaceful life at level NC0, disregarding whatever is in the wider neighborhood, suddenly "fancies" venturing out into that neighborhood and moving, say, one meter to the right or left, then going back and trying the same thing again. If so, it needs something more than its *g*-boundary – the system must establish certain *conditions* that must be satisfied so that the things it is going to meet along its one-meter journey do not pose a threat to its integrity. For example, suppose that the system is submerged in a water solution (which was actually the case in the Ediacaran) and sets the condition that the pressure exercised on it cannot be higher than a certain value. This is of course "decided" by the material and composition of the system's non-interactional *g*-boundary, e.g., its membrane. However, it is not *just* a property of the membrane, for it must also take into account the solution surrounding it. So it *already* belongs to a different level; NC1, therefore, is already not only about how this barrier playing the function of the system's *g*-boundary is composed, how it participates in the internal structure and functioning of the system – the very possibility of acting and moving to another surroundings introduces a new aspect at the NC1 level, so to speak. An analogous claim was made by van Duijn et al. (2006) in reference to cognition. They speak of the meta-metabolic level which clearly serves metabolism but is *not part of* metabolism. So, these new conditions *determined for the occasion of movement* are associated with the emergence of a *new* boundary, and this boundary is of a new type – it is an *interactional* boundary, thus one that is "designed" to maintain the system's integrity and delineation from its surrounding *when the system acts in a particular milieu*.

Therefore, at the NC1 stage, we have some initial patterns of S's self-maintenance *vis-à-vis* its surroundings which are there *for the sake of interaction*, but still no patterns *of interaction* themselves, and therefore still no stable environment. The surrounding at this stage still "looks" to the system like an indefinite flux. Of course, certain things in the surrounding world *matter* to the system in the most basic sense (see van Duijn et al. 2006 again), yet this is not sufficient to speak of *i*-boundaries *on the side of the surrounding realm*. For example, when certain molecules dispersed in the medium selectively cross the simple system's *g*-boundaries (the cell membrane, in real-life cases), one can hardly assign any sense to the idea of *patterns* of interaction in this domain. Let me reiterate: at this stage what is being enacted is the future niche tenant, but its neighborhood still lacks any *interaction-related* structure.

Now, once the possibility of interaction arises for S *as a whole* as a result of having established its first interactive closure, there may also be a growing "need" (to put it in a somewhat anthropomorphic way) for *stability on the neighborhood side*, i.e. a "need" for certain interactional patterns *there*. This is to make the interactions more efficient. When it comes to actual natural history, we can localize this stage of evolution somewhere between the Ediacaran and the Cambrian. Godfrey-Smith writes:

> In the Cambrian, animals became part of each other's lives in a new way, especially through predation.
>
> (Godfrey-Smith 2016: 34)

Predation certainly involves highly advanced interactive structures (note that interaction does not signify cooperation, and comprises predation), which requires certain structural patterns not only on the part of the system, but also on the part of its neighborhood. I therefore propose that the second step of niche construction results in a relatively stable interactional layout of F (this includes other systems *as seen* from the perspective of our fixed S, but I shall not problematize inter-system relations here, undertaking a somewhat "solipsistic" approach for the sake of simplicity).

I propose:

(NC2) At the second step of co-determination:

(a) There is a new setup of *interactive* boundaries on the S side (*the second interactive closure* of S, strictly speaking).

(b) There is a setup of interactional boundaries on the F side too, which signifies the first interactive closure of F.
(c) The (second) interactional closure of S is externally connected to the (first) interactional closure of F; in other words, the newly emerged first setup of F's *i*-boundaries *is identical to* the second layer of S's *i*-boundaries.

Note that although some diversification within F can momentarily appear at this stage, cutting F into segments or pieces relative to S's needs, there is *no stable structure* thereof yet. This is unlike in our familiar world, thus in *our cognitive niche*, which is cut into discrete things, events, processes, etc. This is only going to emerge at further stages.

The new interactional boundaries of the system's neighborhood F may be regarded as historically the first "surface" or "appearance" of reality. However, this surface, first, lacks internal diversification, as mentioned above, and second, it is inseparable from S. Once again, this makes these first *i*-boundaries of F dissimilar to the surfaces *we* are familiar with in *our cognitive niche* which are – we usually assume – still there even when we aren't acting and perceiving them. Here, with regard to (NC2), the existence of the first interactive closure of F is fully dependent on S. We may also say that (NC2) defines the first proto-niche structure, to be further developed.

The innovation introduced by NC2 is quite consequential, however. This is because from this point on, we can begin thinking of *two* distinct clusters of interactional boundaries, and therefore of two distinct evolutionary developments thereof. Admittedly, the interactive boundaries of F arising at the NC2 level fully depend on S (its second closure, to be exact) since in fact we have a single setup of boundaries playing two roles – interactionally closing the system's neighborhood *in addition* to providing the second-layer interactive closure to the system itself. However, since there is a *functional* distinction, this opens the door for an ontological distinction too. In other words, further steps in the evolution of niche construction may take advantage of this functional distinction and actually produce two ontologically distinct setups of boundaries.

This point of divergence is also the right place to (re)introduce the distinction between niches whose purpose is to preserve the system's autonomy, strictly thought of as the mechanisms responsible for the system's integrity, and cognitive niches; a distinction provisionally introduced in Chapter 5.

The divergence must be introduced stepwise, however. First, S's neighborhood, which at the NC2 level is still an internally undiversified mereological fusion, must be decomposed into relatively stable segments. This is going to be possible owing to the fact that already in NC2 we have a system that moves or acts in a certain way.

One thing needs to be clarified before we proceed further. Recall that the system's neighborhood was defined as a fusion of relevant entities $o_m,...o_n$ in the universe. One might therefore think that the decomposition of the undiversified neighborhood F into discrete segments simply "reproduces" $o_m,...o_n$, as if reducing the fusion back to its original building blocks. This is not the case though. For note that $o_m,...o_n$ were assumed as the default universum of our ontology, but they are not what the system S is "familiar" with. In other words, they are postulated by *us qua observers*, as if we were taking a glimpse at S *and* its surroundings from a God's eye perspective. Meanwhile, the ontological "reconstruction" we are pursuing here is an attempt to "see" the world the way S "sees" it over the course of its activity and – to stay with the same S for simplicity's sake – over the course of a much longer evolution of co-determination between S and what S *takes as* its neighborhood. Therefore, for S itself there is no $o_m,...o_n$.

However, the relationship between $o_m,...o_n$, these *Dinge an sich*, as Kant might put it, and the objects S *itself carves up in its neighborhood* F is, indeed, a puzzling issue that we shall tackle in the final part of this chapter. For the time being, let us focus on reconstructing the already mentioned process of "carving up."

To proceed further we need to start by introducing the concept of relocation:

(62) Entity x relocates with respect to y between moments t_1 and t_2 when the relative location of x with respect to y or parts of y at t_1 is different from the relevant relative location of x at t_2.

Having established the above, I propose a further step which is quite natural:

(NC3) In the third step of co-determination the following conditions are satisfied:

(a) S is capable of relocating itself with respect to F;
(b) As S relocates itself with respect to F, S distinguishes $f_1,..., f_m$, in accordance with its *p*-determined capacities and needs, which are proper parts of the interactive closure of F (which NC2 talks about);
(c) For each f_i belonging to $f_1,..., f_m$, there is a moment t in the process of S's relocation when the interactive closure of S and f_i share a boundary and this is the only boundary possessed (momentarily) by f_i;
(d) Each f_i, is in *locative connection* to the interactive closure of S *after* the moment t described in point (b), and this fact makes f_i, although it was *factually* distinguished only for a moment, a *distinguishable* part of the interactive closure of F.

Several remarks need to be appended here. First, the intuitive sense of (b) is that $f_1,\ldots, f_m$ are parts of the neighborhood's interactive closure carved up by S's movements. Actually, the very idea of S's relocation makes no sense without the relativization to $f_1,\ldots, f_m$ or a different carve-up, while, on the other hand, speaking of the emergence of $f_1,\ldots, f_m$ or any other such carve-up of parts would make no sense without S's relocation or some other factor actually singling them out from the somewhat homogenous F. So the two notions are conceptually inseparable here.

Second, (c) and (d) together mean that even if there are no *stable* boundaries attributable to parts $f_1,\ldots, f_m$, themselves, thus independently of what the system is doing at a given moment, S's movements – of course without any intention on S's part – *define a new domain*; i.e., the one uniquely identified by the locative connections between $f_1,\ldots, f_m$ and S. This means that even if the *actual* delineation of $f_1,\ldots, f_m$ is momentary, it nevertheless makes sense from that point on to speak of $f_1,\ldots, f_m$, as at least *distinguishable* parts of the interactive closure of F. This already makes a significant difference, I hold, by determining a certain *domain of possibilities* for the future actions of S. For comparison, think of, say, a wall with a homogenous structure and color, and of someone *momentarily* delineating a part of it by specific hand movements and saying "here we are going to make a window." This momentarily delineated part of the wall has not actually been singled out, not even for a moment, nonetheless, it *does* begin to *function* as a *distinguishable* part, thus as a reference of some future statements (e.g., "she said that the window will be made here") and acts (like making a real hole in the wall), despite the fact that the delineation itself only lasted a moment and did not even involve making any visible lines.

Third, the domain of possibilities composed of $f_1,\ldots, f_m$ has a fixed resolution, relative to S. This refers to a property of niches/environments that was left somewhat unresolved in representationalism (recall the pontoon bridge argument from Chapter 3).

Finally, NC3(d) provides a blueprint for a more substantial connection between S and selected entities in its environment. It was named "access" and "remote connection" by Newell (1980), but its character remained undecided, whereas now we are at least on a path to a proper conceptualization of what this "remote connection" might be.

On this basis, I propose to continue the story by introducing the following step:

> **(NC4)** The fourth step of co-determination satisfies the following conditions:
>
> (a) If $f_1,\ldots, f_m$ are *distinguishable* parts of the interactive closure of F, S is capable of *repeated* relocations with respect to $f_1,\ldots, f_m$;

(b) If S realizes the capacity described in (a), S becomes *a point of reference* for $f_1, \ldots, f_m$.

We can think of this step as the first time when the system leaves something like a "locative trace" in the world; like a trace in the forest which at the same time may start to function as a trail for future walkers. This new network of relations does not mark a spectacular change in the world. Actually, nothing changes in the world when looked at "from above" by an external observer. Yet the step is quite consequential. For from this moment on, it makes sense to say that S not only is *in* the world, but also that the world is *a certain way for* S, that S has a perspective on the world. In consequence, it *begins* to make sense to speak of S as a "center of activity." Prior to that moment the very notions of "perspective" and "centeredness" were empty, but now there is a graspable locative architecture in place. At the most fundamental level it is about a living creature *becoming* a point of reference in its neighborhood, thus about its having a certain locative capacity in its neighborhood.

Ontologically speaking, this is a pivotal moment. All the trouble we had with the locative commitment of the representational system, but also, to some extent, of the autonomous system, essentially boils down to the following issue: How is it possible that these systems maintain actual *system-specific bonds* with a particular domain of entities, and therefore are not just thrown into the domain and made to represent it, to act, to consume the information, or to utilize the affordances waiting there, like a soldier parachuted onto an unfamiliar battlefield (Varela's et al 1991 parachuter comes to mind again). Here we have an emerging *system-specific realm* which we can finally begin to treat as *an environment* (it is not a proper environment yet, but the first step has been made).

This domain, i.e. this system-centered neighborhood, is now going to become the system's *niche*. Actually – two niches: one dedicated strictly to self-maintenance and one dedicated to cognition. How so?

7.6 A niche comes about

First of all, I would like to recall the *container-frame* distinction from Chapter 6, which proves crucial now. While the boundaries of containers, resp. containing boundaries, make some (or all, in the radical scenario) connections impossible for the contained entity (they disable connections), those functioning as frames make some (or all) such connections possible (they enable them).

In this context, I propose:

(63) S is self-contained if a closure of S *contains* S with respect to some elements of $f_1, \ldots, f_m$.

(64) S is self-framed if a closure of S *frames* S with respect to some elements of $f_1,\ldots, f_m$.

This allows us to define the next step in niche construction, which will then be specified in two different directions:

(NC5) The fifth step of co-determination satisfies the following conditions:

(a) There is an *i*-closure of S that renders S self-contained and self-framed with respect to selected elements of $f_1,\ldots, f_m$ (this means that, strictly speaking, we have the third interactive closure of S, relative this time *not* to F as a single bulk but to $f_1,\ldots, f_m$);
(b) If $f_i,\ldots, f_j$ is a subset of $f_1,\ldots, f_m$ consisting of all those *f*s that S is *self-framed* with respect to, then the sum of $f_i,\ldots, f_j$ is S's *niche medium*;
(c) The interactive boundaries for S that function as frames also serve as the interactive boundaries between S and its niche medium (i.e., as the *internal* *i*-boundaries of the niche medium defined in (b));
(d) There are also interactive boundaries between the niche medium and all other *f*s (meaning $\{f_1,\ldots, f_m\}$ minus $\{f_i,\ldots, f_j\}$) which serve as *external* boundaries of the niche medium;
(e) The external boundaries of the niche medium *contain* the medium with respect to all *f*s that do *not* belong to it (this stands for a more intuitive notion of securing certain resources for the privileged use of S only).
(f) The niche for S is the sum of the niche medium and its internal as well as external *i*-boundaries.

What we arrive at is a container–frame complex resulting from the system's active engagement in its neighborhood. It turns out that, metaphorically speaking, niche construction is tantamount to setting up connections and thereby drawing boundaries in the world, while its product, the niche, is a specific bounded locus for the system which is itself a bounded locus.

We can now better understand what Wittgenstein (1922) meant when he said "the world is my world," which was also a point stressed by 4E, namely that "living beings and their environments stand in relation to each other through *mutual specification* or codetermination" (Varela et al. 1991: 198). Moreover, Varela, Thompson and Rosch explicitly ask, "how are we to specify what counts as a surface? How are we to specify its edges, boundaries, texture, and orientation, if not in relation to some perceiver for whom these distinctions are relevant? (Varela et al. 1991: 167). The NC0–NC5 story is at least a certain abstract approximation of how this "specification" comes about.

This means, in my vocabulary, that all the boundaries constituting the niche are eventually *i*-boundaries *and p*-boundaries (they are determined by the niche tenant's core principle of integrity *p*). Of course this is a gross simplification, first of all because speaking of one principle is a theoretical fiction subsuming a large variety of conditions associated with living creatures. Nevertheless, the reference to *p* – one might say a stubborn insistence on *p* – stands for a crucial point, namely that we have been continually dealing here with a certain *system-relative world* or a *system-specific presentation of* the world, very much in the spirit of Kant, Husserl, von Uexkull, Wittgenstein, Merleau-Ponty, and others, including Varela, who put enormous stress on the fact that living creatures, including cognitive systems, are not "parachuters," but instead they *enact their lifeworld.*

The concept of enactment has been a source of friction from the moment it was proposed by Varela, Thompson and Rosch (1991). Here we can finally get closer to a better grasp of it. I propose that speaking of the enactment of *a* world by a living/cognizing creature refers to that creatures' *and all its evolutionary predecessors'* pursuits of niche construction in the sense spelled out in (NC0)–(NC5).

One might say that this is not a very illuminating posit, and, indeed, it does not seem to be. However, we are not saying simply that enactment is niche construction in the standard sense of the term, meaning that an animal comes to some place, reshapes it, e.g. by building a nest, and the like. Instead, the term "enactment" may be understood as referring to the whole long evolutionary process "reconstructed" in NC0–NC5 and in the further steps to be described shortly, in which our individual constructive efforts are just tiny parts. Again, enactment is not "worldmaking" from scratch.

Going further, let us focus on the variety of the system's interactive boundaries, thus on its many interactive closures. Once S becomes capable of relocation, which equals – in this grossly simplified vocabulary – the capacity for action, we can draw a distinction between two *roles* that the interactive boundaries play for the system, both determined by S's governing principle *p*, of course. One role, the evolutionarily older one, has to do exclusively with S's self-maintenance as a system, with its integrity. The second role is evolutionarily newer for it has to do exclusively with S's actions.

So, assuming pluralism with respect to boundaries, we can draw a distinction within the interactional boundaries which emerged over the course of niche construction, between *i*-boundaries determined *solely* by S's pursuit of maintaining its integrity (in real-life cases – by the organism's metabolism) and *i*-boundaries determined *solely* by S's pursuit of relocation (which is a "microscopic form of aboutness," as Fitch 2008 nicely put it). This does not yet add anything to NC0–NC5, but clarifies a distinction already in place.

While in the first case the *i*-boundary crucially contributes to the system's very existence as an autonomous compound, in the second scenario the *i*-boundaries are drawn for the sake of action and contribute exclusively to S's dealings with parts of its neighborhood.

If the *i*-boundaries can play these two *in principle* different roles already at the relatively "primitive" level of NC5, then from that point on it is possible to speak of two different subsystems of *i*-boundaries of S, developing over the course of evolution in different directions: one designed to contribute to S's self-maintenance and the other designed to contribute to the efficacy of S's dealings with its surroundings. Put in a different way still, they are "architectural plans" *of* different things. While the former establishes the most fundamental architecture of the processes of maintaining the integrity of the system, the latter *i*-boundary establishes the most fundamental architecture of the system's actions.

To be clear, speaking of two architectures does not mean that they must actually be separated and that they evolved separately. Insofar as they have different tasks, they need to be *conceptually* distinguished, although they naturally co-exist.

7.7 Making room for the emergence of a cognitive niche

The key idea I draw on is that the two subsystems of interactive boundaries of our target system S, as interconnected as they are, may develop in two (conceptually) different directions, so that the maintenance-related role is played by such advanced and complex subsystems of *i*-boundaries as, e.g. the immune system, while the action-oriented role is played by specific boundary-drawing interventions in S's surroundings.

I therefore propose a certain amendment of (NC5):

> **(NC5*a*)** If all the connections referred to in (NC5) are direct connections in the sense defined by (17), thus cases when S shares a boundary with an entity or overlaps with it, then (NC5) defines S's *autopoietic*-niche; i.e. a niche dedicated to maintaining S's integrity, resp. autopoiesis.

The pivotal point is the *directness* of S's connections. The absorption of certain substances by the organism is a good example. Defining a niche in these terms is a far-reaching simplification, perhaps suitable only for such relatively "primitive" cases as Ediacaran creatures, but certainly not for complex animals. If we take more intuitive examples of niches, such as the bear's cave with a snail referenced earlier, it becomes clear that even if it makes sense to distinguish the purely autopoietic part of the bear's niche from its cognition-related segment, the former cannot be only about direct connection (the bear is not directly connected with the snail, at least unless the latter is eaten by the former). Therefore, speaking of the autopoietic niche *as a distinctive realm* is a kind of theoretical fiction again. As for the example given, the snail must be considered part of the bear's autopoietic niche as a potential source of nutrients required for the bear's self-maintenance, however, this relationship must involve a cognitive element. After all, the bear can see its edible roommate. Thus, in reality each niche of a complex living creature is a complex mix comprising autopoiesis- or autonomy-oriented and cognition-oriented segments.

However, I believe that the aforementioned theoretical fiction can still be useful. Namely ($NC5^a$) defines what the autopoietic niche is *in principle*, which also makes it easier to properly grasp what constitutes a *cognitive* niche. And the latter is my main focus here. I will not be talking about the autopoietic niche so much. In other words, ($NC5^a$), set as a background or contrast, makes it easier to see and recognize specific properties of niches dedicated to cognition. Let me then start uncovering these properties stepwise.

As I said before, there may be a growing need for stability on the part of the system's surroundings if S's actions are to become increasingly efficient, and this stability evolves, beginning with the first system of interactive boundaries introduced to F and shared with S and developing together with the beginning of F's segmentation into $f_i, \ldots, f_j$.

Yet, another step in niche construction is the emergence of the niche medium's internal *i*-boundaries that are *not* shared with the system S. Hence – the emergence of something new built on the NC5 ground. Recall that according to NC5(c), the interactive boundaries of S *also* serve as the interactive boundaries between S and its niche medium, thus as the internal interactive boundaries of the niche medium. Now, I propose, we need to introduce the internal boundaries of the niche medium that are still determined by the system-governing principle *p* (this tie cannot be broken), but nevertheless belong to the niche medium *itself*. This refers to relatively S-independent boundaries on the part of S's neighborhood, thus something much closer to how we see things in *our* world.

The latter move is motivated by a certain peculiarity attributable to cognition, at least as we experience it. Tim Crane gives a fitting formulation of what I mean when he writes that "reflection on what it is like to have an experience does not reveal properties of experiences themselves, but only of their objects" (Crane 2006: 128). This phenomenon is known in the field of philosophy of perception as the *transparency of experience*. To put it in the plainest terms, the world seems to simply be there, *present to me* in a certain way, in a certain guise, displaying certain *surfaces*, while my senses seem to be transparent windows onto it (meaning – I am closed *as* an organism but I am fundamentally *open* to the world *as* a cognizer). There is, therefore, a certain genuine experience of passivity in being *presented with* the world. In my assessment, 4E is right to stress that this passivity is not constitutive of cognition, although it cannot be ignored either. Within the conceptual framework proposed here, we can account for this *being presented with the world* as a relatively stable *product* of niche construction, thus a *product* of a certain *activity*. Yet, as a product, it is *not* an activity itself – a subtlety which in my view is not sufficiently accounted for in the 4E paradigm.

It is here that the real battle over the plausibility of introducing the concept of the cognitive niche unfolds. Someone may argue that speaking of the passive state of being *presented with* the world goes against the very spirit of 4E. In reply, I return to an observation I made in Chapter 1: we think of ourselves not only as doers but also as understanders. As understanders we seem to be capable of "slackening" our intentional bonds with the world, as Merleau-Ponty (1962/2005) put it, and thus to some extent of distancing ourselves from worldly goings-on in order to reflect on them as simply being there, given to us. Therefore, denying this passivity goes against a fundamental phenomenological recognition, which is not something that at least Varela, Thompson and Rosch would recommend given their insistence on taking experience seriously. We must somehow account for this passive quality of experience, and one of a number of possible ways of doing it is by postulating certain relatively system-independent (yet still system-specific, which is spelled out in terms of *p*-boundaries) setups of boundaries/surfaces in the system's surroundings.

There is another crucial thing in this context, related to the issue of "being presented with." Namely, the issue of *productivity*, already cited when I was talking about products of niche construction. To see what is at stake and recognize its significance, let us focus on 4E's appeal to history: what is so special about the *history* of interactions or structural coupling, as highlighted in the 4E literature? My point is this: history is *just a history*; temporal processes are just processes; there is no creative power in the flow of time *alone*. These temporal processes must *produce* something. And this condition is ontologically non-trivial, for acts and products are characterized by different features and there is *no* a priori *necessity* for *all* acts to result in products (see Twardowski 1912/1999). I can run and even break world records, but there is no genuine thing or entity that would last longer than the process and could be recognized as *a product of me running*. Therefore, the bare fact that there *are* interactions or structural couplings does not mean that something is brought forth or enacted by them.

A proponent of representationalism might at this point propose that over the course of evolution organisms acquire an ability to *produce* certain *models* of external reality out of the firings of neurons (as Tooby & De Vore 1987 might say). And, as we already saw, it is not the case that representationalism neglects action. On the contrary, the ability to act within changing environments and to integrate different stimuli plays a crucial role in many representationalist accounts, as seen in Ramsey (2007), Gładziejewski and Miłkowski (2017), Shea (2018); also in Burge (2010) or Feinberg and Mallatt (2016) who study the natural history (evolution) of cognition and consciousness. Hence, we cannot commend 4E solely for highlighting the significance of action because representationalism does exactly the same thing.

Therefore, 4E needs a different account of what is *produced* by the history of interactions or structural coupling. However, it must not be solely about the production of organisms or cognizers themselves, thus a process of making the system a bounded and internally coordinated unity. It must also account for how the environment – which is *not assumed* as given by 4E! – comes about as a relatively stable structure.

My argumentation in favor of the concept of cognitive niche is thus based on the assumption that there is no *a priori* link between patterns of self-maintenance "inside" the living system and patterns of the system's interactions resulting in a relatively stable layout of the world which, in turn, determines and facilitates further interactions. Living systems might have thrived in a medium consisting of a flux without any patterns, yet they likely would not have been able to develop much.

Here is the point: evolution "needed" to find a way to "conserve" certain patterns, not only on the side of living systems, but *also on the side of their surroundings*. And this is where the concept of the cognitive niche comes up. Hence, it is not clear why the history of interaction or structural coupling alone is supposed to result in anything, but *if* this coupling is the construction (production, we might say) of a cognitive niche, then the appeal to history becomes plausible: this is the history inscribed, so to speak, in the structure of cognitive niches, just like the history of states is, in a sense, inscribed in institutions such as parliaments, supreme courts and the like.

The guiding idea here is that over the course of their ontogenesis and of evolution as a whole cognitive systems seek to *conserve* their cognitive efforts and achievements. To achieve this aim, they seek relatively stable structures (for more on seeking conservation as a well-recognized phenomenon when it comes to evolution at large, see e.g., Kovác 2000).

All these caveats having been made, let me repeat my proposal: what is being produced over the course of the development of niche construction is a setup of internal interactive boundaries of the niche medium that are *distinct* from the interactive boundaries of the niche constructor S. And this pivotal moment of divergence of the two *i*-boundary structures marks the birth of the "first" cognitive niche. These structures can be taken *as given* in further steps of cognitive niche construction by future generations of constructors. These *i*-boundary structures, therefore, constitute the world *we* are "awaken" in, "not made but found," as Varela et al. (1991) nicely put it; the world *we* will be able to occasionally "slacken" our "intentional threads" with, seeking a safe refuge for reflection.

7.8 A blueprint for the cognitive niche

All that being said, here is the next step in the locative-ontological reconstruction I propose:

> **(NC6)** The sixth step of co-determination satisfies the following conditions:
>
> (a) For $f_i,\ldots,f_j$ which is, as before, the subset of $f_1,\ldots,f_m$ consisting of all those *f*s that S is *self-framed* with respect to, there emerges a domain consisting of the interactive closures of all these separate *f*s.
> (b) The interactive closures of the *f*s defined in (a) are all *p*-closures (where *p* is, as before, the principle of S's integrity);
> (c) The interactive closure of S and the interactive closures of the *f*s defined in (a) are disjoint;
> (d) The *f*s are self-contained with respect to S;
> (e) The interactive closure of S and the interactive closure of each of the *f*s maintain *direct locative* connections (their *locations* are *directly* connected).
> (f) The sum of the interactive closures of the *f*s is a niche medium.

Each point requires comment. To begin, while (a) and (f) describe the emergence of a new domain of entities and a new niche medium irreducible to what previous points referred to, (b) states that we are still talking about the world that is strictly *relative to the system* (the niche constructor). However – and this is the pivotal point – (c) states that the boundaries of the new interactive closures of *f*s, while still being interactional and, therefore, relative to S, are attributed to *the things* S interacts with, to our *f*s, and *not* to S or *its* closure. They are the boundaries possessed by the *f*s themselves. This means that they, in a sense, persist whether a given *f* is interacting with S at a given moment, or not. Previously, S, for the sake of interaction, "lent" its own interactive boundary to the partner entities, meanwhile here the whole point is that niche construction has now attained a level of productivity at which the partner entities have *their own* interactive boundaries. This accounts for what I referred to as the relative stability of the domain of S's actions; a domain that S enters or faces, but does not create with each individual interaction.

Further on, (d) and (e) are no less significant, and yet the former may cause some confusion. For (NC4) and (NC5) already state, and (NC6) repeats, that the whole set $\{f_i, \ldots, f_j\}$ consists of *f*s that S's connection to is made possible by S's interactive closure. So what is this containment condition in (NC5d) doing there?

Let me begin by stressing that we are talking about a *new* setup of boundaries, this time attributable to the *f*s themselves – to each single one. Although relative to interactions with S, these new boundaries define new standards, so to speak, for these interactions, imposing certain new limits on them. The *i*-boundaries emerging at earlier stages of niche construction are still at work but in addition now the *f*s also "have a say" by establishing their own interactive closures (conditions of interaction) and by limiting S's access to them (which is spelled out in terms of containment).

To get a better intuitive grasp of this dynamic of framing and containing, let us go back to the example of perception, already explored above. Note that the familiar surfaces of things in our cognitive niche are Janus-faced in the sense that on the one hand they make things perceptually accessible, perceptually given to us, but at the same time they always "present" things only to a certain degree, with a certain finite resolution, thereby also concealing the enormous complexity these things are actually composed of. Look at the wall in front of you – it is composed of a hardly countable number of grains of concrete, plaster or what have you; these grains are composed of certain chemicals, and we can go all the way down to elementary particles dancing in space more or less vividly. Now, all this is "masked" by ordinary perceivable surfaces and their limited resolution. I see the wall, not the grains or the smaller chemical complexes. The latter are basically obscured from my view. Now, although such limitedness sounds bad, it is a great advantage that we can enjoy these limited-resolution surfaces which "wrap up" the enormous complexity of any material entity, for otherwise our surroundings would hardly be navigable.

This should give us some idea of what the dynamic of framing and containment described in NC5 and NC6 is about. Its purpose is exactly to do justice to this Janus-faced character of the manifest image of the world we are in touch with.

No less pivotal is (e), and no less controversial. And it actually spells out *what I propose to see as the core locative mark of cognition*. Namely, it speaks to the system's capacity to maintain some kind of direct connection with things *despite* the fact that they are not in the system's direct proximity. It may even seem paradoxical, for how can it be that two entities are directly locatively connected if their exact locations are not directly connected? And yet, I propose that this is precisely the locative peculiarity of cognition, namely that it transcends the limits of exact location. This is what Newell (1980) called "remote connection," and what finally captures the ubiquitous but rarely problematized references to "distal" or "external" things in the Cartesian cognitive science, where the said things are assumed as somehow *accessible*.

Here is what the latter claim stands for. First, it is conceptually useful to emphasize the distinction, already made explicit but not utilized properly so far, between the system itself, defined primarily by its *g*-boundaries together with the exact location of its *g*-closure, and *its interactive closure* (actually many interactive closures) whose exact location may be vastly different from the exact location of the system *as* seen through its *g*-boundaries. Now, the whole point in (e) is that *cognition creates a very special interactive closure of the system*. Putting this in first person, this is an *i*-closure of mine that *makes it possible for me* to set up locative connections with things far from the exact location of my body! *I* am not my body alone in this new context; instead "I" refers to the whole interactive compound, the whole physical-behavioral unit, as Smith (2001) might say, consisting of my body (my biological basis) but also a realm of actual and potential interactions. In this sense, the embodiment condition stressed by 4E not only points to the somewhat obvious fact that cognitive systems are actual biological individuals, a fact acknowledged by more recent developments within representationalism, too, but to embodiment in a more derivative, but also – I believe – more profound sense referring to the creation of peculiar units as defined in (NC6).

Let me again propose an analogy to a more real-life and thus perhaps more intuitively understandable case. When we think of distal perception, a specific feature of it, which marked a great turning point in the evolution of cognition somewhere between the Ediacaran and the Cambrian, is that it somehow puts us "in touch" and makes us "acquainted with" things without the need to abut or actually touch them. It was fittingly recognized by Plotnick et al. (2010) as the Cambrian "information revolution." The evolutionary advantage of this possibility is clear (see e.g. Hsieh et al. 2022). However trivial and simplistic it may sound, it is much better to see a tiger approaching than to have to touch it in order to know that it is there. As already stressed throughout this book, this may seem obvious, and yet it deserves more attention – it is a phenomenon deserving of philosophical problematization that perception enables us to "move closer" to a thing without any physical relocation. Therefore, perception's locative mark is highly peculiar, and a proper articulation of it – without any predetermined assumption about what the term "distal perception" stands for – is a challenging endeavor which I have here tried to at least partly accomplish. And what goes for perception goes for cognition more broadly.

Cognition proper (I remain neutral with respect to where it begins and rely on standard and uncontroversial exemplifications thereof such as vision or hearing) is here portrayed as the capacity to "manipulate" our locative footprint in a manner that is not available to pre-cognitive functioning, as a result of which a new domain – the cognitive niche – comes about.

To shed more light on this locative specificity of cognition, let me invoke an even more "advanced" phenomenon – one that is perhaps surprisingly remote from what we are trying to tackle here, since it relates to the social and economic sphere. Take it as a useful heuristic then.

The economic geographer David Harvey once said that the emergence of capitalism made space less relevant or effectively irrelevant in the pursuit of the exchange of goods and especially of financial capital; he even speaks figuratively of the "annihilation of space by time" (Harvey 1990). For time is the actual force in capitalism, not space. Think of bank transactions which take just few seconds, transferring capital from Asia to America at an ontological level where physical space is almost completely irrelevant (it is effectively negligible). This causes certain tensions due to the trivial fact that actual human lives are highly dependent on space – workers are located, their work is located, their households are located, etc. Meanwhile, the capital enabling them to make their located living is almost free of such locative commitments and free to move from place to place at almost no cost. It is all possible, of course, due to various institutional and technological advances.

The heuristic I propose is as follows: what applies to capitalism as a system of exchange (which by the way may be considered a very high-level development of human cognitive niches; see Frolov 2023 in this spirit) applies at the most fundamental level of cognition: the latter's basic locative architecture. For cognition itself, along with its locative peculiarity, rests on the capacity to *as if* "annihilate" space, as Harvey might say, through the establishment of specific interactive boundaries, interactive closures, and therefore *through new kinds of locative connections*.

This peculiar capacity is grounded in a particular physiological/neurological/computational machinery characterized by a certain sensitivity, reactivity, information processing mechanisms, etc. These are all empirical puzzles which I am not even trying to do justice to. But what they give rise to does have – as I am trying to show – *a unique locative mark*. And this is what I have tried to elicit here and throughout this book.

This is not the end of the story, however. The development described in (NC6) should be considered pre-cognitive, one step before the cognitive domain proper, so the final step is still ahead. Note that NC6 concludes with (f) which says that a *new* niche medium emerges when the closures of each of the *f*s are summed up (which is different from the closure of the entire *set* of *f*s, taken as one, which NC5 referred to), but it does not specify what kind of niche it is, thus *what the system is doing* with this new niche medium. I shall propose that one more condition is needed to supplement NC6.

7.9 The cognitive niche is finally here

Here is another mark of cognition which, however obvious it may sound at first, constitutes an important problem in the philosophical literature and also requires some treatment from the perspective proposed here. Namely, cognition can be successful to varying degrees. A belief is something that may be false; a representation is something that by definition may turn out to be misrepresentation; an intentional act can miss its target; action itself, considered perhaps the most fundamental form of cognition by some 4E advocates, can simply fail. How so?

Cognition seems to have as one of its constitutive features something J. L. Austin (1953) and then John Searle (1983) aptly called "direction of fit." There is something on the side of the cognitive system and something on the side of the cognized part of the world, and the two either "fit" each other to a degree, or not. Traditionally, if one has a belief, it is supposed to "fit" what is going on in the world; whereas when one has an expectation, the world is supposed to "fit" what the system wants.

This aspect is somewhat neglected by 4E and, on the other hand, exploited extensively by Cartesian cognitive science. The notion of representational content does the job well here: the said aspect of cognition, which might be called "epistemic," is defined in terms of some kind of "correspondence" (or lack thereof) between the content on the one hand and the external state of affairs on the other. However, this is not a solution that 4E generally accepts, and, even aside from 4E's hostility toward traditional epistemology (nicely unpacked and nicely argued for by Johnson & Tucker 2021, Chemero 2009 and Rowlands 1999), it is also quite problematic a stance from the niche construction perspective. For how can a niche be "wrong" in any sense of the term? Is a niche "about" anything in the first place? "About" its own base perhaps? Some considerations are very much in order here.

First, distinguishing between internal and external states or entities, which seems to define the very idea of "direction of fit," does not have to entail the whole baggage of Cartesianism. After all, it is trivially true that the table at which I am currently sitting is different from my thought about it. However, the problematic aspect of Cartesianism is that Descartes and his followers seem to adopt monism with respect to boundaries, while there are good reasons to claim that we can have many *internal versus external* divisions drawn by different "subsystems" under different circumstances. A large part of this investigation was dedicated to unpacking and arguing for pluralism with respect to boundaries. That said, I claim that there is no good *a priori* reason not to reintroduce "direction of fit" into this new pluralistic context.

Second, the idea of "direction of fit" is not by definition solely about how "fit" or "accurate" beliefs are, thus about truth and falsity. Instead, not only beliefs but potentially also actions can be bearers or vehicles of the quality of being more or less "fit" or "fitting." Moreover, the said quality is not by definition about structural resemblance or isomorphism. Note that the very idea of "fitting" is rather metaphorical and I keep it that way for a reason: any technical rendering of it would require a well-defined conceptual framework, e.g. formal semantics, and many of these frameworks would likely not be acceptable to 4E. For that reason, I would like to keep to the intuitive understanding at this point, before proposing a formulation that should in principle be acceptable to those who, like me, align with the ecological approach to cognition.

Let us return to the idea of *models* and modeling the environment discussed by Tooby and De Vore (1987) as a defining factor of the cognitive niche. I will not reference Tooby and De Vore's original posit, however; instead, I shall refer to the notion of embodied models provisionally characterized in Chapter 5. The main idea put forward there was that certain interventions within a living creature's surroundings can serve to model cause–effect chains. I shall unpack this concept below. This will finally introduce the proper cognitive niche to the story.

Let me stress once again that given the limited scope of this investigation my goal is obviously not to provide a comprehensive account of how such embodied modeling is actually executed by cognitive systems, for it is in large part an empirical job. The goal is not even to come up with a complete theoretical treatment; my aim is more modest. Namely I wish to elicit the locative architecture of *the capacity to model* an environment possessed by the environmentally plugged-in or embodied system (the niche constructor), thus provide an account of how the pursuit of embodied modeling involves location and boundaries.

Crucially, we are no longer vulnerable to the argument from pregiven environment, i.e. an environment assumed as simply being there, awaiting a creature to "parachute" into it, for the whole conceptual machinery rolled out in this chapter was supposed to account for how niches, and therefore also larger environments come about (the final word shall be said in this section).

What could it, therefore, mean for a niche as defined by (NC6), which might be regarded as a blueprint for the cognitive niche, to work as a model? When we have the answer, we shall finally have the characterization of the cognitive niche that we are seeking. I propose that the key thing is the relation between the interactive closures of the *f*s, thus the entities delineated within the cognitive medium over the course of the system's interactions and evolution, and $\{o_1,\ldots o_n\}$, i.e. the objects, our *Dinge an sich*, which the system's neighborhood was originally summed up from. The latter refers to the assumed niche base which somewhat faded from view over the course of this investigation. Yet, it faded for a reason: we can say nothing about the niche base without touching on the niche built from it. This, however, does not mean that we cannot define a relation that *is at least possible* between the base *o*s and the carved-up *f*s.

In a sense, if we think of "being a base" or "providing a base" as a relation directed from $\{o_1,\ldots o_n\}$ to the niche built from it, I propose to take modeling as a "reply," thus as a relation going in the opposite direction: from the niche as a product, to its base.

This means:

(65) S may use the interactive closures of $f_i,\ldots, f_j$ which are, as before, those entities that S is *self-framed* with respect to, as a model of $o_1,\ldots o_n$ if for some *f* and some *o*, the location of the *i*-closure of *f* overlaps with the location of *o*.

This may sound somewhat artificial, but note one thing: one of the ways to refer to the structure of an entity is to refer to its boundaries, to *where* they are and how they relate to one another (their relative locations), which includes the *i*-closures of that entity (if it has any). For example, I can describe the structure of the tree outside my window by pointing to the perceivable edges differentiating the branches from one another, differentiating the branches from the leaves, and this whole compound from the background, as Gestalt psychology teaches us. If so, the relation of overlap between the *locations* of the closures of two different things can stand for the fact that the things somehow structurally have do to with each other. This is the intuition behind (65).

Speaking of intuition we can imagine the relation defined in (65) the following way. Think of the kind of paper cut-out that kids used to play with, or any package with a line drawn where you are supposed to cut it open to take out the contents. The lines can be considered as boundaries with a fixed location, and the actual cut you make is also a boundary, although a different one. You will never make the cut exactly as the line indicates, but if you do a good job, the actual location of the cut-boundary will overlap with the location of the drawn-line-boundary. We experience something relatively similar, I argue, in the process of cognitive niche construction.

All that said, I propose:

(NC7) The sixth step of niche construction is the emergence of a niche described in (NC6) *such that* S can use it to model the niche base. If a niche can be used in the capacity of a model, the niche shall be called S's cognitive niche.

The question now is: how we can even *know* that our internal-to-the-niche constructs model ("fit") the base appropriately? With this in mind we come back to the issue of success and failure. A cognitive niche is the domain enacted over the course of a long process of co-determination, such that the system can not only *act* there, but it can also *succeed and fail* in these actions. Crucially, success and failure are not inherent to the action itself; they are not qualities possessed by the action alone. An extra condition is needed to make sense of the distinction. Survival or lack thereof are not sufficient. To put it in a very simplistic way, the fact that a given organism was eaten by a bigger one does not itself mean that the former failed in some action; things such as being eaten happen every day. Failure in action is a richer concept, I argue, and I suppose it is clear at least to all representationalists, and should be seriously taken into account by the advocates of 4E as well. One of the ways in which success and failure can be defined makes reference to the pursuit of modeling: here an action is successful if it is *based on* an accurate model – as representationalists would say; or if the action *itself is* an accurate model, or if the enacted domain in which the action occurs is an accurate model (where accuracy is a matter of degree, of course).

The key point here is that (NC7) allows us to speak of models as something actually *embodied* – embodied in action and embodied in a particular environment – thereby freeing it from the Cartesian baggage. For note that we are not dealing with "copies" or "pictures" of an allegedly objective, external realm stored "in the head." Instead, the cognized world is itself its best model, in step with Brooks's (1991) famous dictum: the things populating our cognitive niches are used as models once they are used at all, thus if they are used for the sake of action (if they are taken as affordances, to use Gibson's term).

7.10 Conclusion

(NC7) is the final moment of the locative-ontological "representation" of niche construction. This is not to say that there is nothing more to be said about the pursuit of cognitive niche construction within ontology, and no further steps to be taken. Let me recall that the goal was just to lay out *the most basic* locative architecture of niche construction, and this, I believe, is what this chapter has achieved. Now is the right time to consider the fruits borne by it, thus to recapitulate the conceptual challenges unveiled over the course of Chapters 1–5 and make an assessment of how the proposed vocabulary clarifies things – if it does.

8 Prospects for Ecological Internalism

In this final chapter I would like to revisit several issues raised in earlier parts of this book and reconsider them in light of the idea presented in Chapters 6 and 7. This will pave the way for my concluding attempt to argue for a new position in the mind-*as*-a-place versus mind-*in*-a-place debate – one that I provisionally call *ecological internalism*.

8.1 A quick recap

To begin with, note that thanks to the vocabulary rolled out in the previous two chapters we obtain a unified framework enabling us to conceptualize both sides of the otherwise problematic mind–world bond. This framework forms a single cluster of concepts capturing essential properties of the cognitive system on the one hand, and of the place in which this system operates on the other. We can, therefore, speak of the exact location of a system as well as the exact location of its niche, of various kind of boundaries maintained by the system and those maintained by its niche, as well as boundaries that the two share or "negotiate." We can refer to connections between parts of the system, between parts of the niche medium, and between the system (or its parts) and selected segments of the niche.

Within this framework it becomes possible to actually substantiate the claims presented or at least hinted at in the 4E literature, arguing that the realm in which the autonomous system realizes its cognitive functions should also be thought of as a *higher-level* autonomous system built *by* and *around* the living creature. The latter in this context may be conceptualized as the *fundamental-level* autonomous system. The construction of such a higher-level system helps the fundamental-level system expand its boundaries and "negotiate" new ones in pursuit of greater stability in the process of maintaining its autonomy.

Coming up with this kind of unified conceptual (ontological) framework is by no means a trivial thing. For within this framework there is no Cartesian *dichotomy* between the internal and the external, although there

DOI: 10.4324/9781003580997-8

is a rich variety of more contextual or situational *distinctions* of a similar kind. There is no contradiction between the notion of mind as a locus and the idea that mind is constituted by a larger locus – the complex nexus of ecological bonds.

Within this framework we should be able to answer the need spelled out in Chapter 1 – stemming from the recognition that we are not only doers but also understanders – for a relatively stable "safe refuge" in which reflection and judgment (epistemic or moral) can be undertaken. Recall Plato who was not wary of the world's perceived flux because of some anxiety, as Johnson and Tucker (2021) suggested, but because he understood that wisdom, to use the most traditional term which has been absent from these reflections so far, needs a moment of solitude to grow.

Speaking of philosophical traditions and standing on the shoulders of giants, let me make the latter point differently. In Chapter 1, I expressed the belief that the bucket theory (derided by Popper) arose neither from a mental habit, as Ryle argued, nor from a strong theoretical conviction, as Popper himself suggested, but was just a provisional postulate for lack of a better option. The conceptual framework designed to capture the ecological aspect of cognition was not sufficiently developed at the time to enable thinkers like Descartes to devise a more nuanced locative narrative about the mind.

Today, I argue, there is another option. We can try to do something that may seem, on the surface of it, quite paradoxical, namely provide *an ecological account of inwardness*. This means re-defining the mind-*as*-a-place approach in terms of cognitive niches so that the postulated inner self becomes the interior of a cognitive niche, not the "Cartesian theatre," to use Dennett's (1991) famous phrasings, established "in the head." This is the crux of the announced ecological internalism.

8.2 Going back to the initial questions, and beyond

To make the above promises more precise, let me recall the three questions I posed in the concluding part of Chapter 1.

The first question problematized whether or not it was possible to conceive of the mind as *a locus*, i.e., an entity or place in which some other entity can be located, and if so, what kind of locus might it be and for what kind of entities? Noteworthily, Plato had doubts about this, while Descartes, following Augustine, said "yes" somewhat cautiously, which answer would subsequently, and this time without hesitation, be taken up by Hume and Locke. This mind-*as*-a-place approach would be "naturalized" in the 20th-century philosophy of mind and cognitive science in the form of the idea of the physical symbolic (representational) system. Now we can add a new layer to this story, saying: yes, it is possible to conceive of the mind as a locus, but this locus that the mind is to be identified with (and deemed responsible for *as a constructor*) is the cognitive niche, not just the computational machinery "in the head."

The second question concerned whether it was possible to conceive of the mind as *a located* entity, i.e., an entity that must be placed somewhere, and if so, what kind of located entity might the mind be and what kind of locus would it need? The 4E movement begun as a new chapter of the externalist story which included semantic externalism and, earlier, behaviorism. Here we can also add a new chapter. Mind is in principle a located phenomenon, just like 4E states, and yet this does not mean that it is something that landed in an environment – a kind of pregiven landing pad awaiting the living creature to come and merely "mirror" its structure or gather the information resources awaiting there. Instead – 4E says – a cognitive system's *being-in-the-world* means that the system and the world are structurally coupled and, therefore, co-determined or co-enacted, which is, in principle, a *constructive* process. However, as I have pointed out throughout this book, the notion of enactment proves to be the biggest source of friction due to its alleged "idealistic underpinnings." The way to resolve this dilemma would therefore involve spelling out enactment in terms of cognitive niche construction and carefully distilling all the conceptually distinguishable ingredients of this process.

The proposed story also makes room for representations, since, as I mentioned, there is no need for the mind-*in*-a-place platform to be a mere vehicle of anti-representationalism. The notion of representation as it is now being defined in terms of structural representations and their "consumption" is very much in line with 4E's grounding in the biological sciences and can, therefore, be reintroduced.

The answer to the second question posed in Chapter 1 is therefore: yes, the mind is co-determined or co-constituted by a specific locus; strictly speaking, it is determined over the course of cognitive niche construction.

The third question dwelled on the nature of the internal versus external distinction and problematized whether it was possible for the mind to have boundaries, and if so, what kind of boundaries. We can now obtain a much more fine-grained image, which shows not a single boundary, an "iron-curtain" type of barrier, but rather a system of boundaries of various kinds. This includes interactional boundaries acting as containers but also as frames. Therefore, while the internal versus external delineation is still in operation (there is no reason to get rid of it completely, after all it makes intuitive sense, given our everyday experience), it no longer serves solely to wall off the objective from the subjective. Instead, we can speak of a complex *system of boundaries* whose function is, among others, to make the world, at least in part, accessible to cognition.

Another point made in Chapter 1 is that once the internal/external divide becomes a metaphysical iron curtain, as it has after years of conceptual evolution completed by Locke and Hume (standing on the shoulders of Descartes) and their modern successors, the very possibility of perceiving and knowing anything about the real world (not just our subjective projections from sensory data) becomes a mystery. Newell (1980) explicitly talked of "access" and "inputs" to the system, as if the latter referred to actual things in the world. However, if one embraces the Cartesian internal versus external dichotomy, one has to optimistically assume (take for granted) the very *accessibility of the external world*, for there is no conceptual tool to clarify *how* the external world (if any) becomes accessible. In contrast, the said accessibility conditions were relatively well-defined in the pre-Cartesian tradition which saw cognition as a kind of participation in a larger rationality. This way of speaking was largely metaphorical, but it was still better than nothing. For example, we have Plato's notion of the rational "light" emitted by the highest idea of the Good, which makes bodily reality intelligible.

Representationalism can, therefore, make reference to flows of information coming to the system (Dretske), the consumption of information within the system (Millikan, Godfrey-Smith, Ramsey, Shea), the semantic functions of representation (Newell, Fodor), and structural representations that are isomorphic or at least homomorphic with respect to external structures in the world (Ramsey, Gładziejewski & Miłkowski), but *the very possibility* of all these posits must be assumed upfront as given. Meanwhile, the profound philosophical conundrum has to do with the issue of whether or not these optimistic beliefs in structural resemblance, information flows, etc. are at all accurate. In other words, *under what conditions is the world accessible to us in the first place*?

Thanks to the niche construction framework it becomes possible to retrace our steps and revamp some key aspects of the pre-Cartesian *cognition-as-participation* approach. For cognition as a process of niche construction clearly transcends the bounds of individual thought and information processing. Instead, it works like "participation" (as the notion of structural coupling makes clear) in a bigger cognitive project, so to speak, developing over the course of millions of years of evolution. This "project" is precisely inter-generational cognitive niche construction.

I shall now dig deeper into these barely touched-upon ideas, devoting each section to a specific issue that has stood out over the course of our investigations.

8.3 The boundaries of cognitive systems: Where's "in" and where's "out"?

The extended mind hypothesis set forth by Clark and Chalmers (1998) brought the question of the boundaries of mind or the cognitive system, and therefore also of its locative footprint, to the fore. Clark and Chalmers invited us to reconsider where mind begins and where it ends.

We can now see how things stand in a new light. First, I agree with Menary, who carries on Clark and Chalmers's idea and holds that "cognition does not have a spatial boundary that lies at the periphery of the brain, or even at the skin" (Menary 2007: p. 4), but this does not mean that cognition has no boundary at all. The thing is that there are several kinds of boundaries attributable to creatures capable of cognition, and therefore cognition can be considered *one of* the factors responsible for the establishment of boundaries – one of the boundary-drawers, so to speak. So yes, cognition is not determined by the boundary of the actual matter composing the body. Yet the body itself, too, taken as a living system and not just a physical thing, has more than one system of boundaries, and its physical barriers differ critically from its immunological barriers (as discussed in Chapter 6). The body itself is a living complex (*Leib*, not only *Körper*, as Buytendijk & Plessner 1936 famously put it) maintaining a variety of interactive boundaries, and the same applies to that *same* body thought of as a cognitive system.

By applying the vocabulary developed in Chapters 6 and 7, we can reformulate the extended mind hypothesis as follows: the cognitive machinery is one of the living creature's many subsystems that draw their own system-specific *interactive boundaries* dedicated to "negotiating" conditions of interaction with selected segments of the system's surroundings. At the same time we need not worry that "anything goes" now, and that freed from the confines of "skin and skull" we can take any entity as part of the extended mind, for all these interactive boundaries drawn by cognition must also be principle-based boundaries in the sense defined in Chapter 6, i.e., they must be determined by a given system's unifying "program" (the system's autonomy conditions, as proponents of 4E would say).

It seems that Menary did not take the option just spelled out into account, although it had been hinted at by Clark and Chalmers. While the immune system already draws its boundaries at a completely different level than the physical barrier offered by the integumentary system, cognition reaches even farther from "skin and skull." In other words, cognition operates even more independently of the "skin and skull" boundary system due to its capacity to establish interactive boundaries that make it possible to set up direct locative connections with *distant* entities. Yet, however special cognition's capacity as a boundary-drawer, it no longer appears as something completely outrageous when we adopt pluralism with respect to the boundaries of autonomous systems and view cognitive boundaries against the background of a variety of other organismic boundaries that exist in nature.

All this means that cognition, as seen within the proposed locative-ontological framework, is, indeed, extended, but this does not mean that its boundaries are negatively characterized as simply *not identical* to the barriers of "skin and skull" while their positive nature remains unspecified. We can now say quite precisely what they are and render them somewhat less mysterious: they belong to a larger family of interactive boundaries.

In my view, the external and internal boundaries of cognitive niches, which are all by definition interactive boundaries, are developments of the interactive boundaries of cognitive (autonomous) systems themselves, and as such they are the "extended" boundaries of mind that Clark and Chalmers were seeking. This does not resolve the controversies around the extended mind hypothesis, especially the empirical controversy as to whether the hypothesis is corroborated by relevant data. However, the proposed framework does spell out the postulated extension in a more ontologically developed manner.

The above discussion also touches on an issue that I raised in Chapter 3 when discussing Ramsey's account of representational machinery, in particular his illuminating revision of the Tower Bridge model of the representational system. Ramsey decomposes the system into subsystems and argues convincingly that certain states "serve as representations because that is how the internal sub-systems treat them, given their job descriptions (e.g. performing addition, assessing chess moves, etc.)" (Ramsey 2007: 74).

As I put it in Chapter 3, Ramsey zoomed-in on the system and made an inventive move by transplanting the Cartesian internal versus external distinction into the system's internal realm. However, if so, then how is it possible to identify the "frontier input," so to speak, thus input that is *not* the output of another *internal* subsystem but comes from the domain that is genuinely *external* to the system as a whole? In other words, the puzzle has to do with how to delineate the external boundary of such a decomposed representational machinery.

An advocate of the extended mind hypothesis might claim that certain bearers of representational content are external to the body, yet they should also be considered subsystems of a larger cognitive system composed of the acting body *and* parts of its surroundings, computers, calculators and notebooks included. So, one "pylon" of Ramsey's Tower Bridge "decides" on what counts as another "pylon" and whether or not the latter plays a representational role. For example, the retinal image as such does not play a representational role within the system *because* it is part of the body, but due to the "decision" of the next "pylon" in the visual system which uses the retinal image if not as a representation proper, then at least as something more than a nexus of physical events, i.e., as material to be exploited by further representational machinery. But if so, then a microscope or an RTG device that causes the said retinal image can *also* be regarded as part of the system, of the representational machinery as a whole, *if* a relevant subsystem "decides" so.

This latter issue was metaphorically referred to in Chapter 3 in the question of where the representational Tower Bridge begins and where the relevant "embankment" ends. As I argued, the weak point of Ramsey's model is that it takes the system's surroundings, its "embankment," as "plain," meaning that there is a complexity of pylons within the bridge, thus within the system, while the complexity of the embankment is not accounted for in any way. It is simply assumed that the bridge is anchored somewhere, and that is all we learn. Meanwhile, if we zoom-in on the system, including *its surroundings*, we should also obtain a more fine-grained picture of the boundary between the two. However, we do not obtain it from Ramsey's model.

Meanwhile, if we are to abide by Ramsey's notion of decomposing the cognitive system into subsystems that run the representational machinery, the boundary between the system as a whole and its surroundings is *also a subsystem* or the product of a relevant subsystem, and therefore must not simply be taken for granted. For it may also result from a certain dynamic playing out between a particular subsystem and its local, subsystem-specific surroundings. As pointed out in Chapter 6, once we zoom-in on actual exemplifications of representational systems, namely organisms, we end up with a huge variety of subsystems responsible for different functions and different boundaries, and what we refer to as the "representational system" actually turns out to be part of that variety. If so, it is not necessary to maintain that the system we are interested in, running the representational machinery, simply "buys" the boundaries produced by other subsystems and does not draw its own boundaries in accordance with its own particular needs.

Therefore, my proposal is that cognitive systems, representational systems included, should be seen as evolutionary products of *system–niche* co-determination as described in NC0–NC7. As such, they are capable of establishing and maintaining interactive boundaries, yet not with any physical thing but with specific parts of their niche mediums. These boundaries largely depend on the kind of task the system is performing at a given moment and the niche medium it must operate in (which means that the "embankment" is not blank). There is not just one interactive boundary, but a variety of them, depending on the medium and the task at hand. Therefore, the answer whether a particular entity or state belongs to a particular representational system may differ under different circumstances, depending on how the "line" in question was "negotiated" between the system and its surroundings.

This approach, however, does not strip the cognitive system from its external boundaries and does not make them irrelevant, contrary to what Menary (2007) suggested. Pluralism with respect to boundaries is not anti-realism with respect to boundaries.

Finally – and this is something that I must highlight again – all the interactive boundaries of representational systems are determined by the principle governing the system's integrity: they are *p*-boundaries, which effectively puts a stop to an "anything goes" strategy that one might be tempted to adopt for the sake of a slingshot argument. Such a slingshot argument would try to make the case that anything anywhere can be part of the system, which effectively makes the idea of extension meaningless. My answer is that it does not. Not anything and not anywhere – only those entities that are selected by the system's unifying "program," and only those remaining in the system's locative capacity as defined in Chapter 6. This means only parts of the system's co-determined niche medium, in which the system plays the role of a reference point, nesting a complex entanglement of locative connections. No slingshot argument then.

8.4 A note on structural coupling and enactment

The notion of structural coupling is ubiquitous in the 4E literature, especially in the branch that follows Varela. However, the concept lacks sufficient ontological treatment. One reason why it does need one stems from the recognition that it is one thing to have a definition on paper, and yet another to actually *understand* it. And understanding depends, among other things, on certain ontological assumptions. To take a different example, if we define *population* the way the *Cambridge Dictionary* proposes, i.e., as "all the people or animals of a particular type or group who live in one country, area, or place," there are the categories of *type* and *group*, to take just two from a larger list, and the reader quite naturally takes them both as referring to a *set* in the standard extensional, set-theoretical sense. But this is a certain ontological presupposition, for actually there is substantial controversy in the relevant area of philosophy as to how we should understand types as opposed to tokens. Therefore, a Platonist could read this definition of population differently in light of their presuppositions (whether it makes a practical difference for science is another matter).

Going back to structural coupling, we must decide, for example, whether the relation in question can be articulated in purely causal terms, or whether there is more to it. Whether it is a *relation* at all in fact, or perhaps speaking of *processes* would be more appropriate, with relations as the ingredients of a process? The suggestion in the 4E literature is quite clear that structural coupling is more than a nexus of relations, and that there is more to it than mere causation. Living creatures maintain a huge variety of relations, causal bonds included, and not all of these are part of their structural coupling. Another option is to read structural coupling as referring to some sort of *connection* or "access" as Newell (1980) would perhaps put it. It may be a mereological overlap of parts, or a tie between boundaries, or something weaker still, such as locative connection. All of these issues would have to be decided as part of the missing ontology of structural coupling.

Closely tied to the latter puzzle is another, more general reason why structural coupling requires ontological investigation. At least some advocates of 4E, including in particular Varela and his branch, strongly suggest that structural coupling has the power not only to alter or modify things that are already there (though without changing their ontological status), but also to actually *bring things forth* (see Rolla & Figueiredo 2023). For we are told that the familiar layout of the world, the one that we "awaken" in according to Varela, is neither objective nor subjective in the Cartesian sense, but results from "enactment," while the structural coupling between the cognitive system and its surroundings is clearly a key part of this process. Therefore, if the standard objective–subjective distinction does not apply to products of enactment, with structural coupling somehow embroiled in this mysterious process, an alternative conceptualization of the system–surroundings (mind–world, in more traditional terms) relationship is very much needed. The Cartesian internal versus external distinction is no longer useful, and therefore a more adequate conceptualization has to be found.

I believe that the framework developed in Chapters 6 and 7, including the locative-ontological "representation" of niche construction, can be taken as the first bid for an alternative *ontological* conceptualization aiming to account for the profound novelty introduced by 4E, i.e., the idea that mind–world coupling can actually bring forth *a world*. In essence, the latter does not mean casting projections, composed of sense data or what have you, from the top of one's head, but the stepwise construction of a cognitive niche through the establishment of a variety of interactive boundaries and more robust structures/patterns thereof (see Werner 2020, 2023). This conceptualization cannot be accused of "idealistic underpinnings," as Pascal and O'Regan (2008) suggested in reference to Varela et al. (1991).

8.5 Prospects for clarifying the ubiquitous talk of "environment"

Assuming that the locative-ontological framework constitutes a plausible contribution to the debate on the extended mind hypothesis, structural coupling and enactment, it can also contribute to a better understanding of what is meant by "environment," whether in the 4E literature or the more recent Cartesian cognitive science, not to mention other currents.

I propose to define *an environment* as a mereological fusion of a fixed set of inter-connected niches (cognitive niches if we want to limit our attention to cognition-specific environments), thus niches that share parts or boundaries. What the term "environment" therefore refers to depends on the *condition* underpinning the fusion, which is either up to an external observer, who decides how large the fusion should be for a specific argumentative purpose, or it is up to the living creature "interested" in delineating, for whatever sake, any areas larger than niches proper. In the latter case, the system's unifying "principle" or "program" (its autonomy conditions, if we apply the 4E terminology) determines the range of niches to be counted as its broader environment at any given moment, with a particular action in mind (if this broader area needs to be delineated by the system at all; I assume that this may be the case at least when it comes to relatively complex cognitive systems, e.g. those endowed with meta-cognitive capacities; or those capable of traveling greater distances, etc.).

This relativization is somewhat intuitive, for on one occasion "environment" may refer to local conditions, for example, in a given part of a forest or city, but, at the other extreme, we also speak globally, for example, of "protecting the environment," referring to the Earth's entire biosphere. *Environment* is therefore an occasional and contextual category with an instrumental purpose, especially when it is the observer or speaker who sets up the fusion condition. *Niche* on the other hand, including *cognitive niche*, is a category referring to actual phenomena on the ground, and here the only delineating or constructing factor that should be taken into account is the living creature, the system, itself – its needs, capacities, autonomy conditions, etc., aside from whatever an external observer might want.

Along these lines, I propose that the provisional term "cognitive environment" refer to the mereological fusion of a fixed set of connected cognitive niches *under a particular investigation*. This is the "environment" that all theories of cognition, on both sides of the Cartesian versus non-Cartesian divide, refer to. And they do it all over the place. Note, however, one interesting thing that shows up if we set things up this way. Namely, in many cases referring to "the environment" in cognitive neuroscience, psychology or philosophy is, in a sense, over the top, for it would be perfectly sufficient to refer to a smaller segment of the world, so to speak, thus to a given system's cognitive niche. This is especially true when we are dealing with a single system placed in an artificial setting, in a lab, or descriptively isolated from the broader context, as when we are observing behavior outside of a natural habitat. For example, when we have a single perceiver, e.g., a predator producing structural representations of potential prey deployed in a meadow, and we are interested in the way visual stimuli are processed by the predator's nervous system, it is sufficient to speak of the cognitive niche of that predator. Meanwhile, if we want to say something about the cognitive processes of the predator combined with those of its prey and responsible for how the actual hunt and escape is executed, or if we plan to investigate the way in which a pack of predators organize their hunt and how the herd of prey organize their escape, it would be necessary, indeed, to refer to *an environment*, for clearly a larger number of cognitive niches (how many exactly depends on the scope of the investigation) are involved. All this makes use of the term "environment" more substantial in cognitive science and philosophy, and not just a *façon de parler*.

8.6 Prospects for clarifying the ubiquitous talk of "inputs" and "stimuli"

Recall Newell who writes that the physical symbolic system's inputs are "the objects in certain locations" and "its outputs are the modification or creation of the objects in certain (usually different) locations" (Newell 1980: 142). As I noted in Chapter 2, this notion of *input* is quite unusual, for if we take it literally the only entity that can actually be *put into* the system is a portion of energy that moves receptors and causes a cascade of reactions inside, and even this articulation is highly imprecise – energy is transmitted but there is no "entity" being relocated from the external to the internal realm, that is if we exclude the microlevel of chemical complexes crossing the cellular membrane.

Newell's language comes from early empiricist presuppositions concerning the existence of specific "things" such as impressions or sense data, but this talk hardly makes sense within the proper context of the modern science of perception. On the other hand, Newell isn't speaking of portions of energy or sense data, for it seems clear that he is thinking of ordinary things such as trees and tables. And he has good reason to do so – after all, cognitive science should tell us something about how we perceive and deal with familiar things. Yet calling them "inputs" is misleading, if not an outright misconception.

Further on Newell says something quite interesting, which suggests, not surprisingly, that he did not ultimately succumb to a simple misconception. Namely, he says that the "larger system of environment plus [the physical symbol system] forms a closed system, since the output objects either become or affect later input objects" (Newell 1980: 142). It therefore seems that, aside from the misleading language, being *an input to the system* somehow has to do with the idea that the cognitive system creates a larger system with some of the entities in its surroundings. In effect, the distinction between fundamental-level and higher-level cognitive systems, strongly suggested in the 4E literature and provisionally introduced above, reappears in this representationalist, thus supposedly environment-blind (as some 4E theorists might hold) account. This substantiates Miłkowski's (2017) point that the enactivist literature does not do justice to Newell's legacy.

Perhaps then the surrounding entities can indeed be called inputs, yet not inputs to the fundamental-level system, whether representational or autonomous (or both), but *inputs to the larger, higher-level system*. Thus – inputs to the cognitive niche, however strange it might sound at first. Therefore, if any intuition derived from the bucket theory of mind, thus having to do with "putting something into something else," is to remain in play here, an entity *x* can sensibly be said to be an *input to the larger system* surrounding the fundamental-level system S. Then S, standing at the center of that larger systemic whole, and within its boundaries, gets "access" to *x*, as Newell might say.

I propose that the larger, higher-level system is S's *cognitive niche*. If so, the "inputs" to the larger system that Newell is talking about are parts of the cognitive niche's medium, and the "access" relationship between S and these inputs means *direct locative interactive connections* between S and the entities within its locative capacity – the entities composing the medium of S's cognitive niche.

Therefore, Newell's phrase "objects in different locations" refers not to the relevant objects' exact locations, and not just to their relative locations, but *to their position within the locative capacity of* S, given that S is the point of reference in its own cognitive niche. To be "in different locations" therefore stands for the things' placement within the nexus of the locative connections nested in S (where S functions as a "center of activity," as Di Paolo et al. 2010 put it).

Alongside the term "input" we can also finally grasp the proper meaning of another word that is ubiquitous in the literature, perhaps even more ubiquitous, likely due to its intuitive appeal. This is the word "external," especially in complex locutions such as "external stimuli." By "intuitive appeal" I mean that the word seems perfectly understandable without a reference to any technical posits. We all know what being "external" means when it comes to the table I am sitting at, for example, which is external in the sense that it is not part of *me* or *my body*. Something is external with respect to the building I live in if it is placed on the other side of its walls – as simple as that. I have already flagged, however, that the devil, as always, is in the details.

When we are told that there is "little doubt" as to the causal processes relating the brain to *external stimuli* (e.g. Roskies 2021), things became more complicated. The table's or the Moon's being *external to my body* boils down to the trivial fact that they are not parts of my body and my body is not part of them. But if *this* is the intuitive sense of "being external," then we find ourselves in a pickle when trying to understand how *stimuli* can be external. First of all, if the term "stimuli" refers to what is happening on the surface of the body, to the firings of receptors, then the mereological criteria applicable to tables and celestial objects become problematic. Stimulation *is* a process or event that unquestionably is part of my bodily processes. It cannot be external in the sense in which the table is external.

A simple answer to this conundrum would be that the said table is external in an intuitive sense, and that it also *causes* a certain stimulation on the surface of my body, and insofar as it does, it can also, in a derivative sense, be referred to as an external stimulus (thus as "the object" that gets into the system, in Newell's phrasing). The latter interpretation is, indeed, preferable if we want to preserve the realism claiming that stimuli are our cues in figuring out what the surrounding world is like.

If this realism is to stand, however, an entity's being "external" and at the same time providing "stimuli" must stand for something substantial, more than just being mereologically disjoint. In other words, by dubbing a thing *external*, we learn nothing. There are plenty of things, say some random rocks on Mars, that *are* external to me, and *mean nothing* to me. One might refer to causal bonds and argue that there must be a causal bond between the body and the external thing if the latter is to be considered an "external stimulus." But this remark, while true, does not suffice to characterize the specifically *cognitive* bond. This is because, as pointed out many times over the course of this investigation, we are in causal relationships with a huge number of things, including the moon and the sun, but this alone does not *make these things stimuli*, i.e., material for cognition.

Therefore, being *external* in the way stimuli are, stands for being disjoint *and* at the same time being *somehow* still bonded to the system being stimulated. This latter bond is something mysterious, unspecified in the standard talk of *external stimuli*, external things, and the external world at large.

This peculiar bond is frequently spelled out in *semantic* terms however. Newell, for example, speaks of *designation*. The semantic bond may be understood as a relation that is identified by the same relata as causal stimulation, but with the opposite direction. This seems to be the case in Newell's account. He defines the context "an expression designates an object" by invoking cases in which "the system can either affect the object itself or behave in ways dependent on the object." This way, he writes, "access to the object via the expression has been obtained, which is the essence of designation" (Newell 1980: 116). Yet, "access" still remains a mystery, which makes this conception subject to the *ignotum per ignotum* fallacy.

Now, from the standpoint of locative ontology, "access" suggests something similar to connection. But connection of what kind? After all, it cannot be about sharing parts or any other overlap between the *entities* involved, for in such a case the thing in question would not be *external*. The idea put forward in this book is that this additional bond is about maintaining *locative connection* with the things composing a niche medium for a particular cognitive system. Hence, it is a very special kind of connection, attributable to *things*, but *defined in terms of their exact locations*. More specifically, it is about a particular system's being a point of reference for a range of things in the world – those that "fill" the system's locative capacity. Almost all the categories defined in Chapters 6 and 7 are directly or indirectly in play here.

I therefore propose to define external *entities* as things that a system does not share parts with, although they nevertheless belong to the system's locative capacity inside its niche medium (inside the "larger system" Newell talks about). Now we can say that external *stimuli* are those external entities, things or states that fire up the system's receptors in the way diligently studied by neuroscience. The latter is now understandable since we know what "external entity (object)" stands for. In other words, there is a certain *unique locative architecture* behind the notions of "external entity" and "external stimuli," among many other such conceptual posits, and the conceptual framework which has been rolled out in this book is in my view an apt tool (presumably not the only one) making it possible to elicit this architecture.

8.7 On the cognitive array, ecological architecture and information

The external realm where inputs or stimuli come from has the feature of *centeredness*, which means that it is the realm *surrounding* a particular cognitive system. In Gibson's vocabulary, it is an *array*, e.g. the optic array. This paves the way for the possibility of the perceived world's informational abundance, contrary to what standard representationalism assumes following Marr (1982). According to Gibson, the perceived world contains very rich contextual information due to the fact that the entities surrounding a perceiver reflect light in specific ways, determining unique arrangements of electromagnetic waves, with a specific length, angle, etc. Therefore, there is no need to postulate representational content. The content is already there, we might say, in the perceived world.

Gibson's insight, briefly discussed in Chapter 5, is crucial to the idea of ecological cognition. However, I argued earlier that it is by no means evident what an *array* is. For it is one thing to say that there are things located relative to a fixed cognitive system, and yet it is more conceptually challenging to make the case that the things in question actually form *an array*, as if anchored or nested in that cognitive system. For – let me emphasize – it is not about being merely perceived as an array by an external observer; it is about actually *being* an array attributable to that particular cognitive system. In other words, if the perspective of the external observer is abandoned in favor of the standpoint of the cognitive system itself, playing the role of the *point of reference* in the said realm is not something that we should assume as given. Instead, it needs to be elucidated in one way or another.

When solving this puzzle, we must first realize that the sought locative arrangement, if approached *from the perspective of the cognitive system itself*, evolving from simpler to more complex forms, is a certain "achievement," for lack of a better word. In other words, *playing the role of the point of reference* in a given realm may seem obvious from the standpoint of the external observer, but if we try to see the said realm the way the targeted system itself "sees" it, it becomes clear that being *arrayed* in the sense we are interested in is not a quality that the world possesses in and of itself. Instead, in principle, this arraying must be the result of an effort undertaken by the cognitive system. I say "in principle," since complex systems such as ourselves in large part inherit the said arrangement (it's part of our "evolved apprentice," as Sterelny 2012 might say), but the situation is different for a theoretically postulated simple cognitive system. Note that NC5 and NC6, when read from the Gibsonian angle, are exactly about this effort – the effort of *making the surrounding world into an array*.

Going further, the concept of a *cognitive* array, generalized from Gibson's optic array, is a pivotal posit, since it allows us to target clusters of physical entities in a system's surroundings as *vehicles of information*. This may not sound particularly illuminating at first glance due to the fact that the "information talk" is so ubiquitous, just like the environment talk and the input or stimuli talk addressed above, but consider this: Gibson says that *being a vehicle of information* cannot boil down to how something is processed by the system, including by the string of subsystems that Ramsey (2007) quite rightly distilled, or to how it is consumed (Millikan 1984) by the system in pursuit of building structural representations (Gładziejewski & Miłkowski 2017). All these things *are* no doubt important parts of the story, but the crucial factor is that this potential vehicle has certain *ecological* characteristics. In the first step, it is *the world itself* that creates a kind of *informational potential* to be actualized by the cognitive system. And this potential, if I read Gibson correctly, is generated by *how things stand with respect to one another*, i.e., by a certain locative architecture.

Now, armed with the conceptual framework rolled out in Chapters 6 and 7, we can elicit this architecture. First, note a certain subtlety, namely that arrays are primarily arrangements of *regions*, not of things. The talk of arrayed things is secondary to the proper talk of arrayed regions in which these things are located. Now, the question is how these relations between regions come about. The basic idea is that some actions undertaken by the cognitive system *make its relative location* acquire an additional function or quality with respect to the locations of other entities and the overall locative architecture of the realm in which the system operates: this is the dynamic described in NC0–NC7.

The key notion that I would like to try out is this: to make an array in the Gibsonian sense emerge, the cognitive system must establish its locative capacity, which means that it must set up locative connections with surrounding entities so that it becomes a point of reference for them. This pivotal moment occurs in step (NC3) of niche construction; actually somewhere between (NC2) and (NC3). It is there, I argue, that we should look for the key factors determining the emergence of arrays, and therefore the emergence of informational potentials, too.

So, here is a benefit to be derived from the proposed ontological "simulation" of niche construction: by making this constructive effort and rendering the ecological architecture produced by it explicit, we can substantiate the talk of information-abundant environments, or, as I prefer to put it, of the *informational potential of environments*. This potential is in principle attributable to cognitive niches, and thereby to environments at large. Of course, NC0–NC7 is merely a blueprint for a more detailed ontology of ecological information.

8.8 Reintroduced affordances

Speaking of the informational potential of environments, another key notion introduced by Gibson is the notion of affordance. It requires some additional commentary too.

As already pointed out, what makes affordances ontologically peculiar is the fact that they are neither objective nor subjective, as Gibson describes them. In a sense, both qualifications apply, yet from a different angle neither of them really fits. Therefore, affordances transcend the distinction itself. It is impossible to take them as mere projections of the mind, for Gibson unequivocally places them on the side of the environment, where they seem to await the cognitive system. On the other hand, however, they cannot be deemed external in the sense usually attributed to this notion in the Cartesian tradition, thus as something clear of *any* influence coming from the cognitive system, given the fact that they *answer specific needs* and capacities of specific systems and are therefore different for different systems.

An analogous problem has to do with Varela's concept of enactment. It is clear in Varela et al. (1991) that enactment is *not* about "worldmaking" from the top our heads. Instead, the concept is grounded in scientific realism of a rather straightforward kind which states that physicochemical stuff lies solidly under our feet. Yet, at the same time, we are told, still on naturalistic grounds, that given what we know about the evolution of structural coupling (the coevolution of organisms and their environments) and especially about the evolutionary diversity of organisms' cognitive machinery, the inevitable conclusion is that this shared stuff under our feet, whatever it is, *manifests itself* in very different ways to different creatures. It is therefore, we are told, *enacted* in a wide variety of fashions.

Going back to affordances, I propose to tie them to the concept of embodied models discussed in Chapter 6 and defined in NC7 (grounded to some extent in the original idea set forth by Tooby & De Vore 1987). To recall some key points, NC7 states that if we have the set $\{f_i,\ldots, f_j\}$ consisting of all the *f*s that the system S is framed with respect to by its interactive closures, which means such *f*s that S can connect to, a new domain emerges on this basis. Namely, the domain of the interactive closures of all the *f*s that S "partners up" with, so to speak. This is due to the fact that *each* of these *f*s "negotiates" *its own* interactive boundary with S.

Now, S may *use* some elements of this new realm of closures *as models* of the assumed niche *base* – the assumed reality "under our feet." The relation of modeling is grounded in at least partial overlap between the location of a boundary of an *f* and the relevant location of a boundary possessed by an entity partaking in the niche base. We do not know any such entity directly, of course, so such an overlap can only be judged by its fruits, that is by how it contributes to the efficacy of action. For there is no external, God's eye standpoint that allows for actual comparison between where the boundaries of things in the niche base are and where the boundaries co-constituted by the cognitive system are located.

This means, in the proposed grossly simplified model, that if the system's boundary-drawing activity happens to at least partly *match up* with a boundary of some of the objects in the base, then this coincidence may be exploited by the system to make its actions more effective or efficient, thereby making the degree of success a touchstone of how accurate the model is.

However, there is no reason *a priori* to assume that all the more or less successful "match-ups" between the locations of the relevant boundaries are actually *usable* qua models, for it depends on the actual needs and capacities of a given system, thus also on its tasks. There can be situations in which there *is* significant overlap between where the boundaries of an entity in the niche base are and where the relevant boundaries are drawn by the cognitive system, and yet there is nothing specific that results from that happy coincidence. And this is where, I believe, affordances come on the scene.

I propose to understand the affordances offered to S as potential embodied models that *do* answer the actual needs and capacities of the cognitive system. In simple terms, *affordances are usable embodied models*; usable boundary "match-ups" in the sense just sketched.

Here is a grossly simplified illustration of what this proposal signifies. Suppose we are physicalists claiming that the underlying niche base is fundamentally composed of elementary particles and complexes thereof (likely quite a widespread view). What cognitive systems do is "draw" boundaries around more or less stable "clouds" of these particles, thereby delineating familiar objects, processes and states of affairs, beginning with the delineation that constitutes the systems themselves. Suppose we have a perceptual delineation in the form we tend to call a "tree" and partaking delineations called "branches." These may be compositions of perceptual invariants in the sense of von Foerster (1976/2003) or Di Paolo et al. (2017). Now, there is no such thing as a *tree* and no such thing as a *branch* at the fundamental physical level of particles, thus in the niche base. However, there certainly *are* clusters of specific particles, i.e, chemical complexes dancing in space, such that in some areas there is mostly oxygen, nitrogen, etc., and there are "clouds" in which there are huge masses and structures made of H_2O and carbon, among many other chemical substances. Cognitive systems "draw" perceptual boundaries around these "clouds," and the *places* where the boundaries are drawn may to a greater or lesser degree coincide with the *places* where the somewhat blurred boundaries between two "clouds" of particles actually are. This is how the familiar layout referred to as *tree*, *branches* and *air* emerges (which is a shape-ground setup according to Gestalt psychology). It is like "drawing lines across the board," to use Varzi's (2016) phrase.

Now, when there is indeed a coincidence in terms of location between the drawn boundaries and the boundaries of the particle clouds, we can speak of an embodied model of certain "objective" (if you like) relations occurring between the physical entities existing in the niche base. Moreover – and this is the climax of the story – it may also be the case that what shows up at the perceptual level, as the product of boundary drawing, "offers" a certain possibility of action (keep in mind that for many such drawings that may *not* be the case, thus the sought coincidence may merely be there, without any influence on potential actions). For example, the cognitive system, prototypically a living creature, may hide in the shadow of the tree "drawn" around one cloud of particles, or it can grab a branch "drawn" around a smaller cloud of particles, and climb on it. These are affordances – usable embodied models. But note that this is possible only if there is a sufficient coincidence between the location of the "drawn" boundaries of what the system *regards as* a tree and a branch, and the location of the actual boundaries of the "clouds" of chemical complexes, however blurred they may be. If for any reason the said boundary coincidence or match-up fails, an attempt to *use* the perceived branch as a solid tool in order to climb may turn out to be rather unpleasant.

Arguably, the illustration just given is childish, but it illustrates the basic idea underpinning the provisional concept of embodied models of the underlying (physical, let us suppose) niche base, and how some of these models have an additional function vis-à-vis action: the function Gibson dubbed "affordance."

Let me emphasize that all the posits introduced in this chapter, as well as their interpretation, are provisional. The proper theoretical framework that this investigation aimed to develop was introduced in Chapters 6 and 7, following detailed preparation in the preceding chapters. This chapter wraps things up and has no greater theoretical ambitions. Instead, I wish to flag how the conceptual framework presented here deals with the problems defined in Chapters 1–4, and thus point to potential routes that can be taken. Each of these routes merits a separate research project.

8.9 Concluding remarks: Prospects for ecological internalism

I would like to go back to the opening problem from Chapter 1 – to the distinction between the mind-*as*-a-place view and the alternative view of mind-*in*-a-place. The distinction unpacks two different heuristics that can be used to imagine human cognitive functioning. The final section of this book is dedicated to amending the said heuristics. It draws on the assumption, that making use of such simplified heuristic devices is unavoidable; it is one of the *metaphors we live by*, as Lakoff and Johnson (1980) very aptly put it.

The two heuristics, mind-*as*-a-place and mind-*in*-a-place, elicit two fundamental qualities of mind and cognition. One has to do with mind's environmental plug-in, to use Noë's (2009) phrase, an aspect somewhat neglected by the Cartesian tradition (although, as we learned, not fully neglected). The other with mind's function as a "safe refuge" for reflection and understanding – this being insufficiently covered by the 4E literature. The amendment to be proposed combines the two.

In simple terms the new heuristic says that the mind is indeed constituted by a specific location – a specific environment in which cognition arises, but also one that is in part brought forth by cognition. But if so, then it is also the case that the mind itself can be considered a specific place. For if we are freed from having to address the mind within the physical perimeter of the body, and thus take it as "extended," understood in terms of the system's interactive closure, the cognitive niche medium now becomes the *interior of an extended mind*.

Chapter 1 argued that the Augustinian inner self was conceived as the necessary safe refuge where the self can "distance" itself from worldly engagements in order to reflect on them and, crucially, to pursue meaning and sense naturally identified back then with a divine aspect of the world. For at the end of the day, cognition was thought of as participation in this greater reality. Now, as I pointed out several times with respect to the whole of pre-Darwinian thought, if there is no ecological sense of location available, the best option to satisfy the Augustinian need was likely to devise a special sphere internal to the subject, the *inner* self. When modern physics was born, with Galileo's notion of mathematical description of the *external* world, the *inward* move became somewhat unavoidable, I believe, for those wanting to preserve the idea of cognition as participation in something more than the physical mechanics of the perceivable/measurable universe (thus as participation in the domain of meaning).

Hume or, in a different style, La Mettrie and Hobbes, i.e., those openly rejecting the commitment to "something more," saw no need for the inner self as a qualitatively distinct realm. Yet they nevertheless kept the locative architecture of the rejected inner self in place. This was the moment the "bucket theory" was born, the moment when the container conceptualization of the mind emerged in its full-fledged form as known to us. The mind was reduced to a vessel awaiting externally (i.e., physically) delivered inputs – a reduction which found a clear articulation in behaviorism. Cognitive science rejected behaviorism, but not the locative architecture behind it.

Unpacking the locative architecture underpinning ecological theories of cognition (4E broadly construed) yields a new understanding of *what kind of place* the mind is, but what it does first and foremost is provide a new formula of what was above designated as "something more." Theologically inspired interpretations are still an option, but they are beyond the scope of this investigation. The key idea here is the evolution of (cognitive) niche construction, which – due to its unimaginably long timespan compared to the lifespan of a single individual, including each of us – provides a blueprint for the "something more" we are seeking.

From the perspective of an individual cognitive system, the cognitive niche it inherits and contributes to, thus a relatively stable structure offering certain opportunities for action (affordances), is definitely "something more," thus a certain cognition-related realm that is *inherently meaningful* and at the same time *given* to the system in the sense that it is not the result of the system's own "starmaking" and created from scratch. Niche construction is a process to which the individual does contribute, and yet its lasting millions of years opens room for the fundamental phenomenological recognition of *givenness* – the world we "awaken" in is indeed "offered" to us.

Based on this evolutionary approach to the "greater reality" which our individual cognitive efforts participate in, the mind-*as*-a-place paradigm can be revamped in the form of a view that I provisionally call "ecological internalism." Its *ecological* qualification should be sufficiently clear now. At the same time, I dub it "internalism" because the reformulated *internal versus external* distinction remains a crucial factor for a proper grasp of cognition. It makes a huge difference *to me* whether something is *inside my* cognitive niche, *available to my* cognitive capacities, *open to my* cognitive (also emotional, aesthetic or moral) endeavors, *or outside* the niche, thus unavailable. That said, we are no longer facing an ontological chasm, but a more nuanced, contextual distinction, or even a certain system of distinctions built upon interactive boundaries. Needless to say, it is not a sharp distinction merely mirroring the "skin and skull" barrier.

But what can ecological *externalism* be then? The difference between ecological internalism and its natural counterpart, ecological externalism, can be illustrated (merely for the sake of this short conclusion) by referring to two versions of semantic externalism, referenced as a backdrop in the very first paragraph of this book. Namely, when Kripke (1980) speaks of the meaning of a word being fixed by the relevant history of its uses, he is not only referring to causal connections, as if between particles bumping against one another, going back to the word's first use; e.g. the first use of the name "Aristotle," uttered by his mother to a crying baby. Instead, he is thinking of a whole complex nexus of developing, evolving social practices, patterns of speaking and behavior, which might be called a linguistic niche. Causal bonds are parts of it, although they do not exhaust the realm at stake.

I would call Kripke's position, somewhat paradoxically, *ecological semantic* internalism, for he takes *being inside* a linguistic niche as constitutive to the meaning of words. Meanwhile, Devitt (1981) reduces everything to causal bonds, thereby situating himself on the side of ecological *semantic* externalism. This is because if causality is the only factor that matters, the whole social architecture determining how speaking and acting in the world is organized, is irrelevant. Thus all references to linguistic niches or similar constructs, and their interior, are redundant – chains of causal bonds, e.g. the one connecting this page with Aristotle's mother, fix the meaning, period.

Analogously, while ecological internalism puts stress on the complex, contextual and evolving distinction between the interior of a cognitive niche and its exterior, ecological externalism would hold that there is no real job that the concept of the cognitive niche does, and the whole story of cognition could be told in purely causal terms – no place for structural coupling, sense-making, "web of significance" and no enactment either.

Therefore, the final word is this: speaking of *the locative footprint of mind* refers to a realm in which mind emerges and acts. It also refers to a realm inside the interactive boundaries of mind which are not identical to the boundaries of "skin and skull." This is the realm that I propose to call the *cognitive niche*.

Bibliography

Ajdukiewicz, K. (1934). Das Weltbild und die Begriffsapparatur. *Erkenntnis*, 4(1), 259–287.

Allen, C. (2017). On (not) defining cognition. *Synthese*, 194, 4233–4249. https://doi.org/10.1007/s11229-017-1454-4

Allen, M., Friston, K. (2018). From cognitivism to autopoiesis: Towards a computational framework for the embodied mind. *Synthese*, 195, 2459–2482. https://doi.org/10.1007/s11229-016-1288-5

Allison, H.E. (2006). Kant's transcendental idealism. In: G. Bird (ed.), *A companion to Kant*. Oxford: Blackwell, 111–124.

Arnellos, A., Moreno, A. (2015). Multicellular agency: An organizational view. *Biology and Philosophy*, 30, 333–357.

Arp, R., Smith, B., Spear, A.D. (2015). *Building ontologies with basic formal ontology*. Cambridge MA: MIT Press.

Aaby, B.H., Ramsey, G. (2019). Three kinds of niche construction. *The British Journal for the Philosophy of Science*. https://doi.org/10.1093/bjps/axz054

Austin, J.L. (1953). How to talk: Some simple ways. *Proceedings of the Aristotelian Society*, 53, 227–246.

Baggs, E., Chemero, A. (2021). Radical embodiment in two directions. *Synthese*, 198(Suppl 9), S2175–S2190. https://doi.org/10.1007/s11229-018-02020-9

Barandiaran, X., Moreno, A. (2006). On what makes certain dynamical systems cognitive: A minimally cognitive organization program. *Adaptive Behavior*, 14(2), 171–185.

Barker, R.G. (1968). *Ecological psychology. Concepts and methods for studying the environment of human behavior*. Stanford: Stanford University Press.

Bechtel, W. (2008). *Mental mechanisms: Philosophical perspectives on cognitive neuroscience*. New York: Routledge.

Beer, R.D. (2023). Cultivating the garden of Eden. *Complex Systems*, 32(1), 1–17. https://doi.org/10.25088/ComplexSystems.32.1.1

Beer, R.D., Di Paolo, E. (2023). The theoretical foundations of enaction: Precariousness. *BioSystems*, 223. https://doi.org/10.1016/j.biosystems.2022.104823

Ben-Zeev, A. (1984). The passivity assumption of the sensation-perception distinction. *The British Journal for the Philosophy of Science*, 35(4), 327–343.

Bertalanffy, L. von. (1968). *General system theory: Foundations, development, applications*. New York: George Braziller.

Bertolotti, T., Magnani, L. (2017). Theoretical considerations on cognitive niche construction. *Synthese*, 194, 4757–4779.

Bohr, N. (1963). The unity of human knowledge. In: N. Bohr (ed.), *Essays 1958–1962 on atomic physics and human knowledge*. Woodbridge, Conn.: Ox Bow Press, 8–16.

Brewer, B. (2007). Perception and its objects. *Philosophical Studies*, 132(1), 87–97.

Brooks, R.A. (1991). Intelligence without representation. *Artificial Intelligence*, 47(1–3), 139–159.

Brożek, B., Olszewski, A. (2014). The mathematical subject and Church's Thesis. In: Brożek et al., (eds.), 397–416.

Brożek, B., Olszewski, A., Urbańczyk, P. (eds.) (2014). *Church's thesis: Logic, mind, and nature*. Krakow: Copernicus Center Press.

Bruineberg, J., Chemero, A., Rietveld (2019). General ecological information supports engagement with affordances for 'higher' cognition. *Synthese*, 196, 5231–5251.

Burge, T. (2010). *The origins of objectivity*. Oxford: Oxford University Press.

Burkhardt, H., Smith, B. (eds.) (1991). *Handbook of metaphysics and ontology*. Munich: Philosophia Verlag.

Burnet, F. M. (1969). *Self and notself*. Cambridge: Cambridge University Press.

Buytendijk, F.J.J., Plessner, H. (1936). Die Physiologische Erklärung des Verhaltens. *Acta Biotheor*, 1, 151–172.

Carnap, R. (1950). Empiricism, semantics, and ontology. *Revue Internationale de Philosophie*, 4, 20–40.

Cary, P. (2000). *Augustine's invention of the inner self: The legacy of a christian platonist*. Oxford: OUP.

Casati, R., Varzi, A. (1994). *Holes and other superficialities*. MIT Press.

Casati, R., Varzi, A. (1999). *Parts and places. The structures of spatial representation*. Cambridge, MA: MIT Press.

Chalmers, D. (1996). The conscious mind. In *Search of a fundamental theory*, Oxford: Oxford University Press.

Chemero, A. (2003). An outline of a theory of affordances. *Ecological Psychology*, 15(2), 181–195.

Chemero, A. (2009). *Radical embodied cognitive science*. Cambridge, MA: The MIT Press.

Chisholm, R. (1996). *A realistic theory of categories*. Cambridge University Press.

Clark, A. (2001). *Mindware: An introduction to the philosophy of cognitive science*. Oxford: Oxford University Press.

Clark, A. (2003). *Natural-born cyborgs. Minds, technologies, and the future of human intelligence*. Oxford: Oxford University Press.

Clark, A. (2005). Word, niche and super-niche: How language makes minds matter more. *Theoria*, 54, 255–268.

Clark, A. (2006). Language, embodiment, and the cognitive niche. *Trends in Cognitive Science*, 10(8), 370–374.

Clark, A. (2008). *Supersizing the mind: Embodiment, action, and cognitive extension*. Oxford: Oxford University Press.
Clark, A., Chalmers, D. (1998). The extended mind. *Analysis*, 58, 10–23.
Clarke, B.L. (1985). Individuals and points. *Notre Dame Journal of Formal Logic*, 26, 61–75.
Coninx, S. (2023). The dark side of niche construction. *Philosophical Studies*, 180, 3003–3030. https://doi.org/10.1007/s11098-023-02024-3
Crane, T. (2006). Is there a perceptual relation. In: T. Szabo Gendler, J. Hawthorne (eds.) *Perceptual experience*. Oxford: Oxford University Press, 126–146.
Craver, C.F. (2007). *Explaining the brain*. Oxford: Oxford University Press.
Cummins, F., De Jesus, P. (2016). The loneliness of the enactive cell: Towards a bio enactive framework. *Adaptive Behavior*. https://doi.org/10.1177/10597123166 44965
Cummins, R. (1989). *Meaning and mental representation*. Cambridge, MA: MIT Press.
Danto, A. (1964). The artworld. *Journal of Philosophy*, 61(19), 571–584.
de Carvalho, F.N., Krueger, J. (2023). Biases in niche construction. *Philosophical Psychology*. https://doi.org/10.1080/09515089.2023.2237065
De Jaegher, H., Di Paolo, E. (2007). Participatory sense-making: An enactive approach to social cognition. *Phenomenology and the Cognitive Sciences*, 6(4), 485–507.
De Jesus, P. (2015). Autopoietic enactivism, phenomenology and the deep continuity between life and mind. *Phenomenology and the Cognitive Sciences*, 15, 265–289.
Deacon, T. (2021). How molecules became signs. *Biosemiotics*. doi:10.1007/s12304-021-09453-9
Dennett, D. (1988). Quining qualia. In: A. Marcel and E. Bisiach (eds.), *Consciousness in modern science*. Oxford: Oxford University Press.
Dennett, D. (1991). *Consciousness explained*. Boston: Little Brown.
Dennett, D. (2013). *Intuition pumps and other tools for thinking*. New York, London: W. W. Norton & Company.
Descartes, R. (2008). Meditations on first philosophy. In: *With selections from the objections and replies*, trans. M. Moriarty. Oxford: Oxford University Press.
Devitt, M. (1981). *Designation*. New York: Columbia University Press.
Di Paolo, E., Cuffari, E.C., De Jaegher, H. (2018). *Linguistic bodies: The continuity between life and language*. Cambridge: MIT Press.
Di Paolo, E.A., Rohde, M., De Jaegher, H. (2010). Horizons for the enactive mind: Values, social interaction, and play. In: J. Stewart, O. Gapenne and E. Di Paolo (eds.), *Enaction: Toward a new paradigm for cognitive science*. Cambridge: MIT Press, 33–88.
Di Paolo, E.A. (2005). Autopoiesis, adaptivity, teleology, agency. *Phenomenology and the Cognitive Sciences*, 4(4), 429–452.
Di Paolo, E.A. (2009). Extended life. *Topoi*, 28, 9–21.
Di Paolo, E., Buhrman, T., Barandiaran, X. (2017). *Sensorimotor life: An enactive proposal*. Oxford University Press.

Dickie, G. (1974). *Art and the aesthetic: An institutional analysis*. Ithaca NY: Cornell University Press.
Dretske, F. (1981). *Knowledge and the flow of information*. MIT Press.
Dretske, F. (1988). *Explaining behavior. Reasons in a world of causes*. Cambridge MA: MIT Press.
Dretske, F. (1995). *Naturalizing mind*. Cambridge, MA: MIT Press.
Elton, Ch.S. (1927). *Animal ecology*. New York: Macmillan.
Emmeche, C., Kull, K. (eds.) (2011). *Towards a semiotic biology. Life is the action of signs*. London: Imperial College Press.
Favareau, D. (ed.) (2010). *Essential readings in biosemiotics: Anthology and commentary*. Berlin: Springer.
Feinberg, T.E., Mallatt, J.M. (2016). *The ancient origins of consciousness. How the brain created experience*. Cambridge, MA: MIT Press.
Feiten, T.E. (2020). Mind after Uexküll: A Forray into the worlds of ecological psychologists and enactivists. *Frontiers in Psychology*. doi:10.3389/fpsyg.2020.00480
Fine, K. (1996). The problem of mixture. In: F.A. Lewis and R. Bolton (eds.), *Form, matter, and mixture in Aristotle*. Blackwell Publishers, 82–182.
Fine, K. (1999). Things and their parts. *Midwest Studies in Philosophy*, XXIII, 61–74.
Fine, K. (2017). Naïve metaphysics. *Philosophical Issues*, 27(1), 98–113.
Fitch, W.T. (2008). Nano-intentionality: A defense of intrinsic intentionality. *Biology and Philosophy*, 23, 157–177.
Fodor, J., Pylyshyn, Z. (1988). Connectionism and cognitive architecture: A critical analysis. *Cognition*, 28(1–2), 3–71.
Fodor, J. (1975). *The language of thought*. Cambridge MA: Harvard University Press.
Foerster H. von (1976/2003). Objects: Tokens for (eigen-)behaviors. In: H. Foerster (ed.), *Understanding: Essays on cybernetics and cognition*. New York: Springer, 261–272 (Originally published in 1976).
Friston, K. (2009). The free-energy principle: A rough guide to the brain? *Trends in Cognitive Sciences*, 13(7), 293–301.
Frolov, D. (2023). Post-Northian institutional economics: A research agenda for cognitive institutions. *Journal of Institutional Economics*, 19(2).
Gallagher, S. (2017). *Enactivist interventions: Rethinking the mind*. Oxford: Oxford University Press.
Gärdenfors, P. (2004). *Conceptual spaces: The geometry of thought*. Cambridge MA: MIT Press.
Gibson, J.J. (1979). *The ecological approach to visual perception*. Boston: Houghton Mifflin.
Gładziejewski, P., Miłkowski, M. (2017). Structural representations: Causally relevant and different from detectors. *Biology and Philosophy*, 32, 337–355. https://doi.org/10.1007/s10539-017-9562-6
Godfrey-Smith, P. (1996). *Complexity and the function of mind in nature*. Cambridge: Cambridge University Press.

Godfrey-Smith, P. (2016). Individuality, subjectivity, and minimal cognition. *Biology and Philosophy*, 31(6), 775–796.
Goodman, N. (1978). *Ways of worldmaking*. Indianapolis: Hackett.
Grinnell, J. (1917). The niche-relationships of the California Thrasher. *The Auk*, 34(4), 427–433.
Gurwitsch, A. (2010). The collected works of Aron Gurwitsch (1901–1973). In: R.M. Zaner (ed.), *Volume III: The field of consciousness: Theme, thematic field, and margin*. Dordrecht: Springer.
Hallet, M. (1994). Hilbert's axiomatic method and the laws of thought. In: A. George (ed.), *Mathematics and mind*. Oxford: Oxford University Press.
Harvey, D. (1990). Between space and time: Reflections on the geographical imagination. *Annals of the Association of American Geographers*, 80(3), 418–434.
Haugeland, J. (1985). *Artificial intelligence: The very idea*. Cambridge MA: MIT Press.
Heft, H. (2001). *Ecological psychology in context: James Gibson, Roger Barker, and the legacy of William James's radical empiricism*. Mahwah, NJ: Erlbaum.
Herbert, Z. (2010). *The Collected Poems: 1956–1998*. New York: Harper Collins.
Herskovits, A. (1986). *Language and spatial cognition: An interdisciplinary study of the prepositions in English*. Cambridge: Cambridge University Press.
Heersmink, R. (2020). Narrative niche construction: Memory ecologies and distributed narrative identities. *Biology & Philosophy*, 35, 53. https://doi.org/10.1007/s10539-020-09770-2
Hoffman, D. (2019). *The case against reality: How evolution hid the truth from our eyes*. New York: WW Norton & Co.
Hofweber, T. (2005). A puzzle about ontology. *Nous*, 39(2), 256–283.
Honner, J. (1982). The transcendental philosophy of Niels Bohr. *Studies in History and Philosophy of Science*, 13(1), 1–29.
Hsieh, S., Plotnick, E.E., Bush, A.M. (2022). The Phanerozoic aftermath of the Cambrian information revolution: Sensory and cognitive complexity in marine faunas. *Paleogiology*, 48(3), 397–419. DOI: 10.1017/pab.2021.46
Husserl, E. (1901/2000). *Logische Untersuchungen. Zweiter Teil: Untersuchungen zur Phänomenologie und Theorie der Erkenntnis*. Halle: Max Niemeyer. Available in English Logical Investigations (2nd ed., 2 volumes) (J.N. Findlay, trans.). London: Routledge, 2000.
Husserl, E. (1970). *The crisis of European sciences and transcendental phenomenology*, trans. D. Carr. Evanston: Northwestern University Press.
Hutchins, E. (1995). *Cognition in the wild*. Cambridge, MA: The MIT Press.
Hutchinson, G.E. (1957). Concluding remarks. *Cold Spring Harbor Symposia on Quantitative Biology*, 22(2), 415–427.
Hutto, D., Myin, E. (2013). *Radicalizing enactivism: Basic minds without content*. Cambridge, MA: MIT Press.
Ingarden, R. (1964). *Der Streit um die Existenz der Welt. Teil 1: Existenzialontologie*. Tübingen: Niemeyer; English translation: Ingarden, R. (2013). *Controversy over the Existence of the World*, Volume 1. Frankfurt: Peter Lang.
Jansen, L. (2007). Aristotle's categories. *Topoi*, 26(1), 153–158.

Johnson, M.L. (1987). *The body in the mind: The bodily basis of meaning, imagination, and reason*. Chicago: Chicago University Press.
Johnson, M.L., Tucker, D.M. (2021). *Out of the cave. A natural philosophy of mind and knowing*. Cambridge MA: MIT Press.
Kant, I. (1999). *Critique of pure reason*. Cambridge: Cambridge University Press. Contains the original German editions A of 1781 and B of 1787.
Keijzer, F. (2015). Moving and sensing without input and output: Early nervous systems and the origins of the animal sensorimotor organization. *Biology and Philosophy*, 30, 311–331.
Keijzer, F., van Duijn, M., Lyon, P.Ch. (2013). What nervous systems do: Early evolution, input-output, and the skin brain thesis. *Adaptive Behavior*, 21(92), 67–85. DOI: 10.1177/1059712312465330
Keijzer, F., Arnellos, A. (2017). The animal sensorimotor organization: A challenge for the environmental complexity thesis. *Biology & Philosophy*, 32(3), 421–441.
Kendal, J.R. (2011). Cultural niche construction and human learning environments: Investigating sociocultural perspectives. *Biological Theory*, 6, 241–250. https://doi.org/10.1007/s13752-012-0038-2
Kirchhoff, M.D. (2016). Autopoiesis, free energy, and the life–mind continuity thesis. *Synthese*. https://doi.org/10.1007/s11229-016-1100-6
Kleinschmidt, S. (ed.) (2014). *Mereology and location*. Oxford: Oxford University Press.
Kleinschmidt, S. (2014a). Introduction. In: Kleinschmidt (2014), xiii–xxxiii.
Kleinschmidt, S. (2016). Placement permissivism and logics of location. *Journal of Philosophy*, 113(3), 117–136.
Koshland, D.E. Jr. (2002). The seven pillars of life. *Science*, 295, 2215–2216.
Kovác, L. (2000). Fundamental principles of cognitive biology. *Evolution and Cognition*, 6(1), 52–71.
Kripke, S.A. (1980). *Naming and nacessity*. Cambridge MA: Harvard University Press.
Kubovy, M., Valkenburg, D. (2001). Auditory and visual objects. *Cognition*, 80(1–2), 97–126.
Lagerlung, H. (ed.) (2007). *Representation and objects of thought in medieval philosophy*. Farnham: Ashgate.
Lakoff, G. (1987). *Women, fire, and dangerous things: What categories reveal about the mind*. Chicago: University of Chicago Press.
Lakoff, G., Johnson, M. (1980). *Metaphors we live by*. Chicago: University of Chicago Press.
Laland, K.N., O'Brien, M.J. (2011). Cultural niche construction: An introduction. *Biological Theory*, 6, 191–202.
Laland, K.N., Sterelny, K. (2006). Seven reasons (not) to neglect niche construction. *Evolution*, 60, 1751–1762.
Laland, K.N., Matthews, B., Feldman, M.W. (2016). An introduction to niche construction theory. *Evolutionary Ecology*, 30, 191–202. DOI 10.1007/s10682-016-9821-z

Laland, K.N., Odling-Smee, J., Feldman, M.W. (2001). Cultural niche construction and human evolution. *Journal of Evolutionary Biology*, 14, 22–23.

Laland, K.N., Odling-Smee, J., Feldman, M.W. (1999). Evolutionary consequences of niche construction and their implications for ecology. *Proceedings of the National Academy of Sciences*, 96, 10242–10247.

Lee, Y.K., Mazmanian, S.K. (2010). Has the microbiota played a critical role in the evolution of the adaptive immune system? *Science*, 330, 1768–1773.

Leibniz, G.W. (1969). Discourse on metaphysics. In: G.W. Leibniz (ed.), *Philosophical papers and letters*. A selection translated and Edited by L.E. Loemker. Dordrecht: Kluwer, 303–330.

Leonard, H.S., Goodman, N. (1940). The calculus of individuals and its uses. *Journal of Symbolic Logic*, 5, 45–55.

Leśniewski, S. (1916/1992). *Podstawy ogólnej teoryi mnogosci I, Prace Polskiego Koła Naukowego w Moskwie, Sekcya matematyczno-przyrodnicza*, Moscow; English version: Foundations of the general theory of sets I. In: S. Lésniweski (ed.), *Collected works*. Dordrecht: Kluwer, 129–173.

Lewontin, R. (1983). The organism as the subject and object of evolution. *Scientia*, 118, 63–82.

Lewontin, R. (2000). *The triple helix. Gene, organism, and environment*. Cambridge, MA: Harvard University Press.

Llored, J.-P., Harré, C.R. (2014). Developing the mereology of chemistry. In: C. Calosi and P. Graziani (eds.), *Mereology and the sciences, Synthese Library*, 371. DOI 10.1007/978-3-319-05356-1__9

Locke, J. (2004). *An essay concerning humane understanding*. The Project Gutenberg, available online: https://www.gutenberg.org/files/10615/10615-h/10615-h.htm#book01

Marr, D. (1982). *Vision: A computational investigation into the human representation and processing of visual information*. San Francisco: W.H. Freeman.

Martin, M.G.F. (2010). What's in a look? In: B. Nanay (ed.), *Perceiving the world*. Oxford University Press, 160–225.

Maturana, H., Varela, F. (1980). *Autopoiesis and cognition. The realization of the living*. Dordrecht: Kluwer.

Maturana, H., Varela, F. (1992). *The tree of knowledge. The biological roots of human understanding*. Boston & London: Shambhala.

McDaniel, K. (2010). Parts and wholes. *Philosophy Compass*, 5(5), 412–425. 10.1111/j.1747-9991.2009.00238.x

McDonough, J.K. (2015). 'Descartes' 'Dioptrics' and 'Descartes' 'Optics'. In: L. Nolan (ed.), *The Cambridge Descartes Lexicon*. New York: Cambridge University Press.

McDowell, J. (1994). *Mind and world*. Cambridge MA: Harvard University Press.

McFall-Ngai, M. (2002). Unseen forces: The influence of bacteria on animal development. *Developmental Biology*, 242, 1–14.

Menary, R. (2007). *Cognitive integration: Mind and cognition unbounded*. Basingstoke: Palgrave Macmillan.

Menary, R. (ed.) (2010). *The extended mind*. Cambridge, MA: MIT Press.

Merleau-Ponty, M. (1962/2005). *Phenomenology of perception*, trans. C. Smith. London and New York: Routledge (quotations from the Taylor and Francis e-Library edition, 2005).

Miłkowski, M. (2017). Situatedness and embodiment of computational systems. *Entropy*, 19, 162. doi:10.3390/e19040162

Miłkowski, M. (2013). *The computational mind*. Cambridge MA: MIT Press.

Miłkowski, M., Nowakowski, P. (2021). Representational unification in cognitive science: Is embodied cognition a unifying perspective? *Synthese*, 199(Suppl 1), S67–S88. https://doi.org/10.1007/s11229-019-02445-w

Millikan, R. (1984). *Language, thought, and other biological categories*. Cambridge MA: MIT Press.

Molnar, G. (2003). *Powers. A study in metaphysics*. Oxford: Oxford University Press.

Moreno, A., Umerez, J., Ibañez, J. (1997). Cognition and life. The autonomy of cognition. *Brain and Cognition*, 34, 107–129.

Nagel, T. (1974). What is it like to be a bat? *The Philosophical Review*, 83(4), 435–450.

Newell, A. (1980). Physical symbol system. *Cognitive Science*, 4, 135–183.

Newell, A., Simon, H.A. (1976). Computer science as empirical inquiry: Symbols and search. *Communications of the ACM*, 19(3), 113–126.

Noë, A. (2004). *Action in perception*. Cambridge MA: MIT Press.

Noë, A. (2009). *Out of our heads. Why you are not your brain, and other lessons from the biology of consciousness*. Hill and Wang.

Noë, A. (2012). *Varieties of presence*. Cambridge MA: Harvard University Press.

O'Malley, M. (2014). *Philosophy of microbiology*. Cambridge University Press.

O'Regan, S., Noë, A. (2001). A sensorimotor account of vision and visual consciousness. *Behavioral and Brain Sciences*, 24(5), 939–973.

Odling-Smee, F.J. (1988). Niche constructing phenotypes. In: Plotkin (ed.), *The role of behavior in evolution*. Cambridge MA: MIT Press.

Odling-Smee, F.J. (2024). *Niche construction. How life contributes to its own evolution*. Cambridge MA: MIT Press.

Odling-Smee, F.J., Laland, K.N., Feldman, M.W. (2003). Niche construction: the neglected process in evolution. In: *Monographs in population biology*, Volume 37. Princeton: Princeton University Press.

Pascal, F.P., O'Regan, J.K. (2008). Commentary On Mossio and Taraborelli: Is the enactive approach really sensorimotor? *Consciousness and Cognition*, 17(4), 1341–1342.

Perzanowski, J. (1990). Ontologies and ontologics. In: E. Żarnecka Biały (ed.), *Logic counts*. Dordrecht: Kluwer, 23–42.

Perzanowski, J. (1993). Locative ontology Parts I–III. *Logic and Logical Philosophy*, 1, 7–94. Perzanowski, J. (2004). Towards combination metaphysics, Reports on Mathematical Logic 38: 93 – 116.

Pinker, S. (2003). Language as an adaptation to the cognitive niche. In: M.H. Christiansen and S. Kirby (eds.), *Language evolution*. Oxford: Oxford University Press, 16–37.

Pinker, S. (2010). The cognitive niche: Coevolution of intelligence, sociality, and language. *PNAS*, 107(11), 8993–8999.

Plato. (2008). *Theaetetus*, trans. B. Jowett. The Project Gutenberg, available online: https://www.gutenberg.org/files/1726/1726-h/1726-h.htm#link2H_4_0002

Plato. (2021). *Republic*, trans. B. Jowett. The Project Gutenberg, available online: https://www.gutenberg.org/files/1497/1497-h/1497-h.htm#link2H_4_0004

Plotnick, R.E., Dornbos, S.Q., Chen, J. (2010). Information landscapes and sensory ecology of the Cambrian radiation. *Paleobiology*, 36, 303–317.

Poli, R. (1996). Ontology for knowledge organization. In: R. Green (ed.), *Knowledge organization and change*. Frankfurt: Indeks, 313–319.

Popper, K.R. (1972). *Objective knowledge*. Oxford: Clarendon.

Pradeu, T. (2011). A mixed self: The role of symbiosis in development. *Biology Theory*, 6(1), 80–88.

Pradeu, T. (2012). *The limits of the self: Immunology and biological identity*. Oxford University Press.

Pradeu, T. (2016). Organisms or biological individuals? Combining physiological and evolutionary individuality. *Biology & Philosophy*, 31(6), 797–817.

Putnam, H. (1975). The meaning of 'meaning'. *Minnesota Studies in the Philosophy of Science*, 7, 131–193.

Putnam, H. (1982). Why there isn't a ready-made world. *Synthese*, 51(2), 141–167.

Putnam, H. (1987). *The many faces of realism*. La Salle: Open Court.

Putnam, H. (1990). Realism with a human face. In: J. Conant (ed.), *Realism with a human face*. Harvard University Press, 3–29.

Ramsey, W. (2007). *Representation reconsidered*. Cambridge: Cambridge University Press.

Ramsey, W. (2017). Must cognition be representational? *Synthese*, 194 (11), 4197–4214. DOI 10.1007/s11229-014-0644-6

Rescher, N. (2008). Ontology in cognitive perspective. *Axiomathes*, 18, 25–36.

Rescher, N. (2013). *On Leibniz* (secondedition). Pittsburgh: University of Pittsburgh Press.

Rolla, G., Figueiredo, N. (2023). Bringing forth a world, literally. *Phenomenology and the Cognitive Sciences*, 22, 931–953. https://doi.org/10.1007/s11097-021-09760-z

Rorty, R. (1979). *Philosophy and the mirror of nature*. Princeton: Princeton University Press.

Roskies, A. (2021). Representational similarity analysis in neuroimaging: Proxy vehicles and provisional representations. *Synthese*, 199(3–4), 5917–5935. https://doi.org/10.1007/s11229-021-03052-4

Rowlands, M. (1999). *The body in mind: Understanding cognitive processes*. Cambridge: Cambridge University Press.

Rowlands, M. (2010). *The new science of the mind: From extended mind to embodied phenomenology*. Cambridge MA: MIT Press.

Russell, B. (1912). *The problems of philosophy*. London: Williams and Norgate.

Ryan, P.A., Powers, S.T., Watson, R.A. (2016). Social niche construction and evolutionary transitions on individuality. *Biology and Philosophy*, 31(1), 59–79.

Ryle, G. (1949). *The concept of mind*. Chicago: University of Chicago Press.

Searle, J.R. (1983). *Intentionality: An essay in the philosophy of mind*. Cambridge University Press.

Sellars, W. (1956). Empiricism and the philosophy of mind. In: H. Feigl and M. Scriven (eds.), *Minnesota studies in the philosophy of science*, Volume I. Minneapolis: University of Minnesota Press, 253–329.

Shannon, C.E., Weaver, W. (1949). *The mathematical theory of communication.* University of Illinois Press.

Shea, N. (2013). Naturalising representational content, *Philosophy Compass* 8/5: 496–509, https://doi.org/10.1111/phc3.12033

Shea, N. (2014). Naturalising representational content. *Philosophy Compass*, 8(5), 496–509. https://doi.org/10.1111/phc3.12033

Shea, N. (2018). *Representation in cognitive science.* Oxford: Oxford University Press.

Simons, P. (2014). Where it's at: Modes of occupation and kinds of occupant. *Kleinschmidt*, 59–68. DOI: 10.1093/acprof:oso/9780199593828.001.0001

Simons, P.M. (1987). *Parts: A study in ontology.* Clarendon Press.

Simons, P.M. (1991). Faces, boundaries, and thin layers. In: A.P. Martinich and M.J. White (eds.), *Certainty and surface in epistemology and philosophical method. Essays in Honor of Avrum Stroll.* Edwin Mellen Press, 87–99.

Sinha, Ch., Jensen de Lopez, K. (2002). Language, culture and the embodiment of spatial cognition. *Cognitive Linguistics*, 11(1–2). DOI: 10.1515/cogl.2001.008

Skrzypulec, B. (2019). Oflactory objecthood. *Philosophia*, 47(3), 881–900. https://doi.org/10.1007/s11406-018-0017-3

Skyrms, B. (2010). *Signals. Evolution, learning, and information.* Oxford: Oxford University Press.

Sloman, S., Barbey, A.K., Hotaling, J.M. (2009). A causal model theory of the meaning of cause, enable, and prevent. *Cognitive Science*, 33, 21–50. DOI: 10.1111/j.1551-6709.2008.01002.x

Smith, B. (1996). Mereotopology: A theory of parts and boundaries. *Data & Knowledge Engineering*, 20, 287–303.

Smith, B. (2001). Objects and their environments: From Aristotle to ecological ontology. In: A. Frank, J. Raper, J.-P. Cheylan (eds.), *The life and motion of socio-economic units*(GISDATA Vol 8), London: Taylor and Francis, 79–97.

Smith, B. (2003). Ontology. In: L. Floridi (ed.), *Blackwell guide to the philosophy of computing and information.* Oxford: Blackwell, 155–166.

Smith, B., Mulligan, K. (1983). Framework for formal ontology. *Topoi*, 2(1), 73–85

Smith, B., Varzi, A. (1999). The Niche. *Noûs*, 33(2), 214–238.

Smith, B., Varzi, A. (2000). Fiat and bona fide boundaries. *Philosophy and Phenomenological Research*, 60(2), 401–420.

Smith, B., Varzi, A. (2002). Surrounding space: On the ontology of organism-environment relations. *Theory in Biosciences*, 120(2), 139–162.

Somorjai, G.A. (1978). Surface science. *Science*, 201, 489–497.

Sprevak, M. (2010). Computation, individuation, and the received view on representation. *Studies in History and Philosophy of Science*, 41, 260–270. doi:10.1016/j.shpsa.2010.07.008

Sterelny, K. (2007). Social intelligence, human intelligence and niche construction. *Philosophical Transactions of the Royal Society B*, 362, 719–730.

Sterelny, K. (2012). *The evolved apprentice: How evolution made humans unique*. MIT Press.

Stewart, J., Gapenne, O., Di Paolo, E.A. (eds.) (2010). *Enaction: Toward a new paradigm for cognitive science*. Cambridge, MA: MIT Press.

Stoffregen, T.A. (2003). Affordances as properties of the animal-environment system. *Ecological Psychology*, 15(2), 115–134.

Stotz, K. (2010). Human nature and cognitive-developmental niche construction. *Phenomenology and the Cognitive Sciences*, 9, 483–501.

Stroll, A. (1979). Two conceptions of surfaces. *Midwest Studies in Philosophy*, 4(1), 277–291.

Swoyer, C. (1991). Structural representation and surrogative reasoning. *Synthese*, 87, 449–508. https://doi.org/10.1007/BF00499820

Talmy, L. (1983). How language structures space. In: H. Pick and L. Acredolo (eds.), *Spatial orientation: Theory, research and application*. New York: Plenum, 225–282.

Taraborelli, D., Mossio, M. (2008). On the relation between the enactive and the sensorimotor approach to perception. *Consciousness and Cognition*, 17(4), 1343–1344.

Taylor, Ch. (1989). *Sources of the self: The making of modern identity*. Cambridge MA: Harvard University Press.

Thomasson, A. (2007). *Ordinary objects*. Oxford: Oxford University Press.

Thompson, E. (2007). *Mind in life: Biology, phenomenology, and the sciences of mind*. Harvard University Press.

Thompson, E., Stapleteon, M. (2009). Making sense of sense-making: Reflections on enactive and extended mind theories. *Topoi*, 28(1), 23–30.

Thurner, S., Hanel, R., Klimek, P. (2018). *Introduction to the Theory of Complex Systems*. Oxford: Oxford University Press.

Tooby, J., De Vore, I. (1987). The reconstruction of hominid behavioral evolution through strategic modeling. In: W.G. Kinzey (ed.), *Primate models of hominid behavior*. Albany: Suny Press, 183–237.

Toulmin, S. (1981). Evolution, adaptation, and human understanding. In: M. Brewer and B. Collins (eds.), *Knowing and validating in the social sciences: A tribute to Donald T. Campbell*. Jossey-Bass.

Turing, A.M. (1950). Computing machinery and intelligence. *Mind*, 59, 433–460.

Twardowski, K. (1912/1999). Oczynnosciach i wytworach. Kilka uwag z pogranicza psychologii, gramatyki i logiki. In: *Ksiega Pamiatkowa ku uczczeniu 250-tej rocznicy załozenia Uniwersytetu lwowskiego przez króla Jana Kazimierza*. Tom II. Lwów: Wydawnictwo Uniwersytetu Lwowskiego, 1–33. English version in: K. Twardowski, On actions, products and other topics in philosophy (edited by J. Brandl and J. Wolenski). Amsterdam: Rodopi, 103–132.

Tyler, A., Evans, V. (2003). The semantics of English prepositions. In: *Spatial scenes, embodied meaning and cognition*. Cambridge University Press.

van Duijn, M., Keijzer, K., Franken, D. (2006). Principles of minimal cognition: Casting cognition as sensorimotor coordination. *Adaptive Behavior*, 14(2), 157–170.

Vandeloise, C. (1991). *Spatial prepositions: A case study in French*. Chicago: University of Chicago Press.

Vandeloise, C. (1994). Methodology and analyses of the preposition. *Cognitive Linguistics*, 5(2), 157–184.

Varela, F., Thompson, E., Rosch, E. (1991). *The embodied mind. Cognitive science and human experience*. Cambridge MA: MIT Press.

Varela, F. (1996). Neurophenomenology: A methodological remedy for the hard problem. *Journal of Consciousness Studies*, 3(4), 330–349.

Varela, F. (2000). Steps to a science of inter-being: Unfolding the dharma implicit in modern cognitive science. In: G. Watson, S. Batchelor and G. Claxton (eds.), *The psychology of awakening. Buddhism, science, and our day-to-day lives*. York Beach MA: Samuel Weiser, Inc., 71–89.

Varzi, A.C. (2011). Boundaries, conventions, and realism. In: J. K. Campbell, M. O'Rourke and M.H. Slater (eds.), *Carving nature at its joints: Natural kinds in metaphysics and science*. MIT Press, 129–153.

Varzi, A.C. (2016). On drawing lines across the board. In: L. Zaibert (ed.), *The theory and practice of ontology*. Cham: Palgrave Macmillan, 45–78.

Varzi, A.C. (2007). Spatial reasoning and ontology: Parts, wholes, and locations. In: M. Aiello, I. Pratt-Hartmann and J. van Benthem (eds.), *Handbook of spatial logics*. Berlin: Springer-Verlag, 945–1038.

Villalobos, M., Razeto-Barry, P. (2020). Are living beings extended autopoietic systems? An embodied reply. *Adaptive Behavior*, 28(1), 3–13.

Virgo, N., Egbert, M.D., Froese, T. (2011). The role of the spatial boundary in autopoiesis. In: G. Kampis, I. Karsai and E. Szathmary (eds.), *Advances in artificial life: Darwin meets von Neumann*. Springer, 240–247.

von Uexküll, J. (1926). *Theoretical biology*. New York: Harcourt, Brace & Co.

von Uexküll, J. (1934/2010). *A foray into the worlds of animals and humans with a theory of meaning*. University of Minnesota Press.

Wallach, E. (2016). Niche construction theory as an explanatory framework for human phenomena. *Synthese*, 193(8), 2595–2618.

Werner, K. (2020). Enactment and construction of the cognitive niche: Toward an ontology of the mind-world connection. *Synthese*, 197, 1313–1341. https://doi.org/10.1007/s11229-018-1756-1

Werner, K. (2020a). Structural coupling and the puzzle of surfaces: Ontology of boundaries from the minimally cognitive perspective. *Adaptive Behavior*, 29(6), 601–615. https://doi.org/10.1177/1059712320937475

Werner, K. (2021b). Cognitive confinement: Theoretical considerations on the construction of a cognitive niche, and on how it can go wrong. *Synthese*, 198, 6297–6328. doi: https://doi.org/10.1007/s11229-019-02464-7

Werner, K. (2022). The problem of presentations: How it is that one object is perceptually given in multiple ways. *Synthese*, 200, 181. https://doi.org/10.1007/s11229-022-03486-4

Werner, K. (2022a). Institutions as cognitive niches: A dynamic of knowledge and ignorance. In: S. Arfini and L. Magnani (eds.), *Embodied, extended, ignorant minds: New studies on the nature of not-knowing (Synthese Library)*, Springer.

Werner, K. (2022b). *The embodied philosopher. Living in pursuit of boundary questions*. Cham: Palgrave Macmillan.

Werner, K. (2023). Enactment. A preliminary study in Varela and traditional metaphysics. *Journal of Consciousness Studies*, 30(11–12).

Werner, K., Kiełkowicz-Werner, M. (2022). From shared enaction to intrinsic value. How enactivism contributes to environmental ethics. *Topoi*, 41, 409–423. https://doi.org/10.1007/s11245-021-09750-5

Whitehead, A.N. (1929). *Process and reality. An essay in cosmology*. Macmillan.

Wittgenstein, L. (1922). Tractatus Logico-Philosophicus. In: K. Paul (ed.), *Quotations from: L. Wittgenstein, Tractatus Logico-Philosophicus*. Mineola, NY: Dover Publications.

Woodward, J. (2003). *Making things happen: A theory of causal explanation*. Oxford: Oxford University Press.

Zahavi, D. (2003). *Husserl's phenomenology*. Stanford: Stanford University Press.

Index

Pages followed by "n" refer to notes.

For Product Safety Concerns and Information please contact our EU representative GPSR@taylorandfrancis.com
Taylor & Francis Verlag GmbH, Kaufingerstraße 24, 80331 München, Germany

www.ingramcontent.com/pod-product-compliance
Ingram Content Group UK Ltd.
Pitfield, Milton Keynes, MK11 3LW, UK
UKHW022350190926
475702UK00015B/2212
9781032946412